A ROADMAP FOR COUPLE THERAPY

A Roadmap for Couple Therapy offers a comprehensive, flexible, and user-friendly template for conducting couple therapy. Grounded in an in-depth review of the clinical and research literature, and drawing on the author's 40-plus years of experience, it describes the three main approaches to conceptualizing couple distress and treatment—systemic, psychodynamic, and behavioral—and shows how they can be integrated into a model that draws on the best of each. Unlike multi-authored texts in which each chapter presents a distinct brand of couple therapy, this book simultaneously engages multiple viewpoints and synthesizes them into a coherent model. Covering fundamentals and advanced techniques, it speaks to both beginning therapists and experienced clinicians. Therapists will find *A Roadmap for Couple Therapy* an invaluable resource as they help distressed couples repair and revitalize their relationships.

"This is one of the best books ever written about couple therapy. Presenting the most comprehensive and thorough compendium of couple therapy interventions ever assembled, Nielsen integrates the many strands of couple therapy into an invaluable coherent framework. Anchored in the author's deep and encyclopedic knowledge of couple therapy and of individual approaches such as psychoanalytic psychotherapy, this is a marvelous resource for both the beginning couple therapist and the experienced practitioner."

—**Jay Lebow, PhD**, editor, *Family Process*; clinical professor, The Family Institute at Northwestern University; author of *Couple and Family Therapy: An Integrative Map of the Territory*

"Art Nielsen has written a great book on couples' therapy that is also highly integrative. It's delightful to read. Based on a wealth of clinical experience and maturity, with excellent scholarship behind it, this book is an important organization of the complexity of and the challenges in doing couples' therapy. It has many helpful examples. The book is also the finest presentation of a modern psychoanalytic perspective on couples' issues and how to help couples with the vulnerabilities each of us inevitably bring to trying to manage having a stable and satisfying close relationship."

—**John Gottman, PhD**, professor emeritus in Psychology, University of Washington; author of *The Seven Principles for Making Marriage Work*

"*A Roadmap for Couple Therapy* is simply a great book, generously delivering on the author's promise of usefulness for beginning and experienced therapists alike. Dr. Nielsen's approach is practical and smart. The book is compelling and readable. Nielsen carries off the impressive feat of integrating concepts and techniques from various therapeutic schools into a unified and usable language and therapeutic plan of action. For the psychoanalytically oriented therapist, he shows us where our perspective is especially helpful in couple therapy, but also wisely offers a broader set of tools for more effective outcomes for our couple patients."

—**Prudence Gourguechon, MD**, past president, American Psychoanalytic Association; faculty, Institute for Psychoanalysis, Chicago, Illinois

"Arthur Nielsen's book is well written, richly researched, and ingeniously thought out. I know of no better account of the range of alternative approaches that contemporary couple therapists actually use. But what really strikes me are the verbatim interventions sprinkled throughout the book—the kind that make you think, 'What a clever way to deal with that particular couple therapy situation. I've got to use that in my own work.'"

—**Dan Wile, PhD**, assistant clinical professor, Clinical Science Program, Department of Psychology, University of California, Berkeley; author of *Couples Therapy: A Nontraditional Approach*

"Drawing upon his vast theoretical knowledge and many years of clinical experience, in this highly readable volume, Nielsen tackles the many knotty problems that couples therapists encounter, navigating us through the sometimes murky waters by providing in-depth, cross-theoretical conceptual understandings of couples' problems and offering a multitude of tremendously practical, creative, and useful exercises and tips to help couples solve problems and change the dance."

—**Rhonda Goldman, PhD**, president, The Society for Psychotherapy Integration; professor, Illinois School of Professional Psychology at Argosy; author with Leslie Greenberg of *Emotion-Focused Couples Therapy: The Dynamics of Emotion, Love, and Power*

"This is a masterful integrative guide to couple therapy. Art Nielsen brings into dialogue psychodynamic, systems, and behavioral approaches, helping the therapist think broadly and deeply. His clinical examples are terrific, his orientation—informed by research and best practices from multiple theories—humane and empowering. A tour de force!"

—**Mona D. Fishbane, PhD**, director, Couple Therapy Training, Chicago Center for Family Health; author, *Loving with the Brain in Mind: Neurobiology and Couple Therapy*

"Even as some portions of our profession succumb to the 'marketplace' strategy of giving their approach a brand label, exaggerating its differences from competing brands, and testing it against an intentionally lame comparison group to get it on spurious lists of 'empirically supported' therapy brands, others, like Arthur Nielsen, aim to improve our service to those we work with in less self-serving and more open-minded fashion. His genuinely integrative approach is to be commended, as is his careful consideration of how each perspective can contribute to the larger effort to help couples change."

—**Paul Wachtel, PhD**, founder and past president of The Society for Psychotherapy Integration; distinguished professor in the doctoral program in clinical psychology, City College of NY and CUNY Graduate Center; author of *Cyclical Psychodynamics and the Contextual Self*

A ROADMAP FOR COUPLE THERAPY

Integrating Systemic, Psychodynamic, and Behavioral Approaches

Arthur C. Nielsen, MD

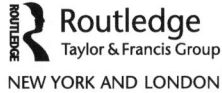

NEW YORK AND LONDON

First published 2016
by Routledge
711 Third Avenue, New York, NY 10017

and by Routledge
2 Park Square, Milton Park, Abingdon, Oxon, OX14 4RN

Routledge is an imprint of the Taylor & Francis Group, an informa business

© 2016 Arthur C. Nielsen

The right of Arthur C. Nielsen to be identified as author of this work has been asserted by him in accordance with sections 77 and 78 of the Copyright, Designs and Patents Act 1988.

All rights reserved. The purchase of this copyright material confers the right on the purchasing institution to photocopy pages which bear the photocopy icon and copyright line at the bottom of the page. No other parts of this book may be reprinted or reproduced or utilised in any form or by any electronic, mechanical, or other means, now known or hereafter invented, including photocopying and recording, or in any information storage or retrieval system, without permission in writing from the publishers.

Trademark notice: Product or corporate names may be trademarks or registered trademarks, and are used only for identification and explanation without intent to infringe.

Library of Congress Cataloging in Publication Data
Names: Nielsen, Arthur C., author.
Title: A roadmap for couple therapy : integrating systemic, psychodynamic, and behavioral approaches / by Arthur C. Nielsen, MD.
Description: New York, NY : Routledge, 2016.
Includes bibliographical references and index.
Identifiers: LCCN 2015049072| ISBN 9780415818070 (alk. paper) | ISBN 9780415818087 (alk. paper) | ISBN 9780203582183 (alk. paper)
Subjects: LCSH: Couples therapy. | Therapist and patient. | Psychodynamic psychotherapy.
Classification: LCC RC488.5 .N538 2016 DDC 616.89/1562—dc23
LC record available at http://lccn.loc.gov/2015049072

ISBN: 978-0-415-81807-0
ISBN: 978-0-415-81808-7
ISBN: 978-0-203-58218-3

Typeset in Bembo
by Keystroke, Station Road, Codsall, Wolverhampton

Printed and bound in the United States of America by Publishers Graphics, LLC on sustainably sourced paper.

To the women who sustain me:
Sheila, my astonishing, magnificent wife, and
Jeni, Katy, and Cindy, our amazing daughters.

The power of love is a curious thing.
Make one man weep, make another man sing.
You don't need money, don't take fame,
Don't need no credit card to ride this train.
It's strong and it's sudden and it's cruel sometimes,
But it might just save your life.
That's the power of love.
—Huey Lewis and The News, 1986*

To recognize that the object of our feelings, needs, actions, and thoughts is actually another subject, an equivalent center of being, is the real difficulty.
—Jessica Benjamin, 2004 (p. 92)

---

* POWER OF LOVE, THE. Words and Music by JOHNNY COLLA, CHRIS HAYES and HUEY LEWIS. © 1986 WB MUSIC CORP., HUEY LEWIS MUSIC, KINDA BLUE MUSIC and CAUSE AND EFFECT MUSIC. All Rights Administered by WB MUSIC CORP. All Rights Reserved. Used with permission.

CONTENTS

Acknowledgments   *xi*
About the Author   *xiii*

PART I
Conjoint Couple Therapy and Marital Challenges   1

1 Introduction   3

2 Couple Therapy 1.0   11

3 What Makes Marriage Challenging   22

PART II
Systems Upgrades   37

4 Focusing on the Interpersonal Process   39

5 Couple Dances Examined More Closely   56

PART III
Psychodynamic Upgrades   79

6 Focusing on Hidden Issues, Fears, and Desires   81

7 Focusing on Divergent Subjective Experiences   108

8	Focusing on Transference	116
9	Focusing on Projective Identification	134
10	Focusing on Acceptance and Forgiveness	152

PART IV
Behavioral/Educational Upgrades 179

11	Teaching Speaking and Listening Skills	181
12	Teaching Emotion Regulation	206
13	Teaching Problem-Solving and Negotiation Skills	219
14	Encouraging Positive Experiences	232

PART V
Sequencing Interventions and Concluding Remarks 245

15	General Guidelines and the Sequencing of Interventions	247
16	Concluding Remarks	262

References	*266*
Index	*280*

ACKNOWLEDGMENTS

I am indebted to the many colleagues and contributors to the field who have shared their ideas, experience, and research findings; to my students who have helped me clarify my thinking; and to feedback from a study group of senior couple therapists with whom I have been able to share safely not only my successes, but my failures and conundrums. Certain colleagues deserve special thanks for their careful reading and resulting helpful suggestions to drafts of various chapters: James Anderson, Mona Fishbane, Charles Jaffe, Jay Lebow, William Pinsof, and Cheryl Rampage. I was particularly fortunate to have the services of my developmental editor, Chava Casper who, though not an expert in the field of couple therapy, brought to the book both her years of relationship wisdom and her meticulous editorial suggestions.

I also want to give a shout-out to my editors at Routledge, Marta Moldvai and Elizabeth Graber, for their encouragement and assistance throughout the arduous process of bringing this book to print.

To my many clients—some of whose stories appear here, in disguised form—I want to thank you for allowing me into your lives, for trusting me with your deepest concerns, for helping me to hone my craft, and for making it possible for me to pass along to the next generation of therapists what we learned together under considerable duress. I wish you well.

And, finally I want to acknowledge the support of my wife, Sheila, whose devotion to her own writing served as a shining star for me, and who has taught me so much about the joys of married life.

ABOUT THE AUTHOR

Arthur C. Nielsen, MD is a board-certified psychiatrist, psychoanalyst, and couple therapist. He earned his undergraduate degree at Harvard College and his MD at Johns Hopkins. He completed his psychiatry residency at Yale, did family therapy training at The Philadelphia Child Guidance Clinic, and graduated from the Chicago Institute for Psychoanalysis. Professor Nielsen is Associate Professor of Clinical Psychiatry and Behavioral Sciences at Northwestern's Feinberg School of Medicine; and serves on the faculty of the Chicago Institute for Psychoanalysis, where he teaches couple therapy, and on the faculty of The Family Institute at Northwestern University. For many years, he has coordinated a for-credit course he developed for Northwestern undergraduates, *Marriage 101: Building Loving and Lasting Relationships*. He is a Distinguished Fellow of the American Psychiatric Association, and the author of over 30 papers in the fields of psychiatry, psychoanalysis, and couple therapy. He lives in Winnetka, IL, with his wife, Sheila, and is the proud father of three grown daughters.

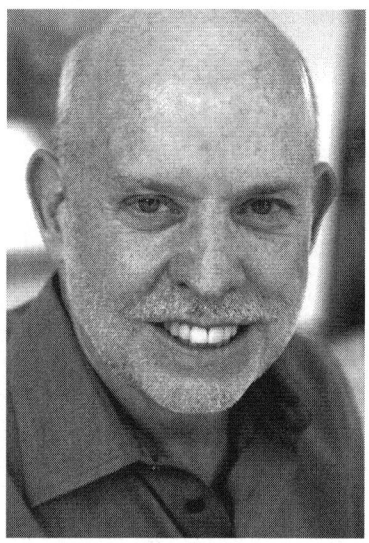

PART I
Conjoint Couple Therapy and Marital Challenges

1
INTRODUCTION

Why Read This Book?

First, because couple therapy is difficult. It is difficult because:

- Therapists must deal with two clients, often at war with each other, with differing psychologies, histories, agendas, and levels of commitment to therapy.
- It involves a mix of many emotions fundamental to the partners' well-being, emotions that run the gamut between rage and despair.
- The subject matter is often loaded and challenging: concrete issues like money, sex, and childrearing, and abstract ones like love, independence, and power.
- Most psychotherapists have inadequate training in it, and the training they have in individual therapy is insufficient to guide them with couples.
- There are many schools of thought on how best to do couple therapy and relatively little guidance concerning how to choose among them.

Second, precisely because it is complex, deals with life's great challenges, and allows us to help people who are suffering, couple therapy can be deeply gratifying, intellectually interesting, and personally rewarding. My goal is that—after reading this book—you will feel less of the stress and confusion and more of the rewards as you practice this challenging form of therapy.

A Roadmap

This book offers a practical roadmap for conducting couple therapy. Covering both fundamentals and advanced techniques, it should prove valuable to both beginning therapists and experienced clinicians. The model is based on my nearly 40 years of experience with more than 250 couples, on an extensive review of the clinical and research literature, and on interactions with others in the field. The book describes in detail each of the three main approaches to conceptualizing couple distress and treatment—systemic, psychodynamic, and behavioral—and shows how they can be integrated into a flexible model that draws on the best of each. Unlike other texts, in which different authors present their distinct brands of couple therapy in separate chapters, this text does not require readers to create their own synthesis. In addition, this flexible, comprehensive model meets the needs of diverse clinical situations, rather than being a one-size-fits-all treatment. Having a straightforward guidebook, therapists will be better able to avoid the disorientation that often accompanies the complexity and emotional intensity of working with distressed couples. I know that my own results have improved as I have worked to refine my ideas while writing this book; I believe yours will too.

The Importance of Couple Therapy

The following statistics illuminate what is at stake.

- Approximately 80% of American women will marry for the first time by age 40 (Copen, Daniels, Vespa, & Mosher, 2012); about 90% of both men and women will eventually marry (Whitehead & Popenoe, 2002).
- Despite the rise in cohabitating couples and single-parent families, most young people want to marry, marriage having "evolved from a marker of conformity to a marker of prestige . . . a status one builds up to" (Cherlin, 2004, p. 855).
- One in five first marriages will fail within the first five years and 40–50% of first marriages ultimately end in divorce (Copen et al., 2012).
- Twenty percent of married couples report significant marital distress at any point in time (Bradbury, Fincham, & Beach, 2000).
- Among clients seeking treatment for "acute emotional distress," problems with intimate relationships are the most frequently cited causes (Swindel, Heller, Pescosolido, & Kikuzawa, 2000).
- Marital success augments general well-being, physical health, and economic success (Doherty, et al., 2002; Proulx, Helms, & Buehler, 2007; Waite & Gallagher, 2000); and relationship success is probably the best predictor of overall happiness (Lee, Seccombe, & Sheehan, 1991; Lyubomirsky, 2013).
- Marital conflict, unhappiness, and divorce cause declines in all the just-mentioned areas and generate similar problems in the next generation (Booth & Amato, 2001; Cummings & Davies, 1994; Hetherington, 2003; Wallerstein, Lewis, & Blakeslee, 2000).

- Marital distress is associated with broad classifications of anxiety, mood, and substance use disorders, and with all narrow classifications of specific disorders (Whisman & Uebelacker, 2006).
- Half of all psychotherapists in the United States do some couple therapy (Orlinsky & Ronnestad, 2005), though many find it daunting or even frightening (*Psychotherapy Networker*, Nov–Dec, 2011).
- On the positive side, couple therapy has been shown to improve marital success and happiness in approximately two-thirds of unselected distressed couples (Gurman, 2011; Lebow, Chambers, Christensen, & Johnson, 2012), with effectiveness rates that are "vastly superior to control groups not receiving treatment" (Lebow et al., 2012, p. 145).
- There is considerable room for improvement in couple therapy, as less than 50% of couples entering therapy reach levels of marital satisfaction seen in non-clinical couples (Baucom, Hahlweg, & Kuschel, 2003); and many couples who improve in therapy later relapse (Jacobson & Addis, 1993).
- There is no consensus on which of the many forms of couple therapy is most beneficial (Gurman, 2008a).

In summary, relationship success matters greatly, is commonly compromised, and improves with couple therapy, a therapy with room for improvement.

The Importance of Integration

My overall approach to couple therapy is synthetic or "integrative," that is, I borrow from different intellectual sources and show how they can work synergistically. The advantages of this method are many:

- **Integrating vocabularies**. The many approaches to psychotherapy employ different terms to describe similar phenomena. This results in a therapeutic Tower of Babel that makes communication difficult among practitioners who might otherwise learn from each other.
- **Improving cross-fertilization**. Disparate vocabularies are partly the result of the lack of cross-communication between practitioners and researchers favoring different approaches. As noted by Lebow (2014), the current separation of professions, journals, and scientific meetings impedes information sharing. In particular, there is little crosstalk between psychoanalytically informed therapists and those writing from a behavioral or social-psychological perspective.
- **Giving common factors their due**. While schools of therapy emphasize differences, they actually overlap considerably in what they consider helpful (Sprenkle, Davis, & Lebow, 2009). Christensen (2010) has identified activities common to most current forms of couple treatment: (a) challenging the individual problem definition that partners favor and replacing it with

a dyadic conceptualization (*systemic therapy*, in the terminology I will be using); (b) eliciting avoided, private thoughts and feelings so that partners become aware of each other's internal experiences (*psychodynamic therapy*); (c) modifying emotion-driven maladaptive behavior by finding constructive ways to deal with emotions (*psychodynamic and behavioral therapy*); and (d) fostering productive communication (*behavioral therapy*).

- **More tools in the toolbox.** The most important reason to integrate therapeutic approaches is that particular therapies propose different and sometimes problem-specific methods for effecting change. As argued by Fraenkel (2009), more options should allow better treatment for the wide variety of problems and clients we see. The expectation that using multiple tools yields better outcomes has been confirmed by studies that obtained superior results after adding psychodynamically informed interventions to traditional behavior therapy (Dimidjian, Martell, & Christensen, 2008).
- **Too many options.** The final reason to *integrate* therapies is to generate a decision tree for choosing among myriad competing options. Having multiple tools may cause confusion if one doesn't know how to choose among them. Couple therapy is complex enough without our having to juggle four or five different schools of thought at every turn. Therapists faced with too many choices may cling for dear life to one theory (even when it isn't working) or throw theories to the winds and simply go with the flow—two errors observed frequently by Weeks, Odell, and Methven (2005) in their study of couple therapist mistakes. A worthy integration of therapies should provide guidance both in selecting among interventions and in determining how to sequence them.

Method, Personal Journey, and Approach to Mental Disorders

The recommendations I make here arise from many sources. In part, they grew from an informal review of 67 couple therapy cases I saw between 1993 (when I started keeping computerized records) and 2003 (when I was asked to give a lecture summarizing my experience as a couple therapist). Consistent with the literature, the majority of my clients improved, though some later relapsed and returned for more therapy or chose to divorce. These couples, like the ones I have seen subsequently and most subjects in the research literature (Lebow et al., 2012), were mostly, though not exclusively, white, urban and suburban, college-educated professionals, ranging in age from their late 20s through their 60s. This book also draws on my earlier and subsequent couple work, from marital issues raised by my individual clients, from supervising cases treated by other mental health practitioners (including clients from more diverse and less privileged circumstances), and from the clinical and research literature (see also Nielsen, 2003, 2005). I have treated a relatively small number of same-sex couples, most from the same demographic as my straight couples, who have presented substantially the same set of problems (see Kurdek, 2004, for a similar conclusion), with some unique challenges, including those due to internalized and societal homophobia. Couples with serious violence, drug, or alcohol issues; some ethnic minorities; and low-income couples have been infrequent in my clinical practice, though less-so for the students I have supervised. Clearly, such couples present unique and challenging complications for therapy. Having said this, many of my clients have grown up in severely impoverished and disadvantaged environments, have suffered from poverty, racism, neglect, and abuse, and now struggle with the scars and mental disorders that follow in their wake.

As argued by Gurman (2008b) and Lebow (2014), two of the most well-respected observers of the field, integrative models can gain epistemological strength from formal research that has demonstrated the efficacy of their various components. Consequently, research reports of success with, for example, Emotionally Focused Therapy and with various forms of skill training should support their value when employed in my more comprehensive treatment model (Lebow et al., 2012). While it is theoretically possible that such mixing might detract from success, this has not been my experience, in keeping with the field as a whole, which appears to be moving to more inclusive approaches, as previously distinct models have been cross-fertilized by their earlier competitors (Lebow, 2014; Gurman, 2013).

Having just asserted my confidence in learning from my own experience, I acknowledge the possible danger lurking there. As a long-time teacher of scientific methods courses, I know it is easy to exaggerate one's knowledge and expertise. (Psychoanalyst Marshal Edelson (1983) has asserted that whenever Freud wrote, "It cannot be doubted that . . ." this reliably flagged Freud's actual uncertainty.) I, therefore, acknowledge upfront that things don't always go as smoothly as I may sometimes imply.

On a more positive note, my conscious awareness of imperfect results has propelled my search for better ways to practice. The "upgrades" I will be describing to the basic format of conjoint couple sessions have all assisted me personally to do better than I was doing before I added them to my repertoire. Just as a new drug that cures a previously incurable illness suggests that that drug, rather than various alternative explanations, led to the cure, so my improved results after adding new interventions have increased my confidence in their value.

This book has been shaped by many additional influences that encouraged my integrative approach. I was fortunate to have begun my psychiatric training at Yale in the early 1970s, where biology, psychology, and social systems were all recognized as important causes of abnormal behavior and mental disorders (Engel, 1980), and where the ideal mental health practitioner assessed all contributions to a problem before suggesting possible treatments. My diverse education and experience continued at some outstanding institutions, including

The National Institute of Mental Health, The Philadelphia Child Guidance Clinic, the Department of Psychiatry and The Family Institute at Northwestern University, and The Chicago Institute for Psychoanalysis.

Two additional experiences strongly influenced my thinking. At many Tavistock Group Relations Conferences (Bion, 1961; Colman & Bexton, 1975), I studied group process in detail, learned the value of projective identification, and saw how highly educated, well-meaning adults—like most of the couples who are the subject of this book—could regress as a function of group process and their current interactions with others (Wachtel, 2014). And from developing and teaching the *Marriage 101* course to undergraduate students at Northwestern (Nielsen, Pinsof, Rampage, Solomon, & Goldstein, 2004), I encountered important research on success in marriage and learned the value of adding a relationship education component to my clinical work.

Terminology

I have chosen to use *couple therapy*, rather than *couples therapy* or other possible variations, by analogy with *individual therapy* (never termed *individual's therapy*) and also because the leading anthologies in the field use that term (Gurman, 2008a, 2010).

For purely stylistic reasons, I sometimes use the more restrictive terms *marital* and *spouse* interchangeably with the more inclusive terms *couple* and *partner*, with the understanding that, in most situations, it makes little difference whether the individuals are formally married or not; what I am discussing throughout are people in committed, intimate relationships.

Finally, I have chosen *not* to give my specific brand of couple therapy a proprietary name. Such names are currently common in the field and include: Emotion-Focused Couples Therapy, Psychodynamic Couple Therapy, Object Relations Couple Therapy, Narrative Couple Therapy, Behavioral Couple Therapy, Cognitive-Behavioral Couple Therapy, Integrative Behavioral Couple Therapy, and Integrative Problem-Centered Metaframeworks Therapy. Having seen how approaches can be limited by their names, I have resisted the urge to create a new "brand"—even an integrative one—so that others can more easily add to the inclusive scaffolding I am proposing.

Outline of the Book

Part I: Conjoint Couple Therapy and Marital Challenges describes the basic conjoint couple therapy set-up: a three-person group consisting of two clients and a therapist that tries to expose and ameliorate the couple's problems by talking about them. This is the unadorned foundation for all couple treatment, which I have termed the Talk-To-Each-Other Model or Couple Therapy 1.0. Chapter 3 ("What makes marriage challenging") describes many of the challenges that couples face, challenges that I will be discussing in the remainder of the book.

Upgrades. The sections that follow describe the refinements or "upgrades" I have discovered to be helpful, and frequently necessary, for obtaining better results. I use the metaphor of "upgrades" to call to mind technological improvements that took the car from the original Model T to the modern automobile, and the earliest computer operating systems to their current, ever-evolving versions. In both cases, the essential form and goals are unchanged—the newer model is recognized as in the same class of objects as its predecessors—while added complexity and functionality have improved performance.

The couple therapist in 2016 resembles the couple therapist of 1960 as he or she meets conjointly with two distressed people and tries to help them to talk to each other to work out their problems. Like automotive and computer technology, couple therapy has advanced considerably since 1960, making this work both more complex and more efficacious. This book describes and categorizes the upgrades and improvements now available to the practitioner of this therapeutic art.

Part II: Systems Upgrades. The first crucial upgrade is to focus explicitly on the couple's interpersonal process: their maladaptive dance. What I refer to as "negative interaction cycles"—in which couples do all the wrong things and gradually escalate to increasing levels of distress and incapacity—usually must be addressed before specific problems about finances, children, or sex, for example, can be tackled. This focus is based on a systems view of couples' problems: that the observed dysfunction is the consequence of maladaptive interaction and is greater than the sum of the contributions of each partner. The first chapter in this section discusses this shift in focus generally, and the second goes into detail about some common maladaptive cycles.

Part III: Psychodynamic Upgrades discusses ways to unpack and gain a deeper understanding of maladaptive cycles by exploring their underlying psychodynamics. Here, the therapist helps partners examine their dysfunctional process from the overlapping vantage points of hidden issues, fears, and desires; divergent subjective experiences; transferences; and projective identification. The outcome is a new narrative and an emotional experience that provides hope and understanding, increases intimacy, and is a prerequisite for discussing additional areas of unhappiness and controversy. A psychodynamic understanding also informs another upgrade: shifting the focus to acceptance and forgiveness, so the partners can move on to a more enjoyable future, rather than remaining stuck relentlessly complaining about past offenses or attempting (unsuccessfully) to get each other to change.

Part IV: Behavioral/Educational Upgrades covers interventions that teach empathic listening, emotion regulation, problem solving, and other communication skills. The section also includes a chapter on encouraging couples to cultivate positive experiences. These interventions have been developed and popularized by behavior therapists, by cognitive behavior therapists, and by therapists focused on "emotion regulation." They share a direct educational approach, as therapists teach clients how best to relate, especially during "difficult conversations" that can turn into maladaptive dances.

Part V: Sequencing Interventions and Concluding Remarks completes the book. The first chapter covers some overarching attitudes about doing therapy and then discusses how to sequence the interventions described previously. The final chapter summarizes the roadmap and offers some additional closing remarks.

2
COUPLE THERAPY 1.0

Fred and Beth[1] consult me for chronic marital unhappiness, having been referred by Beth's psychiatrist. They are intelligent people, tastefully dressed, he more casually than she. Fred is an industrial engineer and Beth an architect. They are in their mid-30s, with three young children who they say are doing fine. They have been unhappy for much of their 10-year marriage, especially since the children were born. They have intermittent verbal battles that end with both of them feeling worse about each other, themselves, and their marriage. They have few good times together and their sex life, which has been an on-and-off problem throughout their relationship, is now nearly non-existent. Both feel guilty, hopeless, confused, and frustrated. Beth has been thinking about divorce.

In their first session, Beth goes from anger to anguish to self-rebuke to hopelessness, as she describes how Fred makes her feel that she is not important to him: "I've got to say this stuff. It upsets me . . . even if it seems trivial. But I don't want to be a nag. Maybe I should just accept my situation and not complain." Beth hates the way she can grow increasingly angry at Fred, something that reminds her of how her mother incessantly nagged her father.

Fred looks sheepish, scared, stoical, and innocent, as his body language seems to say, "What could I have done to stir this up?!" He doesn't dispute Beth's descriptions of their problems, but never quite addresses her concerns. He tries to appear level-headed and calm, but he is clearly upset and insecure, as he notes that Beth's criticism makes him feel she doesn't love him and regrets having married him.

Beth says when they are home Fred tells her she is overly insecure and needy, and sometimes even calls her a bitch. Because she also sees herself as excessively insecure, Beth can freeze up when Fred responds to her criticisms by telling her that she is over-reacting. This "flight" response, coupled with Fred's pervasive avoidance of conflict, leaves them unable to address important external problems in their lives, such as how to spend money, share household tasks, and parent their children.

Beth and Fred are fairly typical of couples who come to me for help. We will return to their therapy as we proceed through this book.

"Just Talk to Each Other"

Had I seen Fred and Beth when I began doing couple therapy as a psychiatric resident in 1975, I would have simply asked them to come to my office and talk to each other while I tried to mediate. I will refer to this unstructured, here-and-now approach as the Talk to Each Other (TTEO) Model or simply Couple Therapy 1.0. It is the Model T of couple therapy, and it still provides the structural scaffold for how I work, even as it lacks crucial modifications that are the subject of later chapters.

The model asks the partners to meet with the therapist *together*, as almost always both of them are part of the couple's problem-maintenance structure. Like psychoanalysis and many other forms of instruction—think piano, dance, or tennis lessons—the model assumes that it won't suffice to just talk about how one interacts or plays to reveal what is going on or to change it. Instead, the therapist, teacher, or pro must observe the client or student in action, sizing up strengths and weaknesses. Such direct observation then informs interventions whose impact on here-and-now action can also be observed by all.[2]

In this chapter, I describe the key elements of the model: what a therapist needs to know in order to get started doing couple therapy, including guidance in getting clients talking, managing the emotional room temperature, and remaining neutral. This should be especially helpful to therapists with experience with individuals, but new to couple therapy. After this nuts-and-bolts beginning, I will discuss the diagnostic and therapeutic utility of this model, while noting its limitations.

The Basics of Couple Therapy 1.0

Let the couple choose problematic topics and attempt to work them out. I begin most therapy sessions by inviting the couple to choose the topic for discussion. This increases the probability of exposing a topic of emotional significance, and correlates with client satisfaction (Bowman & Fine, 2000). Once started on this task, the couple soon reveals not only the topics that give them trouble, but also their maladaptive manner of discussing them.

I do this also in conjoint *diagnostic* sessions. After asking each client to describe his or her concerns, I allow time to observe the couple discussing some problem with as little input from me as possible.

Observe and interrogate the silent partner. The conjoint format allows the therapist to hear and observe spouses' reactions to what their partners say. This means keeping one eye on the body language of the partner who is *not* speaking, which provides a running commentary on the speaker's account. This input is then supplemented by the therapist's eliciting a verbal response from the listener, including his or her emotional reactions to what has been said.

Assist clients who don't want to talk to each other. The first problem therapists encounter when using the TTEO model is that most clients prefer to tell *you* their problems, rather than to talk directly to each other. They want to convey to us how they see things and why their partners are wrong or bad or mentally ill. They rationalize this preference by pointing to the undeniable truth that if they could talk to each other successfully, they wouldn't be here!

A related problem is that we therapists, unconsciously wanting to keep things under control, may collude with the couple and allow them just to talk to us about how they talk to teach other. As we shall see shortly, sometimes there is a legitimate need for such control. Nonetheless, keeping the observational and therapeutic advantages of the TTEO model in mind, the therapist should more often persist in encouraging couples to interact with each other.

To counter the couple's desire to talk only to the therapist, give them a rationale: Explain that, "As with music, tennis, or dance lessons, I need to see you doing what you do, so I can help you do it better. My goal is to make myself obsolete as soon as possible." This phrase "obsolete as soon as possible" also helps solidify an alliance with reluctant or cost-conscious clients.

Manage the emotional room temperature. The ideal session has the couple engaging emotionally significant issues, and doing so in a respectful manner. In this regard, exposing feelings is necessary, but risks being only destructive. Think of Goldilocks and the porridge: A session should be neither too hot nor too cold. In the early history of couple therapy, these poles were represented by Virginia Satir (1967), who encouraged clients to disclose their authentic feelings in the service of creating intimacy, contrasted with Jay Haley (1976) and the early behavioral couple therapists (see Baucom, Epstein, Taillade, & Kirby, 2008), who taught that strong feelings regularly interfered with couple collaboration. Both sides are right: We will need some interventions that heat things up and some that cool things down. Therapy must be safe, but not too safe.

Some couples will find a workable emotional temperature on their own. Such couples are rare in my experience. More common are those whose exchanges become increasingly loud and intense, but no more effective. Without intervention, these encounters spin out of control, exacerbating the pain the couple hoped to alleviate. Other couples, understandably fearful of such escalation, play it too safe. Our illustrative couple, Fred and Beth, did both. Often Beth would angrily guilt-trip Fred into silent, sullen submission. Other times, sessions would go nowhere as neither partner wanted to risk rocking the boat.

Several interventions are especially helpful for adjusting the emotional room temperature. I present the basics here; more techniques are provided later in the book.

Calm things down by putting yourself in the middle. According to a recent issue of *The Psychotherapy Networker* devoted to the subject, "Who's Afraid of Couples Therapy?: Stretching Your Comfort Zone" (Jan–Feb, 2011), therapists identified calming things down when emotions ran high as the biggest challenge when working with couples. This is the individual therapist's nightmare, when you wish for only one client in the room at a time. So what can we do when things are too hot and the partners are trading increasingly extreme insults?

First, you must deal with yourself: *You must be comfortable breaking into an ongoing discussion (or tirade or yelling match)*, and *you must be comfortable taking action, even before you know exactly what to say*.

One particularly useful way to cool things down is a corollary to the fact that clients generally prefer to talk to the therapist: *When things are spiraling out of control and the room's emotional temperature is too high, the therapist must step between the clients and return to an individual therapy model, where the clients talk to an empathic therapist or, more soothing still, listen as the empathic therapist talks to them.*

Sometimes, to interrupt the pathological process, I have to call a time-out by literally making the T-sign with my arms. In extreme situations, I will make this "louder" by standing up and getting physically between the partners. More often, I interrupt the process with words alone. Here, my empathy offers the partners what they aren't giving each other and helps to calm them.

Having stopped the escalation, rather than talking to *both* partners about what I see, *I find it more effective to talk to each person separately*. Of course, both will hear everything I am saying, but it is still more powerful to address them in turn. As concerns content, there are two options. In one, *I speak to one partner about his or her distress*, making an effort to validate it and convey empathy. This is nearly identical to how I might provide empathy to a client in individual therapy. But as I do this, the partner will be "listening in" and will hear the issues stated by me with less anger and more insight. After doing this for one partner, I switch and do the same for the other.

The other option is to *speak directly to one spouse and explain what I see as the other's message or distress*. As I will discuss in detail later, Dan Wile (2002) has made this central to his "doubling" technique, but it is something most experienced couple therapists seem to have learned to do. Susan Johnson (2008), another master therapist, calls it "talking through the therapist" (p. 79). When I do this, I am acting as a model, a more articulate, less inflammatory spokesperson for one partner (who can feel my empathy), with the hope that the other partner can listen better as I talk respectfully to him or her. I can then hear any rebuttal or distress and relay it back to the first partner—like an interpreter translating what each would otherwise fail to understand. At the same time, I am modeling a less reactive, more differentiated stance toward each other's distress.

Heat things up by moving out of the middle. At the other extreme, the "porridge is too cold," the emotional heat is too low, and the defenses are too high. When this happens, it helps to employ interventions used in psychodynamic individual therapy for dealing with anxiety and resistance (self-protection). These interventions aim to create greater safety so that clients can risk more authentic emotional exposure. They consist of gentle encouragement coupled with inquiries about the calamities clients fear would occur should they become more emotionally present and forthcoming. Once clients begin to open up, the therapist must help prevent those dreaded outcomes from materializing.

Almost all clients in the throes of marital unhappiness and conflict fear that opening up will only make a bad situation worse, and most have experienced just that! Clients will periodically slow things down and retreat behind defensive walls of their own design.

As David Shapiro noted in his wonderful book, *Neurotic Styles* (1965), therapists should customize their approach to each client's individual defensive style. Following Shapiro, constricted clients should be encouraged to identify their *feelings*, and emotional, histrionic ones should be encouraged to express their *thoughts*. This is usually a stretch for both types, but it tends to advance the therapeutic process, which always requires a healthy combination of both feeling and thinking.

Most couples try to avoid the intensity of interacting with each other directly, hoping that the therapist will do the work for them. So, in addition to using psychoanalytically informed methods for dealing with resistance, the couple therapist can also move out of the middle and instruct the partners to interact more directly with each other. *The directive to "talk to each other" will have to be repeated frequently and persistently. One of the most important skills for the individual therapist beginning couple work is to learn how, literally, to point the partners toward each other,* virtually forcing them to make eye contact and speak to each other, rather than referring to each other in the third person.

Therapists must learn how to forcefully encourage such here-and-now encounters, which are central to the TTEO model. *"Can you say/repeat that to your partner?" is one of the most common and most powerful interventions that I use.* When clients say the very same words to their partners that they have just said to the therapist, they have a far greater chance of having an emotionally significant encounter. Many spouses feel relieved, almost instantly, when the fear that their partner will not listen turns out to be false. And if they *are* rebuffed, the work continues.

The therapist needs judgment, based on experience, to know when and how much to press a particular couple to talk directly to each other. He or she must continuously monitor and facilitate a workable emotional ambience positioned somewhere between too much safety and too much danger.

In general, work to stay neutral. Another essential role requirement of the basic TTEO model is that the therapist not be perceived as consistently biased in favor of one of the partners, a situation that correlates with poor outcomes (Lebow, Chambers, Christensen, & Johnson, 2012). Paradoxically, partners *fear* that the therapist will take sides, but simultaneously hope the therapist will side with *them*! When asked at the close of successful therapies what made for success, my clients—in keeping with those in large-scale studies (Sparks, 2015)—almost universally mention my ability, over time, to remain neutral.

Early fears about therapist bias are often related to transference assumptions and should be addressed directly. Sometimes I find the wife believes that I, as a man, will side with her husband; or the husband may think that I, as someone in the intimacy business, will side with his wife, who is complaining that he is not communicating more deeply with her. One partner may assume I will side with the other because we have similar professional degrees, or because we are from the same hometown, or because of some detail concerning the manner of referral. Therapists may also be suspect based on their appearance or demographics, and need to be familiar with likely scenarios. While the details will vary, anxieties about therapist bias are common, and must be addressed explicitly and early . . . and usually later, as well. They cannot be dispensed with once and for all because their true source is each partner's sense of culpability or inadequacy, attributes they fear the therapist will confirm in their nightmare fantasy of therapy as marital court.

In individual therapy, it is far easier to convey empathy and a sense of shared purpose with the client, but *couple therapy provides the constant challenge of conveying to the partners that you are working for the interests of both.* In individual therapy, when the therapist asks a client to examine some less-than-admirable trait, there is a risk the client will see the therapist as more critical than helpful. In the couple setting, there is the additional danger that such scrutiny will heighten one partner's shame or guilt because it supports the accusations of the other. This can be made still worse if the partner "piles on" by agreeing with the therapist ("See, that's just what I've been telling you all these years, you jerk!").

Another difficulty unique to couple treatment is that if the therapist spends too much time and too many consecutive sessions focusing on the symptoms or defenses of one spouse, he or she may feel (understandably) that the therapy has become too tilted against him or her. In such cases, the therapist may have to sacrifice thematic continuity in order to sustain a neutral position and the therapeutic alliance.

Take sides when necessary. Remaining neutral does not mean that the therapist does not challenge clients' views or side with one or the other from time to time. Partly through my training at the Philadelphia Child Guidance Clinic, I came to appreciate the power of sometimes taking sides and shifting alliances, of "unbalancing," as it was termed there (Minuchin & Fishman, 1981). So I have often found myself challenging partners, questioning them, or translating their partner's concerns to them, all of which deviate from the image of a non-participating "neutral" person commenting "objectively" from outside the system. Surprisingly, partners who have had trouble standing up for their rights will sometimes become anxious when the therapist articulates what they have been reluctant to say, even as they see they can actually demand more of the relationship than they had imagined.

When taking sides, it helps to be explicit that one is doing so, since it flags this as an exception in the service of bridging the gap between the partners. A therapist might say, "I'm going to take Paul's side now, just to see if I can convince you that he might be appreciating more about how you're feeling than you think" (Wile, 1981).

Side first with the less likable person. There are several important exceptions to the principle of maintaining *overall* neutrality. One is captured by what I term, "The Rule of Siding First with the Less Likable Person." In operating in the psychological space between partners, we sometimes think that one of them is more obviously the wounded or wronged partner, victimized by the psychopathology of the other—and we feel inclined to say so. And sometimes the therapist should do just that, by focusing on the blatant psychopathology of the more difficult spouse, whether the issue be drug or alcohol abuse, physical violence, or some other obvious disorder.

Over the years, however, I have learned the merits of resisting my reflexive countertransference and working to assist the partner who seems most obviously offensive. This strategy stems partly from systems thinking: a whining, depressed, or stridently defensive spouse is the one holding the fewest cards, having the least power, and, therefore, acting the most symptomatically. In couple therapy, the squeaky wheel is usually the partner who is not getting needed psychological grease.

Systems thinking aside, the principal rationale for siding with the less likable person first is pragmatic: It is usually the quickest route to therapeutic benefit. In general, this is the person who is either hurting more or is more defended, and is more likely to need encouragement. Often, though not invariably, this is the person with one foot out the door, the one who needs to be encouraged to return for more sessions.

Although it makes sense to empathize with such people, it is not easy, especially when you are witnessing that person abusing or traumatizing another in front of you. So a final reason to take sides this way is that it will interfere with your reflexive inclination to act out (sometimes unconsciously or via body language) negative countertransference feelings and thereby lose the crucial position of therapeutic neutrality.

What the TTEO Model Offers

The TTEO model offers a regularly scheduled forum; safety, containment, and hope; and some mediation, translation, and coaching.

A scheduled occasion to talk. Almost all the couples I see have been avoiding serious discussion of their problems, either because they hate the emotions stirred up or because prior attempts have created more problems than they have solved. Most distressed couples think there is no good time to talk. If they are temporarily in a good place, they don't talk for fear of rocking the boat, whereas if emotions are boiling over, no one wants to risk making things worse by talking. Looked at the other way around, being able to talk comfortably, spending more time talking, and having no "taboo" topics correlates with marital success (Pines, 1996); so helping people in this area, even nonspecifically, is likely to help them.

At the most basic level, the couple's weekly appointment is like a weekly, scheduled session with a personal trainer—sometimes it matters more that the workout occur than that the trainer provide specific expert knowledge about workout machines or exercises. In this model, the partners have finally agreed to meet to talk about what they have been avoiding, and they may succeed in doing that. If they fail to do so expeditiously, all may agree that they require professional assistance.

Safety, containment, and hope. Beyond representing the scheduled task, I also symbolize a sort of "container," in that clients view me as an experienced, idealized professional, committed to mature problem solving in a safe forum. Here I represent their wishes to behave maturely and safely when talking about unresolved issues. Sometimes this is sufficient to allow people to exert some restraint in the service of the task. More often, symbolization of this commitment to fair play and problem solving is insufficient, so I have to work actively to maintain a safe atmosphere, including by employing the interventions described above.

Just as severely depressed clients who see their futures as unremittingly black and view suicide as the only way out, distressed couples frequently feel hopeless and see divorce as their only escape. *Since therapy is often a slow process, when hope seems to flag, I offer explicit reassurance.* I do this by pointing to some combination of real progress achieved so far and my experience with similar situations. Such interventions are consonant with the abundant literature that identifies providing hope as an important common mutative factor in successful psychotherapy (Frank, 1961; Alarcón & Frank, 2011).

Mediation, translation, and coaching. In this pared-down TTEO model, there are times when therapists must translate what each person is saying into language that the other can comprehend and work with. In general, it is the couple's inability to do this when emotions run high that has led them to come for assistance. This involves a certain amount of "reframing" as deeper concerns are identified, so that the couple can understand what they are "really arguing about." Therapists can also restrain partners from both talking at once, while helping them to speak for themselves and express their needs openly. Therapists can encourage clients to let their guard down by asking, "What would it be like to tell her [him] how lonely [hurt, sad, etc.] you feel when she [he] is distant [angry, defensive, etc.] like that?"

Some simple coaching is also part of this model, as the therapist sometimes suggests alternative ways of approaching the spouse, encourages partners to try new ways to express their fears and desires, and provides information about the skillful management of some life problems.

The Therapeutic Potential of the TTEO Model

The *diagnostic* utility of the TTEO model is pretty obvious: We get to observe couples directly as they show us their problems being close and settling their disputes. Similarly, the *therapeutic* potential of the model rests on our working with couples as they try to work out their problems in the here and now. Much of the psychoanalytic literature emphasizes that it is insufficient for clients to merely *talk about* their problems; they must have a chance to *experience* them in the room, often intensely, with the therapist, so as to have "corrective emotional experiences." We reach a similar conclusion when we recall that much learning is state-dependent: Couples will have to do more than just talk *about* their problems; they will have to try out alternatives when they are upset (Greenberg & Johnson, 1988).

To the couple therapist, it often appears that most couples only want to complain or to find a third party to rule in their favor—if they do not just want to run for the door. But this is precisely the reason couples are in our offices and the reason why helping them avoid their natural tendencies is likely to help. This wish to complain to a sympathetic third party also explains some of the pitfalls of individual therapy: that therapists will fail to understand the other (non-attending) partner's side, that partners will fail to engage each other expeditiously, and (worse) that marriages may deteriorate unnecessarily (Gurman & Burton, 2014).

Whenever I despair and wonder about the value of what I do (see Wile, 2002, for thoughts on the ubiquity of such doubts), I return to this fundamental fact: There is no other way to improve troubled relationships than for the partners to "encounter" each other directly—to use a very 1960s term—and I am providing the opportunity for them to do just that. Partners must face each other—and themselves—in order to work things out, and they clearly need help in doing so.

When Does the Talk to Each Other Model Work Best?

In reviewing my own cases, I saw that the unadorned TTEO model worked fairly well when couples had to resolve important disagreements, but were not impeded by serious character pathology or entrenched maladaptive patterns of relating. Common situations were debates over whether to have a child, whether to relocate, or how to handle a difficult situation with a child or other family member. This makes intuitive sense because the conjoint therapy format can provide a safe forum for facing difficult external decisions and working out sensible approaches and compromises. Rapid success is contingent on these conflicts not being proxies for deeper, more longstanding issues. In such situations, therapists can improve on Couple Therapy 1.0 by becoming familiar with structured methods of problem solving and "getting to yes" and by knowing more than their clients do about how to manage certain life challenges.

Another situation in which the TTEO model worked well was when couples needed help venting their feelings and sharing the details of some current life difficulty. Many couples have trouble doing this and, instead, either distance themselves from each other or take out their frustrations on each other. Examples were couples distressed by the uncertainties and disappointments of infertility treatment, cancer chemotherapy, relocation to a new city, or caring for an ailing parent. Here, the therapist's role is not so much to assist the couple in problem solving, as to help them express their distress and support each other through stressful times. Unsurprisingly, some successful couples benefitted from assistance with *combinations* of ventilation and problem solving.

When Does the TTEO Model Fail?

Although the Couple Therapy 1.0 model worked for some couples, often it did not work. Instead of resolving here-and-now problems or improving their interaction, couples went week after week doing the same old thing—with me sometimes pointing it out and sometimes interrupting it—but with everyone having an experience similar to writing on sand, as the same painful arguments were replayed time after time.

In such cases, superficial conflicts about external events turned out to be embedded in deeper, life-long concerns about intimacy. In addition, although Couple Therapy 1.0 was offering some holding, hope, and empathic glue to bring the parties together amicably, many couples needed me to be physically present for them to stay on task. Outside my office, such couples lacked the ability to manage either their emotions or those of their partners.

Alan Gurman (2008b), perhaps the scholar/therapist most knowledgeable about the research on the efficacy of couple therapy, summarized what has also been my experience:

> Some couples (with basically flexible styles of interaction, a more robust degree of self-acceptance, etc.) facing "situational" problems can rather rapidly be helped with direct, concrete problem-solving guidance . . . The great majority of couples seeking therapy, however, present difficulties that are much more complex both in origin and maintenance,

and require a therapist's intervention at multiple levels of experience, using a rather broad array of techniques.

(p. 402)

Doing Couple Therapy 1.0 With Fred and Beth

Couple Therapy 1.0 got us off to a good start, allowing me to witness, in person, how Fred and Beth would get stuck. Without much encouragement, Beth would criticize Fred, who would then withdraw. Or sometimes he would counterattack, and she would retreat in tears. Then both would fall silent and wonder about the value of the therapy. Each week, they would bring up different areas of conflict, but they made no lasting headway. I was able to establish an alliance where each felt I was neutral and empathic, but just helping them talk about surface issues didn't do much for their self-defeating process, their chronic lack of connection, or their inability to solve external problems. More would be needed.

In subsequent chapters, I describe the modifications and refinements (the "upgrades") that I have found to be useful when added to the neutral, hopeful forum for couples to talk to each other. Before doing so, I will present some thoughts about what makes marriage and other intimate partnerships such a challenge.

Notes

1 All of the couples I describe are disguised and some are composite versions of couples I have treated.
2 As concerns this "here-and-now" therapeutic format, Wachtel notes that traditional behavioral therapy can be seen as "experiential" in that it forces "exposure" to feared situations and offers opportunities to unlearn the fears that power maladaptive behaviors (2014, p. 89). In a similar way, individual psychodynamic therapy and psychoanalysis resemble Gestalt Therapy's "experiments" as they encourage clients in an "experiment in intimacy" with the therapist (Nielsen, 1980). Even more obviously, conjoint couple therapy provides a chance to "experiment" in intimacy and conflict resolution with precisely the person who has become almost a phobic object.

3
WHAT MAKES MARRIAGE CHALLENGING

Marriage is challenging, even as the reasons remain mysterious to most people. In order to improve on the results obtained with Couple Therapy 1.0, we need to understand the challenges and impediments that make intimate relationships difficult and so frequently turn love into virtual war. These challenges can be subsumed under three categories: *personal challenges* due to problematic expectations, "human nature," and immaturity; *interpersonal challenges* due to inevitable differences/incompatibilities and the need to settle conflicts; and *external challenges (stressors)*.[1] These categories are not entirely orthogonal since they overlap and influence one another. For example, some *unrealistic expectations about marriage* are a type of *emotional immaturity* that limit a person's *ability to manage conflict*. Nonetheless, the categories used here are easily recognizable and practically useful. We will want to keep them in mind as targets for the interventions to be described in later chapters.

PERSONAL CHALLENGES

Problematic Expectations

Three types of expectations make marriage challenging: (a) high societal expectations for the "love match," (b) unrealistic romantic wishes, and (c) unconscious wishes for a cure for emotional problems.

High societal expectations for the love match. *Perhaps* the most obvious reason that marriages run into trouble is that society has currently set the bar so high. Stephanie Coontz (2005), the noted historian of marriage, describes contemporary expectations and historical attitudes this way:

> Married couples should be best friends, sharing their most intimate feelings and secrets. They should express affection openly but also talk candidly about problems. And of course they should be sexually faithful to each other. This package of expectations about love, marriage, and sex, however, is extremely rare. When we look at the historical record around the world, the customs of modern America and Western Europe appear exotic and exceptional . . . Never before in history had societies thought that such a set of high expectations about marriage was either realistic or desirable.
>
> *(pp. 20, 23)*

The many studies cited in Chapter 1 showing that happily married people fare better in almost all areas of life encourage us to aim high, but we can also benefit many couples by helping them to accept less than perfect.

Unrealistic romantic wishes. More than half a century ago, the psychoanalyst Edmund Bergler wrote, "The difficulties of marriage are mostly caused by irrational expectations" (1949, p. 167). More recently, Alan Gurman, the preeminent couple scholar of our day, wrote that "utopian expectations" are at the heart of much couple unhappiness (2008b, p. 390). Bergler's and Gurman's assertions are well supported: Bradbury and Karney (2010), for example, found that couples fare less well when they believe that they should not have to ask for things, that there should be no fights, and that sex should always go well.

Many couples believe that the romance and happiness that began during their courtship will be self-sustaining, and that they need to give little attention to actively managing the stresses of married life. Although initial romantic attachment does predict later happiness, excessive idealizing of a partner with little basis in fact and/or believing in such romantic truisms as "love at first sight" or "matches made in heaven" do not bode well (Pines, 1996; Niehuis et al., 2011).

Couples too often buy into the plot-line of our culture's romantic comedies and romance novels: After overcoming a complicated succession of obstacles, the partners are finally united and ride off into the sunset to live happily ever after. This script takes as a given that passion never wanes and assumes that relationships can continue to thrive without attention, effort, and work, as reflected in such naive, wishful notions as:

- "My partner should be more like me," which would eliminate conflicts before they arise.
- "Our time together should be free of competition from other areas of life, especially work and children."
- "Although I must put up with stress and strain during the day, at work or on the home front with children, the time after work with my partner should be stress-free."

- "Although I must show restraint and tact in other settings, I should be able to say whatever I feel like to my partner."
- "My partner should know me so well that I don't have to tell him what I want, and if he does what I want *after* I tell him, it doesn't count, because I had to tell him."
- "Love means never having to say you're sorry" (as in the 1970 movie, *Love Story*). In fact, as we will see in Chapter 10, research shows that apologies are *essential* to marital success.

Ideally, and contrary to these romantic misconceptions, couples learn that "love" is an active verb, not a passive state of being. Love means accepting differences, relating with sensitivity, apologizing often, and proactively attending to the needs of one's partner and marriage.[2] That said, therapists should, nonetheless, handle these unrealistic wishes with care, lest we come off as cold or judgmental and thereby shut down exploration of unmet longings.

Seeking a "cure." Some individuals choose partners they unconsciously hope will remedy an emotional problem they have been unable to solve on their own. These marriages are a "search for healing" or a "delayed developmental thrust" (Hendrix, 1988; Lewis, 1997). Although this is not universally a hopeless quest, it can be a major source of marital unhappiness; I discuss it more extensively in Chapter 9 on projective identification.

The original theory—based on clients observed to be pursuing partners who uncannily resembled parents who had caused them pain in childhood—was that these people were motivated by an unconscious wish to redo the past and produce a different, happier ending. For instance, the daughter of an alcoholic father who had felt unloved and neglected by him might choose an aloof man with a drinking problem. Unfortunately, her wish for repeated declarations of love from this surrogate father is unlikely to be satisfied.

This model is a version of Freud's "compulsion to repeat," described in *Beyond the Pleasure Principle* (1920) as a seeming exception to the idea that humans seek to maximize pleasure and minimize pain. The self-defeating nature of such a pursuit is now understood not as an exception to the pleasure principle but, rather, as a wishful attempt to gain mastery over past traumas by restaging them so as to produce a better ending. In such restaged attempts, the partner typecast to resemble someone from the painful past commonly turns out to be unable to fulfill the other's longstanding needs.

People can also attempt to heal themselves through marriage not only by restaging past traumas, but by finding partners they perceive as being able to compensate for their personal deficiencies, such as playfulness or organizational skill. Such deficiency-correcting scenarios are also usually doomed because the idea that someone can simply confer capacities on you that you do not possess is as irrational as believing that a rock star can confer fame or success on a groupie follower. Instead, such efforts routinely have the reverse effect, interfering with individuals' developing their own abilities: Thus, the woman who thinks she needs a big strong man to speak for her is unlikely to make the effort to develop her own assertive capabilities.

Attempts to get intimate partners to heal us burdens them and strains our relationship. As Terrence Real (2007) put it:

> Perhaps you married your mate to steady you, or to be successful for you, or to give you value, abundance, culture, standing, or friends, or to stop you from drinking or start you having fun, or simply to give you the gift of not draining you dry. And all these things are wonderful; they're great—as gifts. But they're poison as obligations. We must stop oppressing others with "the mad agenda" that they heal us.
>
> *(p. 76)*

Having shown that attempts at "cure by marriage" not only fail, but are counter-productive, I would also point out that, as with unrealistic romantic wishes, identifying what a client is hoping for—whether restaging or self-completion—is extremely useful for all to know. It can help to explain the appeal of extramarital affairs and—less dramatically—to identify capacities that a person needs to develop. And sometimes, when the demands are not too intense, the partner can become a valuable helpmate who can facilitate growth.[3]

"Human Nature"

Based on our evolutionary psychobiology, the following human inclinations ("human nature") commonly cause trouble in our intimate relationships:

- We tend to attribute changes in internal states to external events or people, rather than to an admixture of internal predispositions and external events ("I was doing just fine at work, until my wife started bugging me about getting a promotion.") This inborn capacity to focus on dangers in the external environment ("Look out for that lion!") is reinforced by its psychological value in helping us defend against guilt and shame, whereas the capacity to bear such emotional states is a developmental achievement.
- The flip-side of denying and externalizing blame is the human capacity to shoulder too much responsibility when things go wrong. Just as some of us externalize blame, others accept too much of it. Feeling excessively guilty, such people may become depressed; feeling undeserving, they may fail to stand up for themselves.
- We suffer from the "fundamental attribution error," the human tendency to attribute responsibility for events to human *motivation* more than to contextual variables (Ross, 1977; Gladwell, 2008). This is exacerbated by our tendency to cut ourselves slack by blaming external circumstances for

our own misdeeds, sometimes termed "actor–observer bias," as in "*I* was late due to traffic, but *she* was late because I'm not important to her!"
- We are more likely to notice and attend to things that are not working (the current back pain, the promise not kept) and lose sight of, and take for granted, what is working well (the functioning knee, the spouse bringing in a steady paycheck). This design flaw is aptly described as the tendency to see the hole, rather than the doughnut, and to notice what is bad more than what is good (Baumeister et al., 2001; Reis & Gable, 2003), a predisposition that may once have provided a Darwinian advantage.
- "Negative sentiment override" takes the salience of the negative a step further: We tend to perceive events increasingly negatively once the ball starts rolling downhill (Baucom, Epstein, Taillade, & Kirby, 2008). This bias makes it difficult for spouses to alter their partners' negative conceptions about them ("He's only being nice so that I will have sex with him . . . or because Dr. Nielsen told him to.") And while it is true that "the pessimist is never disappointed," expecting the worst tends to be self-fulfilling.
- Humans sometimes get a perverse pleasure from "getting even" or from holding grudges. This is perhaps the principal route through which love turns to virtual war. As partners disappoint and wound each other, they may continually escalate in an attempt to "even the score."
- When our self-esteem is undermined or our moral goodness is questioned, we tend to react defensively.
- Because human defensiveness can occur outside our awareness, we can deny responsibility for our misdeeds not only to others, but also to ourselves.
- There are many marital challenges related to our powerful sex drive. Many mammals mate only once a year, but human sexual desire is more omnipresent. Whatever the true nature of the unsocialized human primate sex drive, for most of human history, most cultures have viewed male sexual desire as not containable by marriage, allowing men to have sex with more than one wife or with women who were not their wives. It is only relatively recently that seeking sex outside of marriage came to be viewed as such a transgressive betrayal. In most societies, women having sex outside marriage has been far less accepted, although the strength of that taboo has weakened. Clearly, the human sex drive, when coupled with powerful negative reactions to infidelity, is a risk factor for marital crisis. Marital problems may also result from the waning of sexual interest or from a mismatch in sexual desire or preferences between partners. The sex drive may also be oversocialized or inhibited, leading to excessive guilt, avoidance, or other forms of sexual pathology that become marital problems.
- Related to the human sex drive is our human capacity to "fall in love," now understood to be encouraged by powerful neurochemicals (Fisher, 2004). While this facilitates initial pair bonding, when "love is blind," this biological potential can lead to incompatible matches. In addition, the

decline of these romance chemicals often creates unease, as couples must seek alternative ways to sustain attachment once the honeymoon is over.

Maturity/Immaturity

While I was describing the personal challenges posed by "human nature," I was simultaneously discussing an aspect of emotional immaturity. This is because the failure to restrain some of our reflexive human tendencies is a form of immaturity. I was also discussing a form of emotional immaturity when I referred to problematic expectations, including wishes to be "cured" by a partner. Clearly, marriage requires a considerable amount of emotional maturity. Sometimes, this is so obvious that we might wonder why states that require drivers' licenses do not require some proof of relational know-how before they grant a license to marry. The topic of what sorts of maturity make for relationship success and what sorts of immaturity lead to problems is very broad and will be an ongoing concern in the chapters that follow.

The earliest cross-sectional studies in this area, by Lewis Terman in the 1930s, showed that "being overly sensitive or grouchy, losing one's temper easily, fighting to get their own way, [and] lacking self-confidence" correlated with marital unhappiness (quoted in Bradbury & Karney, 2010, p. 250). Subsequent longitudinal studies have found a greater likelihood of divorce in couples with one partner who rated high on neuroticism (exhibiting negative affectivity, including a tendency to interpret the partner's behavior more negatively), rated high on impulsiveness (in husbands), rated lower on "agreeableness" or "conscientiousness," and rated lower on self-esteem, including doubting their partners' compliments and expressions of love (Bradbury & Karney, pp. 251–255). Because therapy aims to improve relevant constructive personal qualities, rather than to simply identify deficits, the following discussion briefly outlines qualities known to aid marital happiness, qualities whose absence frequently causes problems.

Self-awareness. When my colleagues and I were designing our undergraduate course on marriage, which was to include a practical component aimed at helping students to succeed in their relationships, we polled 15 experienced couple therapists about what they thought we should include in the curriculum. What topped the list was "opportunities to improve self-awareness." Why did these therapists put self-awareness first? Quite simply, if you don't look inside, you will experience your problems as coming from outside. If you don't recognize your own issues, sensitivities, and values, you will tend to see life's inevitable problems and irritations as caused mostly by external circumstances, including by (what you perceive as) the insensitive, frustrating, and generally poor behavior of others, including your spouse. You will resort too easily to blaming others and to oversimplifying situations, and you will experience yourself as more of a victim than is fair or realistic. Blaming, oversimplifying, and seeing oneself as victimized are all common characteristics of partners in unhappy and unsuccessful marriages.[4]

Self-awareness also plays a key role in most of the other positive capacities (virtues) that I will briefly define and discuss.

Relativism and subjectivity. This is the understanding that others can see the world differently. One must know that much of "reality" is not simply "true," but, instead, is subjective and dependent on our current needs, wishes, fears, and sensitivities.

Personal responsibility. This is the willingness to accept responsibility and apologize for mistakes and injuries, nondefensively, and to tolerate the guilt, shame, and vulnerability that can ensue when offering apologies.[5] Absent these qualities, people not only function poorly in intimate relationships, they have difficulty falling and remaining in love, and allowing themselves to be invested and intimate with their partners (Kernberg, 2011).

Self-esteem and resilience. This includes the ability to manage stress without undue self-criticism, anxiety, or depression, and without resorting to alcohol, extramarital sex, or other maladaptive home remedies. It includes the capacity to maintain self-esteem without putting excessive pressure on others for reassurance or requiring that they never threaten it.

Self-assertiveness and mature dependency. This category includes the ability to communicate one's needs, complaints, and injuries forthrightly, without shrouding them in self-righteous blame, guilt-trips, or simplistic declarations ("The only reasonable way to do this is..."), or by putting the other down ("Only a plebian wouldn't want to go to the opera!") Deficiencies in this area are common: In Olson and Olson's (2000) national sample of 21,501 married couples (of whom 60% were "satisfied or very satisfied" and 28% were "dissatisfied or very dissatisfied"), 75% agreed that, "I have trouble asking my partner for what I want."

Comfort with sexuality. This entails accepting one's physical appearance and being relatively free of sexual guilt, disgust, or inhibitions.

Comfort with self-exposure. Just as one should be comfortable taking off one's clothes in front of one's partner, so partners should ideally be comfortable exposing their thoughts and feelings. Such exposure can be one of the great pleasures of courtship and is also one of the frequent casualties of marriage: Olson and Olson reported that 82% of their sample wished that their partners were "more willing to share their feelings."

Empathy and concern. Many of the above capacities depend on the ability to put oneself in one's partner's shoes, to decenter from one's own immediate concerns, to feel one's partner's pain without being overwhelmed by it, and to take steps to assist the "life project of the other" (Kernberg, 2011).

Avoidance of gender polarization. Maturity includes freedom from internalized injunctions that create excessive polarizations around gender, as in the following condensed summary from Goldner (2004):

> [G]ender casts masculinity as an illusory state of omnipotence from which dependency must be externalized by being projected onto a female Other, and femininity is reciprocally constituted as the site of all that masculinity repudiates ... [T]hese pathogenic gender injunctions produce women who existentially recognize, depressively idealize, and unconsciously envy the agency of the men they cannot be. In the same way, men are constituted to refuse recognition to women as independent centers of subjectivity in order to deny the reality of their profound dependency on them ... [G]ender undergirds a commonplace form of relational splitting in which the universal psychic tensions between dependency/connection/sameness and autonomy/separation/difference default into a gendered exchange of projections. The woman, cast as the "dependent object," evacuates her own subjectivity and desire into the man through her submission to his psychic (and sometimes physical) domination. The man, in turn, sustains his position as the "autonomous subject" of the pair only because he is projecting his vulnerability and dependency into the woman, a subject who has become his object.
>
> *(pp. 350–351)*

This list of desirable personality capacities is long, and would be even longer if I had included other terms and theoretical vantage points also known to facilitate marital harmony ("secure attachment," "differentiation," "agreeableness," "reality acceptance"), or if I summed them up under the capacities for teamwork and love. Many signs of maturity also share the characteristic of "waking from the spell of childhood" (Fishbane, 2013), whereby sensitivities to parents as controlling, prohibiting, burdening, disappointing, criticizing, or otherwise disturbing become reduced, so that the predictable challenges of adult life are not seen as so toxic or burdensome.

No matter how labeled, these many components of maturity are desirable and tested in marriage. These are also capacities that can be lost under the stress of marriage, and if they are lost or glaringly absent, this will severely limit the power of couple therapy to heal. But as will be discussed in later chapters, they are best seen not as immutable and unchanging personality givens, but as dynamic capacities, capable of being strengthened and developed in the therapeutic setting.

INTERPERSONAL CHALLENGES

Managing Incompatibilities

Many studies show that the more partners agree on various subjects, the better their chances for marital success (Pines, 2005). Nonetheless, after marriage, couples will find that no matter how careful they have been, incompatibilities and differences that already existed or that emerge may threaten their harmony. In Olson and Olson's survey, 79% agreed that, "Our differences never seem to get resolved." Even couples who are highly compatible on a particular variable (e.g., on how much to socialize) might not be on the same page on a given day.

The areas of relationship differences and incompatibilities span the spectrum from trivial to fundamental, from getting partners to put their socks in the hamper to persuading them to take responsibility for their health. Differences will stir disputes over how much money to save, how often to have sex, how strict to be with parental discipline, how neat to keep the home, and how timely to be with appointments, to name some of the more common sources of marital conflict. Many arguments seem to stem from ingrained differences between men and women—differences somewhat normalized by John Gray (1992) in his books on men being from Mars and women from Venus—although how much these differences are due to biology or socialization remains hotly debated. On average, men have been socialized to focus more on work and women on relationships, so that differences in priorities in these areas are common. Some part of normal married life, and much time in couple therapy, is spent trying to discover which differences are worth fighting about and which should be accepted. If they are to be happy, spouses must eventually stop trying to change each other and/or stop refusing to change. Successful relationships require not only accepting differences, but making sacrifices. That may mean you go to the ballet because the person you love wants to go to the ballet, or it may mean you put off your professional dream to allow your partner to pursue his or hers.

Managing Conflict

Critical sources of difficulty in marriages involve determining how to share power equitably and how to work out inevitable conflicts, including over the differences in the previous section. The overwhelming majority of couples struggle in these areas, as illustrated by the following statistics from Olson and Olson's sample: 93% reported "trouble with leadership," 87% described their partners as "stubborn," 83% described them as "negative/critical," 79% agreed that "I go out of my way to avoid conflict with my partner," and 79% felt that "Our differences never seem to get resolved." These statistics are particularly worrisome because one of the best predictors of couples' success is how well they manage conflict (Fincham & Beach, 1999; Gottman, Coan, Carrera, & Swanson, 1998; Stanley, Markman & Whitton, 2003).

Although many couples come to therapy complaining of "communication problems," often they *have* communicated their positions . . . repeatedly. Their real problem is that they have remained unmoved by their partner's stated request or, worse, have become rigidly entrenched or vindictively passive-aggressive. Sometimes, they have just stopped listening. Unable to find common ground, they may try to coerce each other to change, or they may simply try to flee the conflict.

The co-captains problem. Optimal functioning in marriage, as in any group, requires rules for setting goals and settling disputes; ideally, everyone perceives these rules as fair. But how do you break a tie in a two-person group? I call this "the politics of two" or "the co-captains problem." While some cultures handle this challenge by granting power on the basis of tradition, religious belief, or gender, such solutions are unacceptable to most modern couples. Absent such a default setting, this structural challenge—how to decide things in a two-person polity—is a powerful reason that couple therapists so often find themselves caught in the middle, entreated to serve as tie-breaking judges. When this happens, I often point out that the problem is not illusory and that it explains why ships have but one captain authorized to act expeditiously when icebergs threaten. No co-captains there! My point is not that marriages would do better with one "captain," but that having two creates predictable difficulties. The problem for the co-captains is to become team-mates, team-mates who can certainly differ, but who never forget that they are on the same team.

Faulty "solutions." There are many maladaptive ways to break a tie. One gives one partner his or her way almost always, creating a chronic power imbalance. The "one-up" partner may dominate by threats of physical violence or verbal abuse, or the one-down partner may dominate by guilt-tripping or through various forms of going on strike. In both cases, the marriage is tilted too much toward meeting the needs of one person, and this feels morally wrong.

Accepting influence. In other situations where the needs of the partners diverge, one partner simply fails to engage. He or she refuses to put aside self-interest when his or her spouse is sick, depressed, or otherwise in distress, leading to a serious erosion of marital trust (Johnson, Makinen, & Millikin, 2001; Gottman, 2011). The resulting marital damage resembles Gottman's finding (Gottman & Levenson, 1999) that husbands who fail to "accept influence" (to take their wives' needs into account) contribute to later marital unhappiness.

Attuning. Gottman (2011) and all psychoanalytic self psychologists after Kohut (1971, 1977) highlight the opportunities partners have to "attune" or relate empathically to one another—or not—and stress that these events have a profound impact on well-being and trust. In the life of each couple, there will be a series of "at bats," or chances to experience the other, not as an adversary in a zero-sum game, but as someone who can be trusted, someone who cares about one's well-being. Such moments of testing will come loudly and acutely in times of crisis, and also quietly and matter-of-factly in ordinary, everyday transactions. Just as the structural "co-captains problem" makes managing marital conflict more difficult, the level of responsive attunement will influence—for better or worse—the couple's capacity to manage their differences.

The corrosive impact of conflict mishandled. Not only does conflict handled poorly erode trust and the marital bond, it can have negative, real-world consequences. Constantly tussling over who will steer the ship will result in hitting some icebergs! And sidestepping conflict will lead to tasks left undone (e.g., a failure to arrive at a sensible budget) or performed inconsistently (e.g., setting limits on children), and problems not faced, let alone not solved, tend to get worse over time.

Avoiding conflict also means increasingly avoiding each other and becoming more estranged from each other's vital concerns. This lack of intimate connection and emotional support may result in even more deficient task performance. Some partners will become psychiatrically impaired or resort to maladaptive solutions that further stress them and their partners. Most will feel increasingly lonely as their lives diverge. It is at this point that many couples seek help.

EXTERNAL CHALLENGES

Life Stresses and Social Pressures

Life presents many external challenges that may erode happiness and drive a wedge between partners. Some challenges are ongoing and highly predictable: setting external boundaries with family and work, dividing tasks equitably, managing finances, raising children, and maintaining sexual satisfaction. Others are tied to specific life events: adapting to the birth of a first child or to infertility, coping with an empty nest or with "boomerang" children, assisting aging parents, or transitioning to retirement. Still others result from contemporary social structure and normative expectations: emotional and time demands on dual-career families with ever more demanding employers, high levels of geographical mobility that leave couples far from their families of origin and supportive friends, and expectations that parents provide rich cultural opportunities for their children. Other serious challenges will come less predictably: illness, unemployment, forced geographical relocation. Some are pervasively built into our present-day culture: racism, sexism, homophobia, "structural" unemployment, limits on affordable childcare, and inadequate mental health resources.

Solving these myriad problems is made more difficult because many couples lack role models for how to manage. In addition, the modern couple's multiple role requirements often cause stress as partners try to do too many things in too little time and, as a result, perpetually experience themselves suffering from what Doherty (2003) calls "time famine."

Ideally, couples faced with substantial life challenges will rally and work as a team to meet those challenges constructively. If, on the other hand, they succumb to stress and become overwhelmed, they will be susceptible to maladaptive sequelae that often make matters worse:

- Endlessly arguing about how to cope with stressful situations, often becoming more and more polarized in their search for sensible approaches (e.g., whether to be tougher or more lenient with teenagers).
- Haggling over the equitable distribution of tasks.
- Becoming sidetracked by minor or tangentially related issues when faced with a core problem that is much harder to control (e.g., fighting over parenting when one partner has just been diagnosed with cancer). The anxious, overwhelmed couple may then turn their frustrated anger on each other, rather than on their real, shared enemy.
- One or both partners coping in ways that create additional problems: Feeling left out as his wife bonds with a newborn, the husband seeks connection by having an affair; then, hurt by her husband's affair, the wife quietly turns to alcohol.
- One or both partners becoming depleted, anxious, depressed, or demoralized by a life challenge (e.g., one of them has been laid-off) leading to the other becoming contentious or burned out.

When such secondary problems follow on the heels of external life stressors, they make difficult situations worse. Typically, couples who seek couple therapy present with a complex mix of real-life stressors and maladaptive solutions to them.

Maintaining Couple Positivity and Identity

One adverse consequence of contending with external life stressors is that couples have less time or inclination to seek out and cultivate positive experiences to share. Such experiences can be as simple as those they enjoyed during courtship: conversation, nice food, time away from external demands, intimate conversation, and sexual connection. Indeed, 82% of Olson and Olson's sample wished their partners "had more time and energy for recreation with me."

Even in the absence of significant external stressors or time demands, there may be fewer positive experiences because of marital conflict and disappointment. Couples can wear each other down—in a kind of "death by a thousand cuts"—as they inflict small, but repeated psychic injuries. When partners fail to alter their behavior after being asked to do so many times, the spouses asking will often conclude (falsely I think) that their partners, deep down, do not really love or care about them.

Not only can couples "torture" each other bit by bit, but they often fail to compensate and heal the damage by neglecting to engage in positive, shared experiences, "to put money in their marriage love bank" or "to cultivate their marital garden," to use two metaphors popular in the field.

So, another reason that marriage is challenging is that many couples take nurturing their sense of "we-ness" (their couple identity) and shared pleasure for granted, not paying enough attention to things that appear to be working . . . until it's too late.

In the chapters that follow, I elaborate on the material in these introductory chapters to show how Couple Therapy 1.0 can be improved, including by utilizing our understanding of the considerable challenges that couples face in marriage.

Notes

1 After reviewing 100 longitudinal studies, Karney and Bradbury (1995) proposed and validated a similar categorization of variables predictive of marital success. Their Vulnerability-Stress-Adaptation model was subsequently validated in a prospective study by Lavner and Bradbury (2010). Our models overlap closely in that their Vulnerability category consists mostly of personal limitations, their Stress category is identical to my external challenges category, and what they term Adaptation (operationalized as how well couples functioned in a Gottman-style conflict discussion) is covered in my model by the interpersonal challenge of managing conflict.
2 Many arranged marriages may be successful because spouses do not have to weather the disillusionment of waning romance, and because they expect success to require effort. Daniel Jones (2014) describes couples in arranged marriages as

> expecting to have to get to know each other, to come to love each other over time, and to somehow make it work. As improbable as it may seem, they very often do. And part of this is surely due to the fact that instead of starting out at a peak of love and then watching in anxious disbelief as the marriage deteriorates over the years into that thankless grind (for some), they begin with the blank slate and, if they are lucky, are able to gaze upon their life in wonder as warmth and affection take hold and flourish in the unlikeliest terrain.
>
> (p. 49)

3 Regarding the benefits of seeking healing in others, Lewis (1997) cites studies showing what all experienced therapists know (and base their practices on): that children with insecure attachment and difficult childhoods can become more mature and do better with their own children if they have had the benefit of "corrective emotional experiences" with spouses, teachers, or therapists (p. 32). He also cites a study by Cohn et al. (1992), who observed that in "the interactions of insecurely attached wives and securely attached husbands . . . the wives behaved like securely attached women" (p. 32). So, the search for a "better object," one who can stabilize us and allow growth, is not necessarily doomed.
4 Our informal study findings on the importance of self-awareness are consistent with several studies by Curran and associates (in particular, Curran, Ogolsky, Hazen, & Bosch, 2011) showing that measures of "insightfulness" in describing one's parents' marriage (including negative memories) predicted greater marital happiness and less involvement of children in parental conflict seven years later. Similarly, many studies

from the perspective of attachment theory find that the ability to narrate relationship stories richly, openly, and coherently—i.e., insightfully—during the Adult Attachment Interview predicts emotional health and healthy relationships (e.g., Paley, Cox, Burchinal, & Payne, 1999).

5 Supporting the importance of this capacity, George Vaillant's well-known longitudinal studies (1993) found that the maturity of a person's defense mechanisms—one measure of responsibility—assessed in young adulthood were robust predictors of emotional and relationship health in later life.

PART II
Systems Upgrades

4

FOCUSING ON THE INTERPERSONAL PROCESS

> Problem sequences are the symptomatic manifestations of the presenting problems and provide the most concrete, accessible, and ultimately changeable aspects of the problems.
>
> Breunlin, Pinsof, Russell, & Lebow (2011)

> When someone loves you, the way they say your name is different. You just know that your name is safe in their mouth.
>
> Billy (age 4)

The first key upgrade to Couple Therapy 1.0 is making the couple's interpersonal process the focus. The pathological dance, in which the emotional music generally matters more than the words, must become the principal concern of both the therapist and the couple. The noted couple therapist and researcher Susan Johnson put it this way: "The novice therapist has to learn not to get lost in the pragmatic issues and the content of interactions, but to focus instead on the process of interaction, and how inner experience evolves in that interaction" (2008, p. 129). Virtually all experienced couple therapists agree. This is a systems theory upgrade because it views much couple behavior as *an emergent property* of individual interactions, where what emerges is more than the sum of the individual contributions.

In this chapter, I will mostly be discussing sequences of "circular causation": A influences B, who subsequently influences A, who subsequently influences B, etc. As with systemic thinking generally, we want to know not just what person A does, but how others respond when he or she does it, and the impact of these responses on A's behavior. In later chapters, we will be interested in systemic thinking more generally, such that, for instance, both A's illness and

B's unemployment may simultaneously influence the couple system, which may, in turn, deal well or poorly with those stressors. Systemic thinking will also alert us to the impact of grandparents, teachers, colleagues, clergy, concurrent therapists, and therapy supervisors on what occurs in the therapy.

Terminology

There are many names that couple therapists use to refer to the maladaptive couple process. Some simply speak of "vicious circles." The term I generally use when speaking to couples is "pathological dance"; with professional audiences, I prefer "negative interaction cycle" (following Greenberg & Johnson, 1988; and Greenberg & Goldman, 2008). "The vulnerability cycle" (Scheinkman & Fishbane, 2004) works for both audiences. In this book, I use all of these terms interchangeably.

Process Precedes Content

Negative process predicts poor outcomes. Although I discovered the value of this statement independently in my own practice, it has been reassuring to find support for a focus on pathological process in formal couple therapy research (Lebow, Chambers, Christensen, & Johnson, 2012) and, most famously, in John Gottman's research in his "marriage love lab" (Gottman, Coan, Carrera, & Swanson, 1998).

In Gottman and colleagues' longitudinal study of 130 newly married couples, measures of negative process in a problem-solving discussion were strong predictors of the future health of the marriage: Gottman's group identified criticism, contempt, defensiveness, and stonewalling—which they dubbed "The Four Horsemen of the Apocalypse"—as behaviors that predicted marital unhappiness and divorce at follow-up, six years later. Similar findings have been reported by others, as well (Karney & Bradbury, 1995; Lavner & Bradbury, 2010; Waldinger et al., 2004).

The previously cited, cross-sectional study by Olson and Olson (2000) also found glaring differences in the responses of "happy couples" and "unhappy couples" to the following questions concerning their interpersonal process: "I am very satisfied with how we talk to each other" (90% vs. 15%); "My partner is a good listener" (83% vs. 18%); "My partner does not put me down" (79% vs. 20%); "When we discuss problems, my partner understands my opinions and ideas" (87% vs. 19%); "We are able to resolve our differences" (71% vs. 11%).

How do we explain these correlations and predictions, and are there other reasons to focus on negative cycles?

Negative process communicates negative attitudes. One explanation for why the process of interacting is so important follows from the work of Bateson (1972) and others (Watzlawick, Beavin, & Jackson, 1967), who noted that communication not only carries content, but also conveys the attitude of the speaker toward the listener. If this attitude is contemptuous, vengeful, or rejecting—as it often was in the clinical or unhappy couples in the process studies above—the listener will feel that the very ground of love and marital connection is shaky.

Negative process interferes with problem solving. For groups of any size to function successfully, members must focus on the tasks at hand. To function optimally, group members have to face their differences, share power equitably, and resist the temptation to cope with anxiety by treating each other badly. Ideally, couples will view facing their differences as not only inevitable, but as potentially beneficial, as emphasized by expert negotiators: "[T]he best decisions result not from superficial consensus, but from exploring different points of view and searching for creative solutions" (Fisher, Ury, & Patton, 2011, p. xiii). Accepting differences and sharing power are not easy, however, and many couples will go off the rails into negative interaction cycles that will impair problem solving.

Focusing on process reduces the number of problems needing attention. Couples routinely bring multiple problems to therapy, but the impediment to solving all of them may be the same, namely, their characteristic negative interaction cycle. *Helping couples improve their process or structuralized ways of interacting facilitates conflict resolution across multiple content areas.* Once their process improves, clients who entered therapy with what seemed like an endless list of problems will often solve many of these on their own, without the need for direct therapeutic attention. Focusing on their process can significantly expedite therapy, which can otherwise feel like herding cats.

Focusing on process improves future problem solving. Since problems will continue to emerge after therapy is over, helping improve process gives couples the tools they need to address future problems.

Correcting system dysfunction is easier than changing personality dysfunction. Personality, by definition, is slow to change. Group process can be surprisingly malleable; in Chapter 11, I will show how teaching couples speaker–listener rules can often lead to rapid improvement in their interpersonal process. This is not to say that it is easy to alter negative cycles or that simple orchestration is always sufficient, but in keeping with many decades of family therapy experience, it is usually quickest to focus first on family structure and process (Pinsof, 1995).

"Solving the moment" strengthens intimacy. Dan Wile (2002) recommends that we "solve the moment rather than the problem," that is, that we prioritize process ("the moment") over content. Working on the here-and-now situation, rather than on surface, external areas of difficulty, can improve intimacy between partners who are feeling very alone in their relationship. If the therapist succeeds in helping them feel closer *in the moment*, they can feel connected, listened to, and important to each other.

Examining negative process is the royal road to underlying psychodynamics. Solving the moment helps not only because it centers attention on process over surface content, but because examining the components of negative cycles quickly leads us to crucial underlying issues. Inquiring why a man clings so anxiously, we can uncover his abandonment fears. Inquiring why a woman defends so angrily, we can uncover her shame. Just as Freud taught us that dreams can be the royal road to the unconscious, unpacking the vulnerability cycle can lead to core psychodynamic issues.

Formal research supports focusing on process. The foregoing discussion has listed many theoretical reasons why focusing on process *ought* to be beneficial. There is also formal research that supports this approach (Cordova, Jacobson, & Christensen, 1998; Sullivan & Baucom, 2005, cited in Baucom et al., 2008). For all of these reasons, the couple therapist is advised to devote attention early to the negative cycles of couple interaction.

Exceptions. Having declared that process should, in most cases, become the early focus of therapy, I must acknowledge that it is impossible to discuss process in the abstract, separate from *some* concrete content. In *Alice in Wonderland,* the Cheshire Cat's smile could exist without the cat, but in real life, "process" will always require some content if it is to be seen. With this in mind, *in order to make the focus on process easier to sustain and more likely beneficial, I try to steer couples early in treatment to discuss more workable, less emotionally charged, content.* This may not always be possible, for instance when the consultation is driven by a serious rupture of trust, such as one caused by infidelity. With such couples, we may have to begin with the topic that is most pressing, even though it is also the most volatile and, thus, may make examination of the couple's process more difficult.

There will also be days when we should follow a rule from Couple Therapy 1.0 and allow the couple to choose the most pressing topic and focus on that content (say, on a family emergency), and assist them directly with that, rather than spotlighting their interpersonal dance. The art of therapy includes knowing when to focus on content and when to focus on process, keeping in mind that, both early in therapy and in the long run, attention to the structure of how couples interact will be more productive.

Another exception to focusing primarily on negative interaction cycles is discussed in Chapter 14, where I note the value of encouraging discussion of positive experiences relatively early in therapy. When successful, such positive experiences (e.g., date nights) will improve the couple's ability to fight fair and make it easier for them to maintain good will toward each other during conflict.

Steps in the Pathological Couple Dance

In this section, my aim is to outline the basics of negative interaction cycles, which I will dissect further in Chapter 5.[1] In general, what the couple therapist encounters is an escalating sequence that runs as follows:

Poor start-ups. The pathological process usually begins when one partner starts a conversation badly, often in an abrupt, one-sided, hostile, or unsympathetic way that conceals his or her own subjectivity and desire. Only rarely do couples use "I-statements" or ask for things politely. In fairness to our clients, however, some of the topics they raise are just not that easy to open up for discussion.

Defensive, one-sided responses, and functional deafness. The other partner responds to this opening move defensively—with assorted varieties of fight or flight, hostility, blaming, swearing, rebuttal, self-justification, and a paucity of validation, understanding, or empathy. (For a detailed catalog of possible defenses, see Wile, 1993, pp. 88–99.) While most spouses understand the defensive nature of such responses, they are, nonetheless, put off by it, and rarely address what it signifies (e.g., shame or guilt). Instead, spouses press on, trying to make their case, to partners who have now become functionally deaf, part of the explanation for the raising of voices and the increasingly simplistic language.

Both partners begin to talk at once (or one withdraws), and invalidation crowds out listening. This may take the form of one-sided arguing, insulting the partner, not letting the partner speak, saying the partner is over-reacting, or "cross-complaining": A admits that he has done something wrong, but counters that B has been similarly hurtful in the past. Both claim to be the victim of the other, the abused rather than the abuser, the "done-to" rather than the "do-er" (Benjamin, 2004). Some partners freeze up after becoming flooded with emotion, and are misperceived as unaffected and uncaring.

Clients are almost always more conflicted about how to respond than they let on, often rejecting more nuanced statements because these threaten to open them up to blame or to expose their vulnerability. This makes matters worse because they present themselves as more adversarial and one-sided than they actually are. Even when they correctly identify circular causation, comments intended as self-exoneration can make matters worse: "I'd talk more if you weren't such a nag!"

Negative reciprocity, escalation, and polarization. The argument escalates and becomes increasingly polarized as each partner meets negative with negative ("negative reciprocity"). This differs from a forceful or angry disagreement, a process that might still be productive. Rather, there is a qualitative "change of state" (as when water turns to vapor): Accusations become exaggerated, voices get louder, and everyone digs in deeper. Neither partner acknowledges what the other has said. Rather, they put their energy into fending off each other's attempts to bring counterarguments into evidence. They shout each other down, point out each other's weaknesses, and voice objections as though they were attorneys at a trial. Neither is able to apply the brakes, and both feel caught in a maelstrom of feelings that they don't understand but which seem somehow to be terribly important, usually more important than the original dispute.

The collapse of interpersonal space: A (k)not. The resulting panic and confusion can be conceptualized as the result of the collapse of the "interpersonal space" between the partners, as they fail to acknowledge each other's subjectivity. Pizer and Pizer (2006) call this failure to acknowledge the other a "(k)not"—conveying simultaneously the tangled obstinacy of a physical knot and the emotional negation of the partner as a "not." Once they have lost the capacity to see each other as individuals, partners will find it impossible to work out differences, and the process will deteriorate further. They often recognize that they are caught in such a (k)not, but don't understand why and see no way to escape.

The absorbing quality of the conversation. Arguments escalate, in part, because the partners have trouble standing down or backing off. They correctly sense that something larger is at stake and become "absorbed" by the process (Gottman, 2011), although they would be hard-pressed to say why it is so captivating. Each one wants to have the last word and sees leaving the confrontation as humiliation and defeat.

Content expands, character is attacked, and the relationship itself is questioned. The content under dispute expands to include (sometimes unrelated) past offenses and each partner's alleged personality flaws, causing another type of escalation, as in "You're too critical!" met with "No, you're too sensitive!" Jacobson and Christensen (1996) call this "vilification," as couples label each other morally or mentally defective. Sometimes, the status of the relationship itself is questioned ("You've *never* loved me!"), and divorce may be mentioned. Couples now go for the psychological jugular: "You're running away, just like your father!" "You can't take the simplest criticism!" We have now reached the highest "level of attack", according to Wile's (1993) scheme:

> Level 1: *Criticizing behavior* ("You never talk to me anymore!")
> Level 2: *Criticizing feelings* ("You should appreciate the good things we have instead of always dwelling on the bad!")
> Level 3: *Criticizing character* ("You're a nag!")
> Level 4: *Making accusatory interpretations* ("I'm tired of you blaming me when you're angry at your boss!")
> Level 5: *Criticizing intentions* ("You're making these problems up in order to make me feel guilty.")
>
> *(p. 109)*

Wile points out that invoking intentions is particularly hurtful and provocative, since it shakes partners' sense of reality. It moves beyond telling them that they should behave or feel differently to telling them that what they *seem to want* is bad and that they are bad to want it. Obviously, threats of divorce are highly inflammatory; in this taxonomy, they might be considered a Level 6.

The couple's worst fears are confirmed. Escalation, invalidation, and polarization stimulate and appear to confirm the partners' worst relationship fears (negative transferences). *Each seems to be acting in the way the other most dreads he or she will act*—what Real (2007) calls "core negative images"—while the motives for doing so appear more negative than they actually are (called "negative interpretation" by Markman et al., 2001). The woman who fears abandonment feels abandoned. The man who fears assaults on his competence feels assaulted. Additionally, *perceiving themselves as unfairly miscast in these negative ways, partners become still more upset, threatened, and defensive.* Feared *self-*images are also activated, so that guilt-prone or shame-prone spouses fear that they have done something immoral or shameful and then defend against that recognition. In such situations of grave threat, partners often believe "that one must either lose the other or lose one's mind" (Ringstrom, 2014, p. 52, citing Davies, 2003).

Vengeful motives emerge. After being injured in such arguments, many partners seek to restore some sense of agency and self-esteem by injuring the other back: "Hurt people hurt people." Couples swear and call each other increasingly cruel names. Sometimes, such vengeance will be wrought via more subtle means, as when partners stubbornly hold to their views and don't allow themselves to yield to sensible arguments. Or they may take a passive-aggressive approach, agreeing to do something knowing they have no intention of following through. In the most serious situations, physical violence not only ends the argument, but exacts self-righting revenge.

Lack of resolution leaves things worse than they were at the beginning. As such cycles come to a close, partners feel some combination of wounded, furious, exasperated, exhausted, and hopeless. Sometimes, one partner unilaterally flees the scene. Sometimes escalation ends in violence or threats of it, and this ends the dispute. More often, the couple simply gives up trying and the partners feel worse than they could have imagined at the start.

Alienation, hopelessness, sensitization, and negative sentiment override. Alienation and additional hopelessness can ensue because not only did the couple fail to handle the initial delimited complaint, but their painful interaction ending as it did will stimulate additional doubts about their relationship. Partners lose good will toward each other and may also view themselves more negatively. (Most of my clients check off "I don't like the way I am with my partner," on their intake questionnaire.) Over time, sensitized partners will need less aggravation to get the negative ball rolling, will fight more fiercely about deeper wounds, and will come to view their relationship progressively more negatively. This "negative sentiment override" will make it harder and harder for them to experience each other as well-meaning or influenceable. Divorce may seem to be the only escape.

Longer-term adaptation and deterioration. Couples whose disputes escalate and end poorly will gradually experience an erosion of the love, respect, and cohesion that are essential for marital happiness and collaboration. Partners then adapt in ways that, over time, will further damage their relationship. Faced with such poor conflict management, they may focus their energies on parenting or work. One or both may lose interest in sex or seek it outside the marriage. Aware of the dangers of "the fight," some partners will make apparent accommodations, but their anger will fester over time. Feeling more irritable, they will squabble more often over trivial matters. The more they do this, the more their marital bond will suffer and their resentment increase, making discussions about inevitable differences and life challenges even more daunting. While the rapid-fire negative cycles I have been describing are easy to see, therapists must also be aware of such longer-term deteriorating processes that occur over months or years and erode feelings of happiness, shared connection, and positive couple identity.

Trying something different and turning things around. Of course, not all marital fights end this badly. Sometimes, couples come to their senses, apologize, and become less defensive, more empathic, and softer, so that underlying issues can be accessed and understood. Problem solving and compromise then become possible. This is a common outcome in cathartic crisis scenes in film and television dramas. As noted by Gottman and Levenson (1999), angry fights per se are not inevitably destructive, and some will force couples to face painful subjects, even if they don't do this smoothly. Indeed, greater confidence and pride in their marriages were outcomes of successfully resolved battles in the "good marriages" studied by Wallerstein (Wallerstein & Blakeslee, 1995).

What allows some couples to come to their senses, regain their emotional balance, and avoid permanent damage? Some care more about losing the relationship than about the issues that had them at each other's throats, and they use this concern to steady themselves and reconnect (Feldman, 1979). Some will reconnect in emotionally gratifying scenes that bind them more strongly together and feel so rewarding that they even reinforce or encourage more of the fights that precede their making up (Goldner, 2004). Many couples will feel relief after having re-established connection, even as they dread a possible return to what set them off. But, of course, most couples who come to our offices will need our assistance to end their battles, heal their wounds, and learn better ways to manage their disagreements.

Interventions That Begin to Alter Negative Interaction Cycles

Focus on the dance and label it as the enemy. The first thing the couple therapist must do to improve couple process is to focus everyone's attention on the process as the core problem. This shift in focus from content to process is the first and most important upgrade to the basic TTEO model of couple therapy. *Focusing on the pathological cycle will usually, in and of itself, improve the process.* It accomplishes this in three interrelated ways: (a) by giving the vague marital problem a diagnostic label ("a systems problem"), (b) by objectifying this systems problem as a common enemy, and (c) by reducing mutual blaming (now attributed to the systems problem).

Having a diagnosis helps. This is clear to anyone who has felt better once a medical diagnosis and its attendant treatment plan have been established. So it is with couples caught in their vicious circles. Beginning to elucidate the components of the pathological dance gives clients a diagnosis and makes clear that others have suffered from similar troubles (normalizing their situation), while assuring them that professionals (researchers and clinicians) have studied such problems and know how to help.

Giving the dance a name also objectifies it and makes it an enemy that the couple can attack jointly, in what Michael White (2007) termed an "externalizing conversation." Some couples will coin names for their dances: One couple called theirs "the morass/more-ass," to describe the quagmire they wanted to avoid when referring to the husband's desire for more sex. Once the enemy has been named, clients can be invited to step back, to take up positions on a shared "perch above the fray" (Wile, 2013a), and to look with "unified detachment" (Jacobson & Christensen, 1996) at their maladaptive process.

Last but not least, focusing on the pathological dance tends to reduce blame (and increase curiosity and reflection), as it counters linear narratives of victim and villain. Reducing blame, in turn, improves couple functioning and morale. Learning that blame itself is an emergent property of their malignant dance is often felt as convincingly experience-near by partners who are quite sure that responsibility can't be solely theirs!

Couple therapists should also take heart. If the regressive blaming and intense defensiveness we see in our clients were truly inherent in the individuals, then meeting with them once a week to cure such malignant negative character traits would be hopelessly optimistic. When we view such behavior, instead, as a function of a pathological process—as a whole transformed into something more negative than its component parts—we, too, can feel hopeful.

Use the chemical reaction metaphor. To convey the idea of a systemic problem—one with additive, circular, and emergent properties—I use the metaphor of a chemical reaction. In this image, the partners are compared to two colorless reagents in two separate beakers that, when mixed, become drastically altered: perhaps freezing cold, explosively hot, different in color, or foul-smelling. One of the reagents might think, "Hey, I was just fine—not cold or hot or red or smelly—before I came into contact with this other chemical. Therefore, this sudden change of state, in which I can't even recognize myself, must be due to that other damn chemical!" This metaphor powerfully illustrates how group process is not reducible to individual behavior and expresses empathy to individuals who feel victimized and then blame their partners for their distress.

As discussed in Chapter 3, humans seem wired to see changes in internal state as caused by external factors, rather than due to a combination of internal predispositions and external events. It is precisely because of this reflexive or default state that couples seem so mystified when they are caught in their pathological processes. Hope can come from gaining a "systemic awareness" (Gurman, 2008b) that is simultaneously a more accurate model of the couple's interpersonal universe and one that reduces personal responsibility, shame, and guilt.

Use the "To the Extent That" Intervention. After describing the situation in general terms using the chemical reaction metaphor, I then apply systemic thinking to what we know so far about the couple and their specific interaction cycle. In doing this, I use what Les Greenberg (personal communication) terms the "To the Extent That" Intervention. I might say, "Fred, to the extent that you fail to engage Beth's requests for help around the house, she tends to intensify her attempts to get you to listen, even at times when you want to be left alone to work." And I might then say to Beth, "To the extent that you approach Fred at times when he is trying to concentrate on his work, he feels unfairly put upon, and then tends to place what you've asked him to do even lower on his to-do list." Or, I may simply say, "The more you . . . the more he/she will . . . and then the more you . . ." This intervention moves beyond explaining circular process in the abstract, as it identifies the specifics of each couple's negative interaction cycle.

Explain the "punctuation" of negative cycles. When I describe the basics of negative cycles to couples, I note that most people "punctuate" their narratives by beginning with some misdeed or insensitive action of their partner's. I then point out that this starting point is usually arbitrary, as it would be when one decides what point to identify as the beginning of a circle. For instance, Beth will say that her anger at Fred is due to his failing to call the plumber as he had promised. Fred will, possibly grudgingly, admit that he failed to call the plumber, but will add that this was because he was angry at Beth for not having sex with him for the past two weeks. Beth will then say that she wasn't in the mood to have sex with Fred because he so frequently fails to keep his promises about household matters, such as calling the plumber. I will affirm that both are right, but that their punctuation is arbitrary. Such arbitrary and self-serving punctuation of circular causation explains why so many arguments concerning "who started it" are both senseless and interminable.

Use metaphors to normalize off-putting demands: the hungry diner and the unresponsive waiter, or the drowning swimmer and the unresponsive lifeguard. Escalation commonly consists of one or both partners speaking increasingly loudly, impatiently, and aggressively, perhaps while whining, nagging, guilt-tripping, or swearing. All of these are ineffective ways to influence a partner, and all occur when the partner appears unresponsive. Several metaphors can help therapists to normalize these unhelpful behaviors by explaining them in systemic terms. One metaphor I use is of a hungry person calling for a waiter who is not responding. At first, the diner waits respectfully, then he tries to signal non-verbally, then he calls out in a calm voice, and finally he might resort to yelling.

Sometimes, I invoke a drowning swimmer calling out to a lifeguard for help. The more the swimmer fears drowning, and the longer the lifeguard fails to respond, the louder and more desperate will be his shouts. This metaphor also helps couples understand—especially those who have had lifesaving instruction—how when you finally respond to a "drowning" partner, you may be met with a kick, rather than a thank you. (Lifeguards are trained to expect this.) Such negativity is a common, seemingly paradoxical, outcome in couple therapy that one sees when one partner rails angrily at the other for offering too little, too late.

In many cases, it helps to characterize both partners as "drowning swimmers." Both are desperate and not getting sufficient "psychological oxygen," and neither is able to assist in rescuing the other. In fact, escalation in negative couple cycles usually requires two drowning partners, even if one may *appear* to be an unresponsive lifeguard.

Use metaphors to normalize flight: firemen and forest fires. Just as increasing anger and loudness can seem sensible in some situations, so can flight. When one client breaks off connection in the middle of an argument, this frequently inflames the other partner who wishes to "settle this once and for all." Here, it helps to have a metaphor that makes flight more comprehensible and acceptable. The one I like to use is that of firemen fighting a raging forest fire. While their ultimate goal may be to battle the blaze, there are times when it is futile, or even self-destructive, to remain in the thick of it. The therapist can then help couples to unpack the perspectives of metaphorical fleeing firemen (Why do they think the situation is hopeless?) and the advancing forest fire (What is making the pursuer so hot and insistent?).

Use the cogwheel or the canoe metaphor. To illustrate how vicious circles work, I show couples a picture of two cogwheels/gears (representing the clients), both of which are connected separately to a third, output gear (whose turning represents the summed constructive or destructive movement in the relationship). In this visual image, not only do each of the client wheels contribute to the final result (illustrating the impact for good or ill of *both* partners on the outcome), but turning one client wheel also turns the other client wheel in the same direction (illustrating their impact for good or for ill *on each other*.) The metaphor is also helpful when discussing the transition to healthier relating, since there will be moments when one person continues to drive things negatively or to oppose positive changes made by the other. At such moments, there may be a "grinding of gears" as the partners are out of sync, with one more willing to change than the other. However, with the therapist's continued help, the gears should start turning again, now both in a positive direction, as when couples offer each other mutual empathy and support. The cogwheel metaphor also allows us to visualize the influence of additional extramarital actors—extended family, friends, bosses—as forces that can influence the movement of the wheels in either positive or negative directions.

Alternatively, you can use the image of two people in a canoe, paddling in the same productive direction, in the same negative direction, or in opposing, nullifying directions. This metaphor is especially useful in situations where couples argue about whether one person is doing an unfair amount of marital work (paddling) or has too much control over the marriage's direction (steering).

Play the improv game. With some couples who are caught in a negative process and have proven impervious to my verbal explanations, I suggest a round of improvisation, to show what a positive cycle—one with the gears turning beneficially—can feel like. As in improv theater, the main rule is that each person must build on what the previous person has said. There can be no rebuttals, only additions. I join the game, as well, and we go around in a circle, each adding to the story that we are co-creating. To lighten the atmosphere, I either start with a whimsical situation, such as, "We are all in a bus on the planet Mars" or let them start after prompting them with, "Once upon a time . . . ." I then intervene only when clients fail to follow the rule of building on what has gone before. It can help to encourage them to begin each addition with, "Good point, and . . ." The goal of this exercise is to demonstrate a positive cycle with everyone "on the same team," but a side benefit is that the therapist may pick up interesting free associations that pertain to the couple's psychodynamics (e.g., one insecure man kept bringing in content related to his accomplishments). After the couple shows they can do this by adding to each other's fictional story, I repeat the exercise with them planning some shared, pleasurable activity. Almost invariably, I am able to show couples what a more positive cycle feels like, how the "music" is different, and how joining together can lead to a positive outcome.

Introduce the goal of "making a short story long." After giving the couple a preliminary outline of the cycle that is simultaneously captivating and torturing them, I explain that we can gain a deeper understanding if we can "make a short story long," using a felicitous phrase from Scheinkman and Fishbane (2004). This involves slowing things down, as in a slow-motion video replay, so we can deconstruct their vulnerability cycle and see where things break down.

A fork in the road. At this point, the therapist can choose to take the therapy in one of two directions, so as to further the task of unpacking the couple's negative interaction cycle. The psychodynamic approach seeks to uncover and address deeper psychological concerns. The educational or behavioral approach teaches couples how to be more skillful and less offensive during difficult conversations. These methods are the subjects of Parts III and IV of this book;

questions regarding how to select and sequence them are discussed in Part V. For now, I will give brief illustrations of each.

Psychodynamic approach: Give voice to each partner's deeper concerns. To deconstruct and reverse the negative cycle, we usually need to uncover the deeper desires and fears that are interfering with productive dialog. As I listen to the recurring fights, I try to discern what these issues are and help clients become more aware of what lies below the surface. When I have a handle on the issues, I try to articulate each partner's central concerns, serving as a translator between the two partners. As noted by Wile (2002), therapists can usually do a better job presenting each partner's case than either of them can. When possible, I also try to help clients speak for themselves. My goal is to reduce their functional deafness so that recurring arguments can be replaced by discussions of the deeper concerns that I hypothesize are fueling the battle. While I am attempting to deconstruct the dynamics of the negative cycle, I am also modeling respectful, collaborative dialog between the partners and between each of them and me, and I am constantly checking to see their reactions to my efforts to speak for and to them. When the process has improved to the point that the couple can talk productively without me, I move out of the middle and let them do so.

Psychodynamic approach: Inquire about families of origin. Partners often assume that the maladaptive ways they behave during negative cycles are their only options. Inquiring into childhood origins of these behaviors can rapidly counter such beliefs. They then become intelligible as roles learned in childhood as ways to cope ("When someone is angry, it's best to just leave the room."), as counter-identifications ("I'll never treat anyone like that!"), or simply as "how all families are or should be" ("We would just yell and the next day it would be over.").

Educational approach: Name the "steps" in the dance and teach alternatives. Just as we can create a name for the dance as a whole, we can give names to separate maladaptive steps and begin to teach more constructive ways to talk during cycles. For instance, I label incidents of *Disputing the Facts* ("I did so tell you to pay that bill!") and ones of *Getting More Votes* ("My mother also agrees that you are too tough on our kids!") as tempting, but almost always inflammatory. Simultaneously, I begin to suggest better ways to respond to criticism, including by trying to remain "calm, curious, and caring," what I call "The Three Cs."

What to Expect at the End of Therapy Concerning Process

Cycle replacement. One obvious goal of working on negative interaction cycles is to replace them with healthier sequences for dealing with conflict and distress—the "sequence replacement guideline" of Pinsof and colleagues (2011). This is sometimes possible and is something to shoot for, even though it may never reach the level we might hope for: Many couples, when sufficiently stressed, will go back to arguing in the same old ways.

Some "sequence replacements" put the passive person in charge of the problem. For instance, when one partner is incessantly complaining about something not happening—be it sufficient sex or involved parenting—the therapist can sometimes make it clear that the noise won't stop until the relatively passive person gets more involved. This can radically change the process into one of mutual collaboration.

Fewer negative cycles. Other times, what one sees are less frequent negative interaction cycles. Cycles still happen, but are far less frequent for many reasons, including that the partners are more aware of the early stages, less sensitive to certain hot buttons, and better able to slow down when things start going south.

Improved repair. Another common, beneficial outcome is that, after having had the same old argument or done the same regressive dance yet again, couples make better efforts at repair, starting them sooner and employing more compassion. Just as couples can become more aware of danger signs and better able to nip negative cycles in the bud, so they can become better at apology and repair by reviewing a fight when passions have calmed. We will discuss how to facilitate such repair in Chapter 10.

Case Example: The Intimidator and the Novelist

Tom, a 35-year-old retired professional football player, and Jennifer, his 33-year-old novelist wife, presented with the manifest conflict of whether to move out of Chicago. There were clear plusses and minuses to this relocation that they had "discussed" endlessly: He used what he considered logical arguments, while she became exasperated and withdrew into confusion, anger, and helplessness. Even when she was not under attack, Jennifer remained unwilling to consider Tom's arguments, as she felt that her needs—though somewhat unclear even to herself—were not being considered. Both were despondent, not only about the deadlocked decision, but about their marriage, and Jennifer was considering ending it.

At our first meeting, they each told me about their difficulties communicating, and when I encouraged them to talk to each other, I got to observe these directly. Watching them talk confirmed for me what they had reported about their frustration and deadlock. Additionally, and not surprisingly, when I attempted to facilitate a productive discussion of plusses and minuses, their negative interaction cycle made problem solving impossible. It was worth a try but, as with most of the couples referred to me, it proved insufficient. We did, however, now have a working diagnosis, as their description, their unaided process in the room, and their imperviousness to straightforward assistance all pointed to their negative interaction cycle as the culprit needing attention.

Tom had gone to business school after ending his professional sports career, and his manner reflected it. He was very competitive and interfaced with the world (including his wife) in a very logical, dogged manner, presenting Jennifer with many charts showing the advantages of moving their family out of Chicago, all to no effect. Her reluctance—not only to move, but to *discuss* moving—remained mysterious, especially since they both knew that Tom was becoming increasingly depressed, as the job opportunities and the recreational activities he loved were only available elsewhere.

Tom and Jennifer had met in college. They had bonded over a love of sports and other shared activities and values. Jennifer had always been attracted to Tom's certainty about how to do things (he resembled her father, who was hard-driving and domineering), but was turned off when he pressured her against her wishes. This was true in the bedroom, as well, where she had initially enjoyed sex with him, but had grown cold when she felt it was imposed on her when she wasn't in the mood. This was a source of frustration for Tom, who felt that while the crowds had cheered for him on the field, his wife failed to be enthusiastic about him in the bedroom. Both his depression and his insistence that they move intensified.

It was now clear that their negative interaction cycle interfered with other important areas in their marriage, most notably their sex life. The opportunity to solve more than one problem simultaneously was then another reason, distinct from our inability to solve their presenting problem, to shift the focus to the pathological dance.

I shifted attention to their negative interaction cycle as follows: "Tom," I began, "to the extent that you press on so forcefully and insistently, attempting to influence Jennifer with what seems to you impeccable logic, Jennifer feels increasingly overpowered and withdraws still more into her angry, confused state of mind. This obvious retreat from engaging with you in a crucial discussion makes you feel unimportant, anxious, and powerless. As a result, you redouble your efforts to force her to come to the table and talk."

My goal here was *to interrupt the negative process* by labeling its steps and showing how these led to their standoff and their escalating unhappiness. Simultaneously, I attempted *to validate their emotional reasons for continuing to dance as they did*. To accomplish this, I empathized with both of them—sometimes speaking to them directly ("Tom, it's hard for you to remain calm when your career and self-respect as a working person are blocked by Jennifer's reluctance to engage these issues.") and sometimes indirectly, as I represented one to the other via the technique of doubling ("Tom, I think what Jennifer would like to tell you, if she could be more direct and less afraid of hurting your feelings, is that when you get all worked up and insistent, it makes her feel like her needs won't be heard. This makes her angry, and then, feeling uncomfortable with her anger, she shuts down.")

Predictably, this combination of labeling the steps in their vicious circle and providing empathy almost immediately helped to slow them down and give them hope. This cleared a space for further exploration of the underlying issues that both powered and were concealed by the cycle. Specifically, by continuing to validate Tom's frustration at Jennifer's indecision and by blocking his guilt-inducing/controlling tactics for dealing with it, I enabled him to be more patient, and made it possible for us to uncover the reasons for that indecision.

As the mood lightened, we found a somewhat telling metaphor for an aspect of their dance: It turned out that both had been known for "intimidating" their opponents *in sports*, but for Jennifer, this was the *only* arena where she had allowed herself this satisfyingly aggressive role. With this in mind, I worked next to help Jennifer voice the anger she felt in interacting with her husband, whom she now dubbed with some humor, "The Intimidator." Previously, she had been doing this only indirectly via characters in her novels who stood up to authority figures. Now, she directly expressed her anger at feeling pushed around. As she did so, she began to reflect on the origins of her difficulties with expressing her needs. We learned of a career-ending sports injury and of how she believed that she had allowed others, including her overbearing father, to bully her into the surgery that only made things worse. We uncovered considerable internal conflict regarding her parents, who lived nearby, and their expectation that she remain in the area to assist them with family responsibilities. Jennifer had trouble speaking up to Tom, just as she had trouble speaking up to her parents, in part, because she really cared about them. She felt their palpable distress whenever she chose a course of action different from one they preferred. This marital short story was becoming long and illuminating.

Tom proved quite "coachable"—not too surprising for a professional athlete—and became almost a co-therapist, drawing Jennifer out about her family and her somewhat unconscious wish never again to go along blindly with plans proposed by others. Just as Tom's more patient and empathic presence allowed his wife to speak up, it also allowed her to listen to him; the cogwheels were now moving in a positive direction. I could now help Tom voice *his* deeper concerns and career aspirations. He told movingly of his fears of being like other professional athletes who quickly ran through their earnings, of the shame he felt at being unemployed, and of his lifelong love of the outdoor sports he couldn't pursue in Chicago. The difference was that now Jennifer could hear him and be moved by his pleas to relocate. More fundamentally, the couple experienced moments of real intimacy and connection in my office . . . and their sex life picked up at home.

With the radical change in their interpersonal process, Tom and Jennifer became a team working together to solve their external problems. On their own, they decided in favor of relocating and, equally important, they worked together to deal with the resulting fallout: their guilt and Jennifer's parents' anger. In addition to solving the specific problem that had brought them to therapy, they developed the ability to manage conflicts in other areas (e.g., over which new house to buy), so that they seemed prepared to handle future episodes of disagreement. The depressed mood that had accompanied them into therapy lifted and was replaced by a profound pleasure in their shared lives together. These improvements were still evident a year later, when they visited Chicago and came in for a check-up appointment.

This is a typical successful case: A couple presents to the therapist with a specific problem and some level of chronic unhappiness. Their sex life is compromised, and they are growing increasingly estranged from each other. They may be considering divorce. What helps, beyond providing a safe forum where they can talk to each other, is directing early attention to their negative interaction cycle, labeling it, and working to discover some of its roots, which, once exposed, will allow them to feel and act more sympathetically and collaboratively with each other. Intimacy and problem solving improve concurrently. All of this occurred for Tom and Jennifer, and it allowed them to agree on an important course of action, one that had been blocked by forces outside of their awareness.

In the next chapter, we investigate the structural properties of some specific couple dances and some interventions tailored to altering them.

Notes

1 I am indebted to the following authors for their perceptive descriptions of couple dances: Christensen & Jacobson (2000); Gottman et al. (1998); Greenberg & Goldman (2008); Greenberg & Johnson (1988); Markman, Stanley, & Blumberg (2001); Real (2007); Scheinkman & Fishbane (2004); and Wile (1993, 2002).

5
COUPLE DANCES EXAMINED MORE CLOSELY

In the last chapter, I discussed the importance of focusing on the pathological couple process. In this chapter, I will go into more detail, elaborating on prevalent issues, common dances, and interventions tailored to these issues and dances. Pathological dances are, by definition, maladaptive or dysfunctional. Couple dysfunction expresses itself most often as spouses failing to work collaboratively in the face of conflict. It is also evident when partners collude to avoid facing problems. We begin this chapter with the topics of anger and blame, since these are so common in all forms of serious couple conflict and tend to be poorly understood.

Anger, Revenge, and Passive-Aggression

Anger as simultaneously valuable and dangerous. Like other unpleasant feelings (boredom, anxiety, or pain from a pebble in your shoe), anger is a signal that spurs us to do something about unacceptable circumstances. Among dysphoric feelings, anger is tasked with increasing our motivation to remove obstacles that block our path. It can be a force behind the healthy assertion of our needs, stirring us to stand up for ourselves. In relationships, anger energizes us to disclose our unhappiness with and to our partners. As anyone past the age of two knows, anger can also get us into trouble and push us into counterproductive actions. As therapists, we try to help clients identify and share the sources of their anger, while simultaneously helping them to use this awareness adaptively, rather than impulsively and destructively—to "report" its presence, rather than to act it out (Greenberg & Goldman, 2008; Wile, 1993).

I often outline these ideas about anger explicitly early in therapy, since clients tend to view anger either as universally bad or as something that cannot be helped and should be unimpeded in its expression. I also find it helpful to examine how anger was handled in the clients' families of origin.

Restraint: Chinese finger traps and tangled shoelaces. In working with couples to identify and communicate their anger or dissatisfaction constructively, I emphasize that being civilized requires learning how to restrain our initial impulses to lash out when we are frustrated or are impeded in obtaining our desires. Being married means frequently *not* doing what comes naturally. I illustrate this with Chinese finger traps (see figure). The secret to freeing your fingers is counter-intuitive: You must resist the urge to pull them out and, instead, patiently move them *toward* each other.

Untangling a shoelace provides a more common example of the need for restraint when faced with a frustrating task: Again, you must resist the reflexive urge to pull on one end since this will most likely create a more intractable knot.

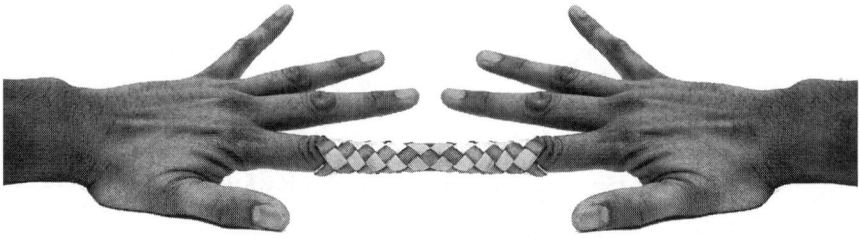

Chinese Finger Traps

Photo Credit: Jose Gil/Shutterstock.com. Used with permission.

Helping clients express their anger. Some clients' anger problem is the opposite: They are so afraid of offending their partners that they suppress their rage and tiptoe around what angers them. Our task here is to help such people feel safe enough to show *less* restraint, so they can express their complaints clearly and productively. Many things can help, including exploring their fears about losing control when they are angry, reviewing past experiences in asserting themselves, exploring how their family dealt with anger when they were growing up, and modeling straight and frank talk ourselves.

Anger as a reaction to injury. We experience anger not only when we encounter a stubborn obstacle, but also when we are emotionally injured. The psychoanalyst Heinz Kohut (1977) famously highlighted the "narcissistic rage" that follows injuries to self-esteem, identity, or "self." In such situations, the therapist is called upon not so much to assist with exposure or restraint (though both may also be needed), but to empathize and to clarify the nature of the injury.

Anger as a defense against other feelings. Related to the idea that anger may be secondary to psychological injury, *expressed* anger can also be used defensively to conceal that injury. Many people are more comfortable hiding their sadness, shame, or vulnerability behind rage. For them, angry, entitled attacks ("I can't believe how you're treating me!") feel safer than their softer cousins ("When you kept me waiting, I felt like I wasn't important to you."). Our task here is to help clients disclose their submerged vulnerability, thereby softening their attacks and making it more likely that they will be heard.

Anger as self-righting revenge. Displays of anger can also be used to hurt the offender and try to restore psychological equilibrium. The "self" that has been hurt or humiliated may seek revenge as a way to regain feelings of power, agency, or equity: "You can't get away with that! Let's see how you feel when I do this!" Revenge used for narcissistic self-righting almost inevitably makes the process worse, as it elicits counter-aggression and non-collaboration.

Passive-aggression and "radioactive" tasks. Anger can also be maladaptively expressed via passive-aggressive behavior. Such behavior usually follows attempts by one partner to dominate or control the other. When Beth makes an insistent request, Fred may (grudgingly) agree to it, but then fail to comply in a timely or conscientious manner. Fred may have *consciously* intended to comply—say, to call a repairman—but his unconscious noncompliance may reveal itself in his continually "forgetting" to get the task done. We call this "passive" because the damage is done by a *failure* to act, and "aggressive," rather than just not completed, because of the predictable damage to the partner who was counting on the action being completed as promised. Such cycles tend to amplify as a person faced with a noncompliant partner grows increasingly frustrated and angry since, not only is the task not getting done, but trust in the partner is being eroded. Typically, the ignored party applies further pressure with repeated requests. The noncompliant spouse—interpreting the repeated requests as criticism—increasingly feels that the punishment doesn't fit the crime. The result is that the task becomes emotionally "radioactive" for that partner, who now becomes even *less* likely to perform it . . . which further enrages the requesting spouse, and around we go.

A serious difficulty in working with passive-aggressiveness is that, because it is in varying degrees unconscious and includes no overt action, clients can easily deny responsibility. When I'm working with clients to access their unconscious aggression (or at least their ambivalent commitment to the promised task), I have found it helpful to share a personal example (see "The Case of the Cat's Fur," below), something that explains the psychology and also makes clear that admitting to such behavior is not the end of the world.

Search your own life for a similar, relatively benign example to relate to your clients, one that shows how some simple task can be rendered emotionally radioactive. You can then fill in the details of your couple's passive-aggressive cycle and begin to examine it with them.

Therapists must be careful here because some noncompliance may be due to external constraints (e.g., unexpected work demands) or to depression, which commonly reduces motivation to perform tasks that are taxing or are

> **THE CASE OF THE CAT'S FUR**
>
> My wife, Sheila, and I have a long-established bedtime routine that includes my folding our bedspread. There's no real reason that it's my job; it just evolved that way. When we got a new cat, Sheila requested that, after I fold the bedspread, I spread a towel over it, in order to prevent the cat from shedding on the bedspread when she slept on it. This seemed to me a reasonable request, even though it was a new one that added to my nighttime duties. Nonetheless, I found myself repeatedly "forgetting" to do it, and each time I forgot, my wife would criticize my negligence. Reflecting on why this was happening, I realized that, although I consciously intended to comply with Sheila's request, actually doing so seemed to be impeded in direct proportion to her reproach each time I failed. Indeed, the annoyance I felt when she got on my case for this minor household crime was part of why learning to do it took far longer than it should have.

not central to the depressed person's needs. In such situations, the couple problem may be less about passive-aggression and more about the couple's failure to explore the impediments to task performance in a realistic and collaborative manner. In my experience, most cases of noncompliance with spousal requests result from a mixture of understandable constraints and passive-aggressive acting out.

Blame

Like anger, counterproductive, hurtful blame is ubiquitous in couple therapy. The excessive attribution of responsibility to our partner grows out of our tendency to attribute adversity to outside causes, coupled with our difficulty conceiving of circular causation. That said, the most powerful reason that blaming others is so popular is that it reduces our shame and guilt. Instead of blaming ourselves and endangering our self-esteem, we find fault with our partners. This explains why people often stubbornly resist accepting responsibility *precisely* when they feel shamefully responsible.

Blaming the pitcher. To characterize blame as a maladaptive and unacceptable defense against guilt, shame, or some other uncomfortable emotion evoked by a spouse, I use the metaphor of a hypothetical batter who, when he repeatedly misses the ball, blames the pitcher. Everyone knows that this is unacceptable, yet often a partner faced with the emotional demands of a wounded spouse blames the spouse for being "too needy." Partners are more likely to feel inwardly justified in doing this when what is required of them is emotional support—though, of course, they will defend their honor in other areas, as well. Distancers generally act under the assumption that everything would be just fine if the pursuer (the pitcher) would just leave them alone. With the "blaming the pitcher" metaphor in mind, the next therapeutic move is to help the blaming partners accept their share of responsibility.

Blame as stalling. When bad things happen, blaming the other is not only a handy way to escape responsibility, but it can also be a magical way to avoid fully experiencing the situation and working to improve it. When a couple I was seeing was faced with the wife's accidentally dropping and losing their house keys in a snow drift during a blizzard, they spent an inordinate amount of time—during and after the storm—trying to assess her level of culpability, seemingly as a way to avoid facing the realistically serious question of what to do next.

In more everyday situations where there is adversity and uncertainty about how to proceed (say, in dealing with a difficult teenager), many couples find themselves arguing over who did what when and who is to blame for the current state of affairs. Many such conversations are efforts to delay the more difficult challenges posed by planning what to do next. Therapists should interrupt and interpret such defensive stalling, while also offering empathy and practical suggestions for coping.

Assigning appropriate blame. Sometimes it *is* helpful to assign blame. By reviewing our mistakes, we may be able to avoid repeating them in the future. And in situations of significant interpersonal betrayal (e.g., an affair), the guilty party must accept responsibility and offer a sincere apology if trust is to be regained and the couple bond is to be repaired.

Tone of Voice

Frequently, in the middle of heated arguments, one spouse will object to the other's (hostile, mocking, sarcastic, or contemptuous) tone of voice. There are two divergent, but equally important, ways to think about this. First, one can see such objections as a defensive way to dodge engagement in the substance of the speaker's words by changing the subject. Sometimes, the spouse complaining about the tone seems to be asserting the illogical idea that, since the tone is harsh, the content of the complaint need not be addressed. Certainly, that is how their partners sometimes react, with still more anger and incredulity: "Who cares how I said it?! This is the thousandth time you've forgotten to pay our electric bill!"

But there is truth on the other side, as well: An angry tone powerfully conveys an attitude of non-collaboration, if not contempt. Tone of voice in problem-solving discussions has been shown to predict marital dissatisfaction and dissolution (Kim, Capaldi, & Crosby, 2007), so complaints about negative tone should not be dismissed as solely an illegitimate ploy to change the subject. Therapists will do well to validate the experiences of *both* spouses—the frustrated spouse who feels that his or her partner is dodging the issue and the partner under attack who is disturbed by the attitudinal harshness conveyed via tone of voice.

In Vino or in Anger *Veritas*?

It is sometimes said that anger, like liquor, makes people more likely to say what they *really* think and feel. Indeed, this can happen when people finally come out of hiding and voice their exasperation about something that has been bothering them for a long time. It is also possible that, in the heat of battle, one partner feels so despondent that he or she mentions divorce (even though that's not what is wanted) or becomes so vengeful that he or she says intentionally hurtful things (known to be exaggerations). In such cases, I suggest that the listener try to "translate" what the speaker seems to have just said: "I don't think you really mean that. I think you're just very angry/hurt." Here the alternative to believing that the speaker meant precisely what he or she said is viewing it as hyperbole, an exaggerated effort to make a point and assure one is heard, similar to yelling. Couple therapists are often called upon to help tease the truth out from the hyperbole.

We now take up some specific couple dances, keeping in mind what I have just said about anger, blame, tone of voice, and the nature of things said in anger.

Taxonomy of Couple Dances

I presented an aerial view of escalating negative cycles in the previous chapter. I would now like to identify some more specific configurations.

In the literature on couple therapy, the most frequently discussed patterns are ones in which (a) both partners engage in usually loud, mostly verbal combat with each other (*conflictual couples* or *adversarial couples*); (b) one partner pursues or attempts to control the other, while that partner distances and resists efforts to be close or to be influenced (*pursuer–distancer couples* or *demand–withdraw couples*);[1] (c) one partner bullies or dominates the other, who more or less painfully and resignedly submits to this abuse of power *(dominating–submitting couples)*; (d) both partners avoid each other and/or their shared problems *(conflict-avoiding couples or mutually-avoiding couples)*; (e) the partners collude to avoid their marital problems by focusing their discontent on a third party, often one of their children (*triangulating couples*); and (f) the partners agree, simplistically or defensively, that only one of them, the "identified patient," has a problem (*identified-patient couples*).

Many couples will move from one category to another, some will present unique forms or combinations, and others will engage hotly and then burn out, like some stars, moving from hot adversarial couples to cold conflict-avoiding/

devitalized couples, couples who have given up on trying to engage each other. Although all of these dysfunctional patterns are sufficient reason to seek therapy, couples often present to us when their pattern has become destabilized: when conflict-avoiding couples must face a problem they can no longer avoid; when dominated, abused wives threaten divorce; or when enabling or caretaking spouses grow tired of their roles.

Roles Exist Independent of the Actors

As we examine the systemic properties of the various dances and the psychology of the various roles, keep in mind that the roles in these dances are somewhat independent of the actors. Each of us has proclivities to interact in certain ways—what Bion (1961) called our "valences"—but once we inhabit a role, we will face predictable challenges, independent of our personal proclivities. For instance, while partners with abandonment fears may be more likely to pursue, *anyone* faced with a partner disinclined to talk, may do so. Most of the maladaptive behaviors we will be discussing make initial sense, even as they fail to achieve their goal, and so can be seen as "ironic processes" (Wachtel & Wachtel, 1986), defined as follows by Rohrbaugh (2014):

> An ironic process occurs when well-intentioned, persistently applied attempts to solve a problem feed back to keep the problem going or make it worse . . . For example, in couples, urging one's spouse to eat, drink, or smoke less may lead him or her to do it more (an ironic cycle), or walking on eggshells to avoid conflict or hide negative feelings can lead to more partner distress (an ironic protection cycle).
>
> *(p. 436)*

Anyone stuck in the pursuer role will notice that some actions only make things worse. Further, most clients in these dances have tried to escape their roles: Pursuers have tried not to nag; distancers have tried to listen when they didn't want to. In the following sections, I will discuss some of the structural characteristics that block escape and then suggest some interventions to help free couples from these painful repetitive cycles.

Mutual Blaming Cycles: Adversarial Couples

The cycles of such couples are reasonably straightforward: Each partner is on the attack, angrily blaming the other. Sometimes, we see the flawed logic of "cross-complaining," as in "OK, I admit I did it yesterday, but you did it last week!" Cross-complaining can also take the form of reminding the other of unrelated sins, in an attempt to make the blame go away. We also see endless, contentious arguments over minute factual details that one or the other thinks are crucial to establishing or mitigating blame, when a simple "I'm sorry" would prove more effective. The major problem in such vicious, escalating cycles is that both parties remain functionally deaf to the truth that the other is proclaiming fiercely and loudly *in response to that deafness*. At such times, *the therapist can interrupt the cycle by noting that both partners have a point and then move on to unpack the underlying issues*.

Desperate attacks often surface when one spouse believes it essential that his or her partner change. Sometimes, we can analyze this desperation and see how it is linked to erroneous beliefs about what the partner needs in order to attain happiness or to move forward after a traumatic experience. *In general, it will help to show couples how their mutual blaming can almost always be deconstructed to reveal both angry criticism and cries for help*. (Recall the metaphor of the drowning swimmer.) Usually, the cry for help is hidden behind the criticism; with our assistance, clients can bring it forward.

In most cases, such episodes of mutual blaming and "negative reciprocity" (Gottman & Levenson, 1999) alternate with periods of conflict avoidance, as couples retreat and lick their wounds. But because some external issue must still be faced, or because the partners continue to touch each other's sensitive nerves, conflict will inevitably break out again.

All negative interaction cycles are susceptible to inertia, so that even when one spouse tries to shift to a healthier form of interaction, the other may resist. With conflictual couples, after the therapist helps one spouse become less combative or more accommodating, the other—rather than jumping for joy— may second the therapist's observations, but in a hurtful manner, "I've known all along that you are just like Dr. Nielsen said, but you're just too weak to admit it!" If this happens, the therapist should not simply lecture the offender for being counterproductive, but should try to encourage him or her to discover and acknowledge why it is so hard to applaud the changed behavior: Is it that it seems like too little too late? That she doesn't trust that the change will be permanent? That he is still angry after so many years of trying to bring about this change? Discussing the possibilities and validating those that ring true will help the couple to become more responsive to change and, over time, will halt the vicious circle of mutual attack and blame.

Pursuer–Distancer Cycles

A recent meta-analysis of 74 studies (N = 14,255) found that pursuer–distancer cycles were common, and were clearly associated with multiple varieties of unhappiness and dysfunction in both distressed and non-distressed couples (Schrodt, Witt, & Shimkowski, 2013). In these cycles, one spouse (the pursuer) tries to get his or her partner to comply with some request—to be more open and intimate or to get some task done—but lacks "relational power" (Fishbane, 2010), because the distancer "controls reward allocations to both partners"

(Rusbult & Van Lange, 2003). Problems arise when the pursuer's efforts to convince the partner to talk or share tasks make things worse or when the distancer's avoidance provokes pursuit, creating a cycle of pursuit, distancing, more pursuit, and more distancing. As happens with mutual blaming, pursuers and distancers become entrenched in their positions, grow progressively more enraged and hopeless, and are unable to discuss the underlying issues that make pursuers so insistent and critical and distancers so wary of engagement. *Each partner has a point: pursuers—that talking is urgently needed, and distancers—that talking is often painfully counterproductive.*

Even though talking things over will ultimately be essential, *therapists must avoid the beginners' mistake of reflexively siding with pursuers.* Doing this minimizes the fact that usually *both* partners contribute to the distancer's conclusion that talking only makes things worse. Of course, sometimes one partner *does* contribute more to the problem than the other, and this may turn out to be the person who hides via withdrawal. My point here is be cautious about assuming that the person who "wants to talk" or "wants more intimacy" is not also contributing to the systemic problem. Many partners who hound their spouses to open up don't really want to hear what they say when they do.

Different attitudes toward talking. Sometimes the roots of pursuer–distancer disputes lie in differing attitudes about the benefits of talking. Some clients want to review recent painful events, while others think it best to let bygones be bygones. Spouses can also disagree about how pressing an issue is, on whether talking will interfere with needed relaxation (say, after a stressful day at work), or on the odds that talking about a particular conflict will help. In all these cases, it is rare that partners join each other in talking about *these* differences, though that is often precisely what we need to help them to do.

Intimacy versus separation. One common version of the pursuer–distancer dance involves one partner who wants more time to talk and share experiences, while the other wants more time alone or away from the partner. Here, we have two people with opposing legitimate needs. This is a common problem, even for couples who are about equally disposed to seek companionship versus solitude since, moment to moment, they may not line up on their preferences. It will be even more challenging for couples with lifelong differing inclinations. To the extent that partners cannot accept their immediate or lifelong differences and work out compromises, they will both be unhappy.

Talking about not talking. Therapists should acknowledge that it can be acceptable and even intimate sometimes to share that one does *not* want to talk. This includes garden-variety talking at the end of the day when one partner is tired and would rather watch TV, but also times when one thinks that talking is not necessary or might well make matters worse. Discussing this issue so that "not talking" is not pathologized may be just the kind of conversation that the prototypical laconic husband might want to do, while some talkative wives may also agree that sometimes talking has made things worse. Having allowed such truths to be voiced, the therapist is then in a position to explore just what it is about talking that has made things worse. Rather than merely pathologizing the avoidance of talking, the couple can look for its hidden logic.

Pseudodialogue: Too much talk met with too little. What often happens is that pursuers, favoring talking and togetherness, go on and on. Fearing that their partners do not want to engage and may exit at any moment, they continue their monologues with hardly a letup for air. As listeners feel hounded and aversively pursued, they will keep their own counsel, waiting politely (they believe) for a pause to get a word in or simply for the other to "talk themselves out." Nonresponsiveness in this pseudodialogue confirms pursuers in their hopelessness about attaining intimacy and distancers in their belief that such conversations are unrewarding. Without intervention, this situation can escalate, with both parties feeling increasingly frustrated.

Nagging and exploding. Pursuers commonly engage in nagging—as well as its close relatives, whining and guilt-tripping—rather than asking for what they want straight out, as they would in, "Honey, please pass the salt." Some pursuers will also be episodically explosive. Nagging, whining, guilt-tripping, and exploding sometimes get results due to their punishing impact on distancers. Unfortunately, this intermittent reinforcement perpetuates behaviors that damage the relationship (Bradbury & Karney, 2010; Jacobson & Christensen, 1996).

When faced with the nagging variety of the pursuer–distancer cycle, the therapist can begin by normalizing and explaining the annoying quality of nagging by comparing it to other situations where a lack of response leads to escalation (e.g., the diner summoning a waiter or the drowning swimmer calling the lifeguard). This fits our therapeutic decision rule to locate the problem, when possible, in the negative cycle, rather than in either individual. After normalizing the pursuit by casting it in cybernetic/circular terms, therapists can begin to explore deeper issues in both the pursuer and the distancer.

Passive-aggressive cycles. Passive-aggressive cycles, as discussed earlier, are a variety of the pursuer–distancer cycle. Maladaptive pursuit evokes noncompliance, usually coupled with increased distance. Requested tasks go undone and become "radioactive."

Overadequate–underadequate cycles. When partners fail to perform tasks, their pursuing spouses may then do more than their fair share, or more than they want, in order to stay current on paying bills, washing dishes, or caring for children. Underperforming partners may enjoy their escape from task performance or may stop trying, based on the belief that "You think I never do anything right anyway!" Overfunctioning partners may be anxious micromanagers or may just be picking up the slack. Pursuit or nagging may become intermittent or even absent, as spouses grudgingly accept their roles. This version of the pursuer–distancer cycle sometimes overlaps with the identified-patient cycle, described below.

More than one cycle. As distancing partners fail to meet pursuers' needs, pursuing partners may also disengage and fail to reciprocate in different areas. A common pattern is the wife who wants more intimate conversation married to the husband who wants more sex. Here, we have two separate pursuer–distancer cycles reinforcing each other.

Skepticism and cycle intransigence. Distancers' initial steps toward change are often met with skepticism by their pursuers. Even when a previously noncompliant partner has performed a task as requested, the pursuer may think, "It won't last. He's only doing it because I reminded him three times. Or because Dr. Nielsen told him to!" When pursuers' criticisms are fueled by a poorly articulated wish for closeness, by a desire for revenge, or by doubt that change is genuine, their attacks can be relentless and extreme. Such behavior will amplify distancers' sense that the attack is unfair and will further reduce their desire to perform better or to connect in a loving manner.

Interventions. This is where we therapists come in. We must "hold" the couple by offering hope, helping each to understand the other's behavior, reminding them that it is normal for change to take time and, above all, encouraging them to open up and reveal their inner lives in all their complexity, rather than continuing the simplistic pursuit and flight that have become their ingrained pattern. *After identifying the systemic issues that maintain these vicious cycles, therapists should move to explore the deeper psychological issues that maintain the cycle for both the pursuer and the distancer.*

Pursuers' issues. Much of the couple therapy literature tends to conflate the two types of requests that pursuers make to partners who are distancing: those for specific task performance and those for emotional closeness. This is understandable because the two so commonly go together. The distinction is important, however, because clients themselves often think that they are *only* trying to get help with the dishes, when they are also asking their partners to confirm that they matter. This is just as true of requests for more sex as it is for more dishwashing. In both cases, the anger of pursuers is not only about task noncompliance or about missed chances for intimacy. This distress often becomes intensified by doubts about whether the partner wants to be with them or "has their back," that is, by attachment concerns. Being repeatedly turned down leads you to conclude that your partner just doesn't like you and wouldn't be there for you in a crisis. Self-esteem declines and panic rises still more, as spouses who nag or intermittently explode disapprove of their *own* behavior, behavior that often resembles that of parents they had sworn they would never be like.

While it is easy to see that *pursuers* are not getting their interpersonal and attachment needs met, we should keep in mind that the same is true for *distancers*. As we will see in Chapter 9 (on projective identification), a man who disowns his dependency needs and then runs from his wife whenever he experiences her as "too needy" will then feel still more "needy" himself (since he is not getting his own interpersonal needs met from his marriage). He will have even more need to locate such unmet, unacceptable needs in her, thus creating escalation in their cycle.

With help from us, pursuers may come to see that their criticisms are not only directed at getting a desired task done (the bills paid or the garage cleaned), but entail hopes for more warmth and caring. When we help clients express such needs less harshly, that will often enable them to elicit the supportive responses they desire. Indeed, studies have shown that "blamer softening" and "intimate disclosure" are strongly associated with improvement in couple therapy (Greenman & Johnson, 2013). Pursuer softening and disclosure then (ideally) allow distancing spouses to show warmth and to re-establish connection, thus restoring the pursuer's confidence in the relationship. As a result, the heat may go out of many arguments about how much time is spent apart (whether at the office or on the golf course), not so much because partners are actually spending more time together, but because pursuers stop experiencing their spouses as running away to a preferred activity, as if to a lover.

It is also useful for therapists to work to uncover pursuers' ambivalence about deserving what they are requesting and their difficulty asking for things, and to teach them more effective ways of asking. Rather than implying that the distancer is morally defective ("What is wrong with you that you always keep me waiting?!"), pursuers can cast their requests in more positive terms ("I really miss you, but I don't know how to bring you close to me" (example from Hazlett, 2010, p. 30).

Distancers' issues. *When encouraging distancers to engage, it is important to learn the specifics of their concerns, rather than merely labeling them as "afraid of intimacy."* A distancer's flight can most often be understood—structurally and sympathetically—as a retreat from unpromising engagement with a critical partner. A normalizing metaphor compares this to a turtle protecting itself from a hailstorm by bringing its head inside its shell. Feeling under attack, distancers believe that they can neither successfully defeat their enemy nor calm him or her down. *Distancers feel more hopeless than adversarial partners, who continue to battle.* For distancers, escape seems a logical and desirable action. Indeed, distancers can sometimes be seen looking entreatingly to the sky for help, as if thinking, "Beam me up, Scotty!" like a character in *Star Trek* might when faced with a threatening alien (Markman, Stanley, & Blumberg, 2001). To the typical distancer, "Beam me up, Scotty!" makes sense, and therapists will often observe that skyward look. This image can encourage us to dig deeper so as to understand why distancers feel so hopeless about engaging pursuers they experience as threatening.

Hopelessness and shame. *The psychology of distancers usually includes the belief that they cannot please their partners, who are some combination of overly needy and impossibly perfectionistic.* As many spouses put it, "Nothing I do will make her (him) stop complaining, so what's the use?" Many distancers feel ashamed of this failure to satisfy their partners. Helping them express this shame will make them more sympathetic characters to spouses who have been doubting that they cared.

Defensive contempt. Sometimes, the inability to make things better leads distancers to a veiled defensive contempt for their partners, communicated via body language and/or occasional verbal counterattacks: "No one could love you! You're just too needy!" *Exposing and sympathizing with distancers' doubts about success allows us to tease apart their sources,* often including childhood failures to please others, not knowing how to satisfy their partners, and the dance itself, which blocks feeling states required for success.

Lack of knowledge and skill. Many spouses faced with a partner demanding "more intimacy" just don't know what is being requested. Many are relieved to learn that such wishes can often be satisfied by sharing the details of their lives in a caring, straightforward way.

The wrong feelings. But even as distancers come to know what pursuers desire and begin to change their behavior, there remains the thorny problem that loving concern cannot simply be summoned by willpower alone. The distress felt by distancers usually leaves them unable to provide the unambivalent emotional warmth their partners demand. Distancers' efforts to perform as requested will often seem forced (which they are) or overly cautious (the husband who checks every detail of a task with his wife to make sure he does it the way she wants). Such behavior may not feel sufficiently convincing or valuable to pursuers, who remain dissatisfied, which, in turn, discourages distancers. For these reasons, *in the transitional period, as distancers are beginning to make efforts to engage, therapists will not only have to help them remain optimistic, but will have to help their pursuers contain some disappointment.*

Distress blocking connection. *Many distancers also have trouble persevering because they become overly upset when their partners are upset.* In contrast to what many pursuers believe, many distancers become too identified with their partners' emotional pain and, not knowing how to make it better, they flee so as to quell this vicarious distress. Teaching distancers how to be more actively engaged *and* how to cope with the distressing feelings that follow will enable them to begin to build the stronger interpersonal boundaries they will need to sustain greater closeness.

Guilt and shame. *Distancers also flee because of difficulty managing self-esteem when it is under attack.* The "Don't blame the pitcher" metaphor is a start on the road to helping such distancers talk openly about how hard it is to hear their partners describe them negatively. With some distancers who are overly sensitive to blame, it helps to show them how to look for the deeper issues that underlie their partner's seemingly unfair attacks. Other distancers will need help facing their own inner demons with less self-criticism.

Wile (2002, p. 302) illustrates this point with the case of a man clearly upset after the birth of his first child. He had been put off by his wife's simplistic attacks on him as "jealous of the new baby," but his feelings were actually far more nuanced, and not as negative: Wile suggests

> that he is angry that his wife is accusing him of this; frightened that she might be right; dismayed that he doesn't like the baby more; upset that he feels left out of the mother-infant dyad; upset about the loss of good will between himself and his wife; and alarmed at times by his wish that they had never had the baby.

Reversals of roles. To add to the complexity just described, we should note that many individuals fear both closeness and distance and may cycle between avoiding and pursuing one or the other. For instance a partner may feel criticized/controlled when the other is close, but guilty/responsible when they move apart. We may then see partners reversing the roles of pursuer and distancer. In other cases, both partners cycle between conflictual (too close) and avoidant (too far) patterns (Feldman, 1979). Such dances are harder to treat because we will have more (and sometimes contradictory) latent issues and fears to expose and work on.

Dominating–Submitting Cycles

Some spouses achieve "power over" their partners (Fishbane, 2010) who submit to their coercion, threats, and bullying. Unlike constructive "relational power," this comes at a heavy emotional and relational price. Submission is frequently only partial or temporary, since many spouses will only have *appeared* to agree so as to end an episode of conflict. Expert negotiation consultants stress that "hard" negotiators risk alienating "soft" negotiators, who will resent unfair agreements and later fail to comply with their terms (Fisher et al., 2011). With couples, the price of "hard negotiating" or dominating can entail not only passive-aggressive noncompliance, but a growing disconnection between the partners, together with depression and other psychiatric symptomatology in the submissive spouse. In order to maintain some power and respect, "submitting" spouses may form coalitions with outsiders (friends, relatives, children, therapists), which may further weaken the marital bond and create additional problems. And most will become secretive, which will fuel suspicion and distrust in dominating spouses.

Perhaps less obviously, dominating partners will not get what they most desire—genuine love and respect—since any positive behaviors they coerce will not count. Positive responses will be no more meaningful than laughter that follows a command to laugh. Worse, if domination is achieved via violence or angry outbursts, there will be a "walking on eggshells" relationship, where submissive partners dread future incidents. Abusive dominating spouses may also be perpetually apprehensive, believing that their outbursts are controlled by the inciting behaviors of their partners (Stosny, 2005). This distress in dominating partners will then increase their need to dominate and control, and the cycle will escalate.

Dominating partners come in many forms, not just the easy-to-spot, violent types who show up more in the newspapers than in my office, but in partners (more often men) who are oblivious to their dominating ways and conceal them behind tradition or logic. Tom, "The Intimidator," was such a man—hardly a psychopathic narcissist but, nonetheless, constantly overpowering his wife. In milder forms, these are people who enjoy taking charge and assuming leadership roles; when their partners view this as legitimate, we see what have been termed healthy "lead-follow cycles" (Greenberg & Goldman, 2008). In pathological forms, dominating partners, like Tom, think that others should just do things their way because it is the "right way" or "the way things have always been done." Often such "privileged partners" are backed up by cultural norms that justify unilateral decision-making (Knudson-Martin, 2013). They frequently assert that because they earn more money, it is only right that they should decide how it is spent. They claim the right to define their cruel jibes as "only jokes" and their partners as "too thin-skinned." Many such putdowns amount to misguided attempts to increase precarious self-esteem by devaluing the partner.[2]

In other situations, excessive control is exerted by partners who "go on strike," such as when partners with less interest in sex control its frequency. Sometimes, an individual with a psychiatric or physical disability will become the coercive partner whose anxieties and special requirements are considered beyond question, so that all other family members must march to his or her tune. Of course, people who feign or exaggerate disability so as to exert control must not have had much power to begin with. Such patterns often emerge as covert tactics to right the balance with partners who have been overtly domineering. Perhaps we should coin a new term for such couples, calling them "dominating–covertly-dominating couples."

A major challenge for therapists when dealing with dominating–submitting cycles is to remain curious and neutral in the face of marital politics that seem illegitimate and unfair. (The case of serious marital violence is an exception to maintaining neutrality, but not curiosity.) There is a strong temptation to confront the obvious abuse of power and to defend the victim, but such direct confrontations will frequently be dismissed as emanating from a naive, left-wing therapist who is threatening the dominating spouse's way of life. Therapists will be assisted in holding their tongues by considering that help for the submissive spouse is unlikely to come from simply lecturing dominant spouses about their misbehavior.

When one partner asserts power unilaterally—over resources, decisions, and definitions of reality and morality—it can help to point out to him or her the costs of such assumed power (Rampage, 2002): People who are into "controlling" or "dominating" others are usually settling for the faux connection and recognition that they can coerce because they do not know how to elicit the genuine articles. Although they will generally be less aware of this than the pursuers in the pursuer–distancer dance who complain so loudly of a dearth of marital warmth and closeness, dominators also live in a chilly emotional climate. Sometimes, I explain this lack of reciprocal warmth by telling the fable of "The Emperor and the Nightingale," in which the controlling ruler can only hear his prized bird sing after he frees her from her cage. Similarly, in order to become "usable" (meaningful) partners, submissive spouses must be free to come and go, to love or not, independent of coercion (Newman, 1996; Winnicott, 1960). Only then can their judgment of the dominator's character be trusted. The metaphor of the caged bird who sings when freed is also helpful in giving a systems account of the depression and devitalization experienced by submissive partners.

After pointing out this lack of efficacy, therapists can begin to enlist dominators' help to explore why they work so hard to control their partners and other aspects of their lives. What idiographic fears take over and lead to excesses of control? Recall that for Tom these included fears of depression if he could not find self-esteem enhancing work and satisfying recreation. Such collaborative explorations can eventually make what is an obviously inequitable political system consciously unacceptable (ego-dystonic) for dominators. Further exploration may uncover unconscious motives that drive dominators, for example, that a man who devalues and teases his wife was beaten and humiliated by his father and is now unconsciously repeating that pattern.

As when working with distancers, we must avoid simplification with dominators. Wile (2002) provides a compelling illustration: Rather than telling a husband, "You're trying to control your wife," he empathizes by remarking, "'What a spot you're in! Your effort to convince your wife not to go back to get her master's degree is alienating her . . . but you're haunted by the thought that her going back is an irretrievable first step toward her leaving you.'" (p. 6).

After we have formed an alliance with controlling partners, we can begin to explore the psychology of their submissive partners. Here, we will be working with the now-familiar challenges of helping clients feel comfortable with angry feelings and with "asking for things." Psychoeducation about how best to raise one's concerns and how to have difficult conversations will help. Submissive people are typically conflict avoiders, the topic of our next section.

Conflict-Avoiding, Mutually-Avoiding Cycles

In many couples who come for therapy, *both* partners are afraid of conflict or of discussing emotionally challenging subjects. We can think of such couples as being composed of two distancers. Some of these have been termed "pseudomutual," where both partners imagine all is well until this fantasy can no longer be sustained (Shaddock, 1998).

Two types of problems bring these clients to us. Most obviously, because they collude to avoid talking about challenging topics, they inadequately address important situations—with children, finances, in-laws, etc.—that require collaboration and deliberation, until those problems can no longer be evaded. Mutually-avoiding couples also present to us due to devitalization and boredom. Afraid to rock the boat, they find themselves unhappy and going nowhere.

But such marriages are not simply the result of the personality limitations or fearfulness of the partners. As with all negative interaction cycles, systemic properties constrain the partners, so that their dance can become self-perpetuating. When Jane observes that Jim is treating topics as too hot to handle, Jane will also come to see them that way and avoid them. Each partner, noting the other's avoidance, becomes still more wary. And each topic avoided increases the likelihood that other topics will be seen as unapproachable. This pattern of avoidance becomes increasingly entrenched as each day that goes by confirms the partners' beliefs that talking is too dangerous. These are the couples we see sitting in painful silence at restaurants, too afraid to open any meaningful dialogue.

Further, when couples persistently avoid engaging in challenging conversations and rely, instead, on hints to convey their preferences, the silence becomes fertile ground for projected fears and for erroneous ideas about each other's desires: One husband, finally opening up in therapy, told his wife that he didn't like how she had seasoned his chicken . . . for the previous 30 years! Those 30 years of misalignment, including in more significant areas, contributed to 30 years of resentment.

When a conflict-avoiding partner can't hold his or her breath any longer about some troubling issue, the resulting interaction is likely to be poorly managed and hurtful, since neither partner is skilled in adversarial conversations. This negative experience will further strengthen the shared belief that open discussion should be avoided.

The devitalization of the marriage can also lead one of the partners to search elsewhere for excitement and warmth. Some will find it in work or recreation outside the relationship, such that eventually the other partner, feeling neglected, will suggest they go for therapy. Or he or she may go outside the marriage to find intimacy. The couple will then present during, or in the aftermath of, an extramarital affair.

When they are finally forced to acknowledge the need for therapy, mutually-avoiding couples will be slow to get into real issues, still fearing making things worse by opening up their Pandora's boxes. Their complaints will be hesitant and vague, as they waver between wanting to be heard and hoping that no one will quite register their complaints. Many clients will be ambivalent about their right to speak up. Sessions may feel boring, but there will also be a pervasive sense of looming danger. Like overly controlled obsessive individual clients, mutual avoiders will frequently find excuses to miss sessions and will often wait until the end of a session to bring up their deeper concerns. Just as they try hard not to discuss difficult subjects with each other, they often don't listen closely to what their therapists say. And some always seem to have one foot out the door. If we offend them or are somehow off base, they usually won't tell us right away. Therapists aware of these defensive tactics should anticipate them and make them subjects for discussion. Therapists can also make use of the "heating things up" interventions described in Chapter 2 and those for distancing partners, outlined above. Exploring family-of-origin attitudes and experiences concerning conflict and open expressions of anger and other emotions will also prove helpful.

While mutually-avoiding couples have certain characteristic dynamics, virtually all couples we see will have been avoiding some assortment of upsetting topics, thoughts, and feelings. They will simply avoid distress by different means. Recall how conflictual couples hide within their angry battles. In this regard, Wile (1993) makes the interesting point that couples may avoid discussions in which compromise will be required, in part, because they have secretly been making compromises all along. Their avoidance consists of not sharing private sacrifices made in the service of marital harmony. He illustrates this with the following example:

> Jim, who did not like Dorothy's staying late at work, asked her to agree to restrict her lateness to once a week and to phone him and pre-prepare his meals when she suspected she might be late. The problem with this solution is that it grafted a compromise to a compromise. Dorothy had already been compromising. She had felt badly about coming home late and, as a consequence, had done it less often than she would have wanted. Now, with the new "official" compromise, she was to stay late even less often . . . Jim too had made a previous compromise. Dorothy's feelings of being suffocated by Jim . . . had led her to withdraw emotionally. Jim's reaction was to accept this withdrawal and to settle for more modest satisfactions: he made a private compromise regarding his original hopes about the marriage. Although it seemed that he was to be deprived of emotional intimacy, at least he could count on a certain measure of companionship and reliability: a wife who would always be here and who would fix his meals. When it appeared that even this was to be taken from him, it became too much.
>
> *(pp. 73–74)*

Such secret compromises must be extremely common, and some are doubtless required to make marriages possible, as we will discuss later under the banner of "acceptance." The practical point here is that once clients have made such secret compromises, they will be more likely to avoid open discussions that might result in further concessions.

Triangulation Cycles

Another way partners avoid facing their problems with each other is by agreeing that their main problem is shared and is caused by someone else. Minuchin (1974) aptly termed this "detouring." Seen from the perspective of group dynamics, this is the psychology of avoiding internal conflict, difficulties, and anxiety by finding an external scapegoat to hold the group's attention and serve as a target for its displeasure. With couples, that external problem or person—often a child—is said to have been "triangulated," with the goal of stabilizing the couple. The discovery and treatment of this problem—when a couple views one of their children as the source of their problems—were central to the development of the field of family therapy. Parents may complain, for instance, that a son is not doing well enough in school—sometimes, despite objectively good grades—as a proxy for shared distress and potential conflict over whether the husband is doing well enough in his career. Other couples will not simply displace their problem (say, about an absent sex life) to a common enemy (a teenager with curfew issues), but may engage in endless, ineffectual arguments over how to cope with that "enemy."

Other parents may encourage the scapegoated child to act out because they vicariously enjoy such behavior, even as they consciously disapprove of it, as discussed by Adelaide Johnson (1949), who noted corresponding "superego lacunae" (holes in the consciences) of the parents and their misbehaving children. Years ago, I saw one such mother in the Yale New Haven Psychiatric Emergency Room. This straight-laced, upper-middle-class woman was there with her 14-year-old daughter, who was suicidal after becoming pregnant. While proclaiming her disapproval of her daughter's premature sexual behavior, the mother eagerly read to me from a pornographic romance novel she had found in her daughter's room, and exclaimed, "I just can't seem to do anything about such things: This is my third daughter who's gotten pregnant before she turned 18!"

In other situations, children may need no encouragement from parents, and will become aggressive or symptomatic as a way to disrupt distressing parental conflict (Minuchin, 1974). This can easily be observed in family therapy sessions when children draw attention to themselves just as their parents begin to disagree with each other. Other children may not act up to curtail parental discord, but may be symptomatic victims of parents who have taken out their frustrations on their children (Fosco, Lippold, & Feinberg, 2014). Still others will be reactively distressed by marital troubles. Others will have problems of their own, independent of their parents.

In my experience, all permutations of defensive displacement, legitimate concern, and concurrent marital problems are possible. Consequently, therapists need to keep an open mind and not be swayed too early by systems theories that preferentially assume defensive parental scapegoating or pleasure in the child's problems. *When couples present to a therapist with their child identified as the problem, it is best to keep an open mind and delay interpreting this as a displacement or triangulation.* Rather, therapists should begin by taking the presenting problem at face value as the best way to establish a therapeutic alliance. They can then explore the individual and group dynamics that might explain the child's symptoms or misbehavior, while attempting to assist the parents in coming to an agreement on an effective parenting plan.

Sometimes, it will turn out that, while the couple does have other "couple problems," the focus on the child is perfectly legitimate, because that problem is sapping the energy that could be going into addressing couple problems and is not simply a handy defense against facing them. In many situations, serious problems in children result from the parents' failure to work together on parenting, just as they have failed to collaborate on other problems. Helping them work on the process by which they discuss parenting issues may then help them more generally.

When working out a parenting plan, we will often be working indirectly on marital issues—say, on the wife's right to have a say in the marriage, or on the willingness of a wife to allow her husband entry into the closed system she has with their children—although we need not always name these explicitly. Many couples of this sort will later transition into explicit couple therapy as the children's problems lessen and the hidden couple difficulties surface; others will thank us and exit therapy.

When couples present in the first therapy session openly acknowledging *marital* problems, defensive triangulation of their children is unusual. More often, they state (frequently inaccurately) that their children are just fine, and that they are the one area of pleasure that holds their marriage together. When they do discuss parenting problems, the process resembles the way they discuss other areas of difference: as an area of conflict, rather than an area where scapegoating is used as a defense. We can, nonetheless, see moments in a couple's therapy when triangulation of children or others (bosses, in-laws, neighbors) does come into play, so that we should be on the lookout for such defensive displacement and scapegoating. When this occurs, it will appear as shared complaints about others, employed to diminish incipient conflict between the spouses. If this is common or persistent, the therapist should interpret it as he or she would any other group defense, "I know you two are very angry at Aunt Sarah for what she said, but I'm wondering if it's somehow safer to unite in berating her than to continue the difficult conversation we were just having about how one of you felt the other acted insensitively . . . in a manner quite similar to your aunt."

Therapists can also become the target of triangulation. Here, couples come together to blame the therapist or the therapy for their troubles with each other. They complain that they are worse after sessions, and sometimes they are. If not addressed directly and sensitively, this sort of triangulation can lead to premature termination of the treatment.

Identified-Patient Cycles

These couples do not blame their unhappiness on an outside scapegoat, but attribute most of it to the emotional failings or mental illness of one of the partners. This partner, at least initially, accepts the diagnosis, thus taking a position dramatically different from that seen in conflictual couples, where both partners shun responsibility. Examples are the spouse who admits to drinking too much, to having had an affair, to an addiction to online pornography, to a lack of interest in sex, to depression, or to outbursts of anger.

Sometimes one spouse is "dropped off" on the therapist's doorstep with instructions that the therapist should "fix" the problematic behavior, and sometimes such identified-patient spouses will comply, identifying themselves as the problem needing fixing, though they usually become more ambivalent about this as time passes. One common situation is the wife who convinces her skeptical husband to try therapy to improve his difficulty being intimate with her and refers him for individual therapy. When I have tried to work this way, without the complaining/pursuing wife present, the result is most often boredom, gridlock, and early termination.

In a situation where the problem is labeled as belonging only to one spouse, it is best to begin the treatment with the complaining, "mentally healthy," spouse present, a tactic supported by extensive research (Gurman, 2011).

When identified-patient couples present for treatment, their cycle is usually invisible to them. In this situation, the most important advantage of conjoint sessions is their ability to assess the contributions of unacknowledged marital problems to the identified patient's symptoms. These symptoms may well be a noisy indicator—a canary in a coal mine—signaling marital problems. While both spouses may agree that one of them should change, they may not yet see how the "well-functioning" partner is also suffering or how that partner may be slowing the process of recovery—"enabling" it in the parlance of Alcoholics Anonymous.

For instance, "unexplained" angry outbursts, where "anger management therapy" is requested, will commonly turn out to be the tip of an iceberg of unmet needs and unvoiced complaints in a partner who, from time to time, can't take it anymore. The same can frequently be said of depression, excessive drinking, and other symptomatic behaviors. Attempts to treat the system's symptom by meeting with only one member of the couple are underpowered and are less likely to succeed because they fail to involve all the players who contribute to symptom maintenance and might assist with improvement (Gurman & Burton, 2014).

It should not surprise us that when treatment involves only the symptomatic partner, it often ends abruptly and unilaterally, when he or she decides no longer to be seen as the only one needing help. At this point, it may become clear that the client has only been going through the motions of individual treatment to placate the spouse (perhaps in the wake of an affair). In most of these cases, therapy would have been more effective if the seemingly well spouse had been involved from the beginning, with that spouse's input and dissatisfaction giving the therapist more to work with and the identified patient spouse more reason to become and remain engaged.

A final reason to treat such couples conjointly is that symptomatic misbehavior that has eroded the offended spouse's trust cannot be treated fully in his or her absence; instead, both partners need to be present so that they can understand the situation, make and receive sincere apologies, and jointly formulate plans to do better.

Even in situations where the identified patient *does* have strong insecurities or unwarranted (neurotic) fears about the other (negative transferences), his or her psychotherapy may be expedited if those fears can be shown to be unjustified in the immediacy of conjoint sessions. Here, the spouse who is already the recipient of the transference concerns may be better able to provide a corrective emotional experience than the therapist whom the patient has just met.

When we have the partners together, we will want to draw them out in a situation of safety, as we try to show them how the identified patient's symptom is embedded in marital issues and process. The main danger with such couples is the therapist getting too far ahead of them, locating the symptom too forcefully in *both* of them. As with triangulating couples who are convinced that the problem lies in an outside enemy, we must build an alliance before we challenge this defensive oversimplification.

Having just recommended a conjoint format for the beginning of treatment, I do not want to minimize the value of intensive individual psychotherapy, which sometimes grows out of a successful couple treatment. Just as many couples enter therapy focusing on their children's problems and then go on to deal with their marital problems, so some spouses who enter therapy with couple problems may discover a need for deeper, more intensive therapy of their own long-standing individual problems.

The "Adhesiveness" of Negative Interaction Cycles

Couples have great trouble escaping their negative cycles. This resistance to change, even when therapists try to alter the process, led some therapists and researchers to propose system homeostasis as an explanation. While some systems and people certainly resist change because of fears of diverging from a preferred (or less-detrimental) norm, this is not a very helpful model for explaining the inertia and resistance of most couple cycles. The most obvious problem with such thinking is that most people caught in these cycles are demonstrably unhappy and *want* to get out. Moreover, these are not stable cycles that maintain their homeostatic emotional temperature. Rather, they are more often characterized by escalation or burnout, the antecedents of painful divorces. This is true even of triangulating and identified-patient couples, for whom the model of systemic defense has some utility.

It remains true that partners caught in such cycles experience what Gottman (2011) calls "adhesiveness," an unwillingness to exit the pathological dance, despite knowing that continuing it will make matters worse. In my view, the best explanation for this adhesiveness and the observed inertia (and escalation) of these pathological dances does not reside solely in the cybernetic characteristics of such "systems"—even as we have shown their tendency to be self-perpetuating (The more she does X, the more he does Y, the more she does X . . .) Instead, cycle adhesiveness derives from the psychological constraints and challenges flowing from the cybernetic characteristics of specific dances (as just discussed) *in combination with* the underlying individual psychological concerns of the partners (the subject of the next section on psychodynamics).

Partners stuck in these dances sense that something larger is at stake, but they are hard-pressed to say what that something is. It is to these largely unconscious psychological issues that I now turn. As we shall see, the adhesiveness and destructiveness of negative interaction cycles hinge on how these cycles prevent important psychological needs from being met, especially the needs to be heard, respected, and supported.

Notes

1 Betchen (2005), who reviewed the literature and nomenclature on such couples, notes that this pattern has been variously termed "the nag-withdraw dynamic"; "the rejection-intrusion pattern"; "the lovesick wife and the coldsick husband"; "the fuser-isolator dynamic"; "close/far polarization"; and (his own label) "intrusive partners [with] elusive mates."
2 Greenberg and Goldman, in their book *Emotion-Focused Couples Therapy* (2008), correctly note that partners who become impatient, dominating, and controlling may be more concerned with what they call "identity issues" (integrity/self-esteem) than with attachment anxiety, the main source of couple distress emphasized by Susan Johnson in her version of Emotionally Focused Couple Therapy (Johnson, 2008). They refer to cycles in which "identity" is at stake as "influence cycles" and include the "dominate-submit" cycle as one variety. This goes beyond seeing all negative interaction cycles as driven by attachment issues alone. Attempts to "dominate" can involve other anxieties, as well. For instance, a female banker was excessively controlling/dominating with her husband in money matters, not so much because of self-esteem concerns, but out of anxiety that she might once again be poor, as she had been as a child.

PART III
Psychodynamic Upgrades

6

FOCUSING ON HIDDEN ISSUES, FEARS, AND DESIRES

Many clinicians have discussed marital problems and couple therapy from a psychodynamic perspective.[1] They (and I):

- believe that understanding and remediating negative *couple* interactions requires uncovering *individual* psychological issues;
- adhere to modern psychoanalytic thinking and research in positing unconscious schemas of self and other in interaction;
- emphasize that abnormal, maladaptive behavior makes sense when examined through the lenses of important, often unconscious, human motives, fears, and defenses;
- attend, to varying degrees, to concerns and conflicts over trust, dependency, autonomy, shame, guilt, identity, honesty, and intimacy;
- focus on sex and aggression, love and hate as highly charged forms of human interaction;
- highlight the formative influence of childhood experiences, as well as later life experiences in intimate relationships, in establishing the structure of personality, including the shaping of expectations, motives, and methods of adapting;
- hold that underlying issues and concerns are often defensively concealed and may reveal themselves indirectly, in seemingly random thoughts or casual remarks (associations), in dreams, in symptomatic behavior, and in patterns of interaction with others (transferences);
- view therapists' emotional responses to clients (countertransferences) as valuable in assessing relational patterns *and* as potential obstacles to therapy;
- believe that curative therapy includes a mix of increasing self-awareness (insight) and experiencing more positive ways of relating to others;

- consider the therapist to be crucial to creating a safe environment for self-discovery and for transformative experiences, some of which involve the therapist–client relationship itself.

Psychoanalytic psychology, though built on Freud's foundation, has moved beyond it, adding new ideas and jettisoning some that have not stood the test of time. Contrary to some misunderstandings of the field that consider psychoanalysis unscientific or passé (see Park & Auchincloss, 2006), most psychoanalytic ideas have extensive research support (Westen, 1999). In the next five chapters, I will summarize contemporary psychoanalytic thinking as it applies to couple therapy. This first chapter begins at the most basic level, by examining some issues that lie below the surface of most couple impasses.

To help couples escape from their pathological dances, we must not only focus on the maladaptive process per se (that when one person nags, the other withdraws, which elicits more nagging, which elicits more distancing), but on what *drives* this maladaptive runaway train, namely, the underlying sensitivities, hopes, and fears of the partners. In most cases, we will find that the cycles are driven by the frustration, and often the invalidation, of basic human needs. The more I have worked with couples whose conflicts seemed endless, the more I have found it critical to focus less on their specific complaints of the moment (the burned toast, the unbalanced budget) and more emphatically on their basic human concerns: their desires for love, caring, appreciation, closeness, and understanding; and their fears and experiences of disapproval, abandonment, domination, and incompetence. This is the first and most obvious contribution (upgrade) of psychoanalytic depth psychology to the Talk To Each Other Model of Couple Therapy 1.0.

When focusing on these underlying fears and desires, I find myself in the company of those who have sought to make "emotion" the central focus of couple therapy, especially Leslie Greenberg and Susan Johnson and their colleagues (Greenberg & Goldman, 2008; Greenberg & Johnson, 1988; Johnson, 1996, 2008), in what has become known as Emotionally Focused Couple Therapy (EFT) or Emotion-Focused Therapy for Couples (EFT-C). In my work, however, I have found it preferable to speak of hidden issues, fears, and desires—and in the next chapters, meanings and transferences, rather than emotions—to cover the amalgam of personal meanings, motives, feelings, and self-and-other schemas that we therapists seek when we look below the surface of couple interactions.

Dick and Tina: Ghosts of Christmases Past

A recently married couple returned to me (I had helped them with some premarital issues) with the vague request that now that Tina was pregnant, I might help them work through some issues concerning how to raise their child. Dick thought there might be trouble since he was a "confirmed atheist" who hated organized religion. Although he began talking in a controlled, rational manner, Dick grew louder and more intense as he detailed his complaints about religion, so that, in the countertransference, I felt uneasy as I recalled earlier sessions when his approach to both me and Tina had been rather fierce.

Surprisingly, Dick's critique concerning organized religion drew no fire from Tina, who said she had not been to church in many years, was unsure about whether she believed in God, and thought their offspring ought to decide religious matters for themselves. She did mention, however, that Christmas was something she had experienced as a rare and special time of family joy and togetherness, and she feared that tradition might end since Dick seemed so strongly opposed to celebrating that holiday at all, even banning a Christmas tree the previous year.

Yet, even as Tina spoke unemotionally and seemed open to compromise, Dick grew more intensely negative, describing all the things about the Christmas holidays that he objected to and would not allow. Suddenly, Tina burst into tears, exclaiming in a little girl's voice of despair, "I wasn't even asking for all that stuff!"

Both Tina and Dick told me that they had gone down this road many times, always ending in deadlock, with Tina sobbing and Dick angry and mystified. Given how cheerful and content they had been just a few minutes earlier and their general level of maturity and levelheadedness, their sudden intense feelings in this dominating–submitting dance were surprising and disturbing.

What I did next serves as an introduction to the therapeutic activity of unpacking negative interaction cycles, where the goal is to discover what lies below the surface so as to begin to heal the attendant disruption in the couple bond. With Dick and Tina, this was rather straightforward.

Just as Freud taught us to solicit associations to dreams, I asked Dick and Tina to step outside their painful discussion and tell me what came to their minds about it. Somewhat predictably, Dick's distress with Christmas—far more intense than with religion per se—concerned many painful memories of Christmases past, ones that included unsatisfying gifts (or no gifts at all), violent confrontations, excessive parental drinking, and, most painful of all, the failure of his parents to mend the long-standing marital rift that led to their divorce when Dick was 10. This was easy to identify as the source of his not wanting to restage Christmas festivities in his new family! Making these connections conscious—as the Ghost of Christmas Past did for Dickens's Ebenezer Scrooge—allowed us to think about what might prevent Dick and Tina from creating alternative, happy family scenes in future Christmases.

But what underlay Tina's tears, tears that conveyed such intense despair? Listening to Tina and feeling my own adverse reaction to Dick's powerful negativity, I hypothesized that her hopelessness was not so much a reaction to the specific content concerning holiday festivities (though these were important to her), but to the negative marital process—to Dick's seeming eagerness to rob her of what, in the here-and-now of my office, had been Tina's enthusiasm as a prospective parent.

So, taking a bit of a leap, I asked Tina what came to mind when she thought of situations where she had been feeling happy and enthusiastic and someone had "rained on her parade." Responding to this question, she told me, for the first time, of her father's severe auto accident. The accident had ended ("rained on") *his* dream, as he was poised to become a professional athlete (similar to her pride and pleasure as she awaited her transition to parenthood) and cast a shadow over his life and his family for many years after. He never fully recovered from the accident, suffering from intermittent back pain and severe headaches for years. It was because of his misery that Tina was often told to tone down her enthusiasm "so that Father can get some rest." Further, Tina's father became a chronically angry, sullen man, venting his unhappiness on whatever target was available. I could see now that Tina's glaring omission of these details from our prior therapy had been an unconscious attempt to keep her grumpy, depressed father out of the room. Though uninvited, he showed up anyway, disguised as Dick, whenever Dick became fiercely negative, as he was now. When this happened, it touched a nerve: her deep fear of being dragged down into a quagmire of negativity and guilt, which destroyed her positive mood in my office, at the holidays, and in anticipation of the birth of her baby.

Hidden Issues

Markman et al. (2001) used the image shown as Figure 6.1 to illustrate how couples encountering life "events" can stumble into progressively deeper psychological trouble when these events connect to their emotionally fundamental "issues" and then, still deeper, to their somewhat unconscious "hidden issues." In this illustration, the hot geysers of surface issues (money, sex, children) are fed by layers of even hotter hidden forces below, such as control, commitment, and acceptance.

For Dick and Tina, these can be summarized as follows:

- Event: Pregnancy.
- Issue(s): How to parent and what sort of family to be.
- Hidden issue, Dick: Avoiding reminders of traumatic childhood scenes.
- Hidden issues, Tina: Avoiding reminders of traumatic childhood scenes, and distress when someone "rains on her parade."

I use this sketch because it explains to couples how fights over seemingly trivial events, like shopping for a new washing machine, can engage deep

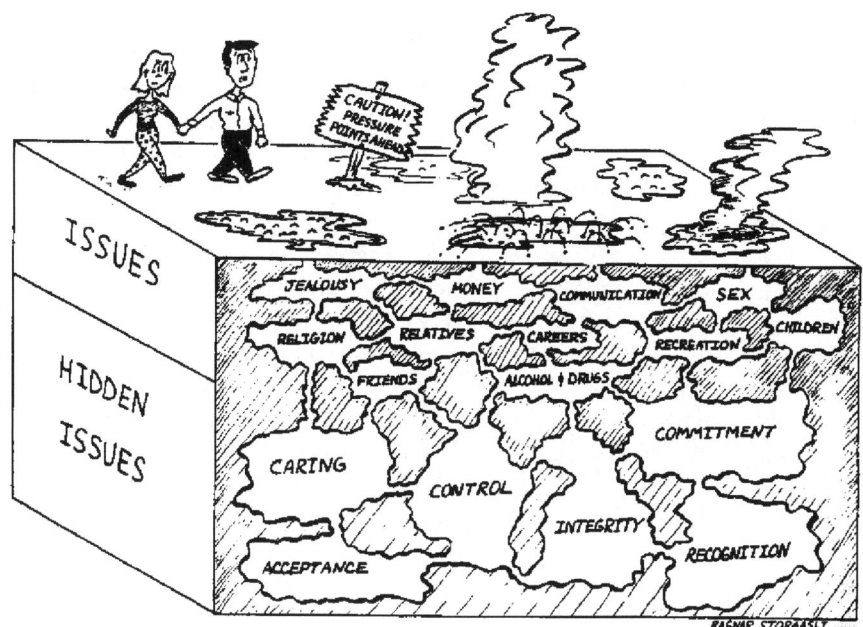

FIGURE 6.1 Hidden Issues

Used with permission. From the book, *Fighting For Your Marriage* (2010), Markman, Stanley, & Blumberg. Artist: Ragnar Storaasli.

anxieties and passions—say, over financial security, control of finances, or responsibility in spending.[2] Understanding this descent from surface events to emotionally significant hidden issues is particularly important, because fights over apparently trivial matters make up the lion's share of couple arguments, as documented by Gottman and Gottman (2010), who wrote:

> Our analyses of over 900 videotaped conflicts in our laboratory and over 1,000 play-by-play interviews about conflict at home have led us to the conclusion that most of the time most couples fight about what appears to be absolutely nothing.
>
> *(p. 144)*

From a psychodynamic perspective, the best way to make sense of escalating negative interaction cycles is to appreciate that "hidden issues" have "come online." Sometimes these deeper issues are what really need attention, even if the couple may stumble on them only occasionally. Escalation results not only from a circular process of hurt and reactive defensiveness, but from each person's awareness that his or her partner needs to hear something of great moment, even as that partner seems to be preventing it from being said.

In such situations, the common advice to focus exclusively on the problem at hand, never to bring up other instances, and never to mention past wounds is usually misguided, since the real problem may be that—across events and over time—one partner has developed serious doubts that his or her needs will be met.[3] An argument that begins with the wife complaining that her husband has failed to change a light bulb and "never helps around the house" will not be settled by advising her on the proper language to employ when she "starts up," for instance, to never say *never*, to confine herself to the current instance, and to use "I-statements." This is because the current instance is the tip of an iceberg, which may concern the division of household labor, power in the family, or mutual assistance and concern. When this is the case, we must not prevent her from engaging these issues and, instead, must work to expose and label them. Once they are exposed, we will be free to advise her on the best ways to talk fairly and nondefensively about these hidden issues.

What about situations where a spouse *begins* with an explicit, rather than a hidden, general complaint, such as, "You've never loved me. You care only about yourself!"? Although it helps to learn what specific events triggered such declarations, it is a mistake to point out that such a general attack is always too global and is unlikely to improve matters in the loving response department. Instead, in agreement with Greenberg and Goldman (2008), who discuss this very example (pp. 64–65), my approach when I believe this a core concern across many incidents is to help the speaker develop that theme. As I do so, I attempt to shift the maladaptive blaming to a deeper expression of the spouse's despair about not having his or her needs met. I try to identify which needs are not being met, but not so concretely as to focus exclusively on clothes not hung in closets or even birthdays imperfectly celebrated. I begin by validating the emotion behind the global attack as the first step toward further exploration. The technical mistake is to call it out too early as an excessive reaction or as a fatally flawed method for obtaining what is wanted.

Core Issues Used Defensively

Sometimes, deep interpersonal concerns about respect, love, and intimacy are raised, but (somewhat surprisingly) are *not* the central "hidden issues." Rather, they serve to conceal other pressing problems that create anxiety or distress. A couple faced with uncertainty about how to make ends meet or how to parent a challenging adolescent may get into an unproductive mutual blaming cycle about duty, love, or respect that takes them away from the anxiety of real problem solving. This is Bion's "basic assumption fight group," where the adversarial process diverts attention from some other anxiety-inducing task (Bion, 1961). Other couples may be mourning the death of a child or feeling guilty about how to handle a declining parent, but instead of facing these profound emotional challenges, they conceal them by fighting with each other over who is more loving or responsible. This is not to say that deeper emotional issues are not real or do not need attention, but only that they can be conveniently invoked in the service of avoiding a difficult discussion. In such situations, the "hidden issue" that should be labeled or interpreted by the therapist is the anxiety over facing some other problem that is even more challenging.

While hidden issues and their idiographic, subjective meanings are many and varied, many can be categorized as specific human fears or desires, the subjects of the next two sections.

Fears

The feared calamities I discuss here are those that commonly arise in marriage. Other fears—of flying, of illness (hypochondriasis), of going out alone in public (agoraphobia), of death—can become the subject of marital discord, and may emerge or be aggravated by deterioration in the couple bond, but my focus will be on fears that commonly emerge during couple conflict and, over time, as partners live together. Because clients can be defensively unaware of such fears or of their role in shaping their behavior, the therapist's task is to identify the fears and their attendant defenses and raise them to consciousness.

As we embark on this discussion, I wish to flag a common misconception: Contrary to common parlance, there is no such thing as a "fear of intimacy" or a "fear of closeness." Both refer to any one or some combination of the feared calamities I will be discussing. This is a practical point, not just a semantic one, since therapists who think people can simply be "afraid of intimacy" may stop their inquiry short of discovering the true, individualized nature of that anxiety.

For similar reasons, we should avoid speaking of people as "fearing things being out of control." If we are to understand people who become anxious when "things" are "out of control," we must not let those labels lull us into thinking we have identified the specific "fears" or "things." A personal example: When we were children, both my wife and I derived great pleasure from organizing our possessions (in contrast to the proclivities, years later, of our children!). Our best understanding of this area of our continuing compatibility is that what we sought was not control in and of itself, but a sort of illusion of control in a childhood world where some family members were unpredictably out of control. Both of us acted as the metaphorical high priests of our own personal religions, religions that might be defined more precisely by the dangers they magically sought to ward off. People who seem unduly "controlling" as adults may fear myriad calamities, not simply a general state of "disorder," as when a mother worries excessively that her children will be injured, or a husband agonizes over the possibility that his wife will cheat on him.

Abandonment/rejection/loss of love. The loss of the loved person, through physical abandonment, rejection, or indifference is the core danger situation highlighted by attachment theory and EFT couple therapists. It is one of the most common underlying fears seen in couple work. The social punishments of banishment from the group and solitary confinement derive their sting from the distress people feel when they are abandoned, rejected, isolated, or unloved.

While the fear of not being "loved" is somewhat broader than the fear of abandonment (and also includes fears of unworthiness that would lead to abandonment), what is generally most dreaded is the *anticipation* of the loss of the loved one. This fear looms large when spouses fear divorce.

Abandonment fears frequently manifest as fears of being psychically invisible to the love object; a potentially life-threatening (attachment) danger for children. Fears of invisibility or non-recognition lie behind the distress we feel when others fail to validate, remember, listen to, or empathize with our experiences. These are "selfobject" functions identified by psychoanalytic self psychologists as essential to maintaining our vitality and functioning.[4]

Shame and humiliation. Fear of feeling ashamed is a core underlying issue powering many negative interaction cycles. Most people find it hard to accept criticism, admit mistakes, or apologize for injuring others. This is especially hard if the person criticizing us matters to us, as partners do. For these reasons, shame is understandably an impediment to managing conflict and maintaining marital harmony. Indeed, it has been suggested that a couple therapist could function just fine by simply helping clients with the human fears of not being loved (as just discussed) and of not being "respected" (Eggerichs, 2004).

Shame is the feeling we have when we fail to live up to an inner ideal, or when we feel our integrity, identity, or self-esteem has been diminished or is under attack from others. It is a double-edged emotion felt both as an interior threat to how we see ourselves and as an external threat to our social group standing, something that can evoke concomitant attachment distress. A certain amount of shame, like guilt, assists social group functioning, but most of our clients do not see shame as beneficial. Rather, they fear shame as though it were a poison that even in small doses might kill them. This is because shame is frequently and reflexively felt as global: not "I made a mistake," but "I'm a failure!"; not "I lost my temper," but "I'm a terrible husband!"

People afraid of shame are usually most afraid of their own self-criticism. This self-criticism often holds them to perfectionistic standards, especially concerning what is expected of them in their idealized adult gender roles. To the extent that spouses (or society) seem to require such perfection, they contribute to shame being felt as poisonous.

Although sensitivity to shame is mostly about self-doubt, it often shows itself in excessive fear that others will publicly expose our defectiveness. This is the psychology we see in gangster movies: The "dis-respected" villain responds in short order by violently striking out at the person who has threatened his self-esteem. Such aggressive responses (Heinz Kohut's *narcissistic rage*) are the stuff of couple conflict, including when it moves to physical violence (Stosny, 2006); they are often based on the pre-logical belief that silencing the accuser eliminates the accusation and banishes the shame.

Fear of shame is central to people who must never lose an argument, who must always be right, and who must always have the last word. Here, the content of the debate is often less important than the person's fear of losing a competition and feeling one-down to an adversary. This psychology drives dominating–submitting cycles that stem from childhood experiences of being excessively shamed or of being valued only when competitively successful. The partners of such dominating spouses frequently give up the fight and then feel ashamed for having done so. Passive-aggression or forming coalitions with others who sympathize may restore some self-respect to the victims of such relentless domination, but at a cost to the relationship.

Jealousy. Jealousy, the painful fear that someone is favored over oneself, can be seen as an admixture of the two fears just described: abandonment, that your partner may leave you for another; and shame, that you are inferior to a rival. In such triangular situations, the third member of the triangle may be a person (a child, another relative, or a potential lover) or an activity (a hobby, a sport, or a career).

Guilt. Guilt is a close relative of shame and is similarly anathema to spouses who fear being called out as insufficiently caring, loving, or ethical. As with shame, guilt depends on the person's own internal standards being questioned; people will not feel guilty if they lack concern for their partners or have not internalized certain ethical standards (e.g., that it is not acceptable to hit someone who has offended you verbally). The usual distinction between shame and guilt is that guilt is experienced when a person violates some internalized *moral standard*, whereas shame is experienced when a person fails to live up to some other component of his or her ideal self. In many cases, however, the distinction blurs as they coexist, as when a person feels guilty after having done something bad ("I did bad") and feels ashamed of being the sort of person who has done such a thing ("I am bad").

Being "controlled" by being told what to do or how to think. While every verbal utterance can be perceived as an effort to influence one's listener, most pass as benign and are not experienced as coercive. The basic objection to being "controlled" is that people don't like being told to do things or think in ways they wouldn't choose on their own. (No one objects to being told to go to the bank to pick up a large lottery check!)

Another reason people dislike being controlled is that it can be perceived as demeaning. The person who is told to do what he doesn't want to do not only suffers from doing X instead of Y, but experiences shame and humiliation at being "pushed around" by someone more powerful. To some extent, we are all sensitive to being controlled, because this hearkens back to when we were children and had to accede to the demands of our caretakers. Adults who experienced their caretakers as having excessively curtailed their autonomy often have trouble with authority or with "accepting influence." Some may also try to reverse their long-ago humiliation by turning the tables and becoming dominating or abusive.

Another common contributor to the sensitivity to authority, specifically at home, is the feeling that, having submitted to authority all day at work, we are entitled to a respite. This break is not only from the demands of our bosses and colleagues, but from those of our internal taskmaster, who expects us to live up to our perception of ourselves as responsible and hard working. The wish for a "vacation" from demands applies equally to stay-at-home parents, who look forward to being spelled or assisted in their duties when their partners arrive home. This is frequently a setup for a collision of wills over what still needs to be done at the end of the day, and over how much downtime each partner will get.

Hypersensitivity to feeling controlled occurs not only following requests to act, but following requests or pressure to think in a certain way. This threat is often referred to as a fear of (psychological) "fusion" or "loss of self" and is fairly common in serious personality disorders and in adults who were subjected to physical or sexual abuse. One explanation for this is that abused children must distort their views of reality and their feelings in order to protect their bond with an abusive parent (Fonagy, 2000). As adults, they may have a fragile hold on certain interpersonal situations and a heightened sensitivity to being told how to see those situations by others who have their own agendas. Such people can become quite anxious in ambiguous situations where there are no hard facts, but only each person's experience of the events, which may be narrated and remembered differently. They can become immersed in endless arguments with their spouses over the "facts" that led to some painful event or argument, and over "what really happened" during the ensuing argument. While there are many sources of such arguments over the facts—including the previously mentioned difficulties accepting blame—what I want to highlight here is the difficulty many clients have in allowing someone else to "dominate their thoughts" or "control their minds."

Losing control of one's emotions or one's mind. People who fear experiencing their own emotions may appear obsessive, overly careful, boring, and, by definition, rather emotionless. The calamity they fear is that their emotions will exceed manageable levels, whether it be anger, dependence, sexual arousal, or something else. The central problem such people present in therapy and in their marriages is that, without having access to their emotional lives, they have difficulty expressing their needs and appreciating the needs of their partners.

In extreme cases, individuals may be afraid of losing control of their minds, having a "nervous breakdown," or "fragmenting" (in Kohut's terminology).

Their partners will then experience them as fragile and unable to fulfill tasks that might push them over the edge.

Being overwhelmed or overburdened by the needs of another. Some people are inordinately distressed when asked to address the emotional demands of others. They fall down on the marital job of serving as an attachment figure or selfobject. Their partners will call them out on this, viewing them as "selfish" or "unfeeling," but we therapists will do better to explore why assisting another person feels so burdensome, distressing, or unrewarding.

Revisiting past traumas. Freud remarked on the reluctance of his patients to comply with his instructions to revisit their painful past experiences; we observe the same hesitancy with ours. The main reason for this reticence is the fear that a strong, painful emotion will emerge. Leading contenders are rage, grief, anxiety, depression, loneliness, or a preoccupation with revenge. Needless to say, this fear interferes with our exploration of the origins and details of other fears.

Tangible negative consequences. For some couples experiencing discord, the most dangerous tangible fear can be physical violence. If talk of divorce is in the air, spouses may fear the loss of financial security or access to their children that a split may entail. Such fears may not be verbalized and, so, may qualify as "hidden" fears (although they differ from the purely psychological dangers already discussed).

Combinations of fears. Fears can combine and interact in myriad ways, and people can be caught between opposing fears. The fear of loneliness combined with the fear of risking intimacy has been termed the "need–fear dilemma," and is common and intense in clients with severe personality disorders. For them, there may be no emotional distance that can be comfortable or sustained: too far and the person loses needed selfobject functions that come from attachment figures; too near and the person feels, among other things, dominated or shamed.

Some fears that emerge in therapy are best seen as a *specific amalgam* of dreaded states of mind. For instance, we may discover that a woman's excessive worry about credit card debt is powered by the fear of the return of childhood traumas that followed her father's losing his job: not only poverty, but also parental discord, paternal alcoholism, inordinate self-blame for parental strife, and shame that she couldn't dress as well as other children.

Desires

Negative interaction cycles are also powered by unmet—and usually poorly articulated— wishes, desires, and needs. A central goal in exploring hidden issues is to help couples articulate what they are really fighting about, including what they really need from each other. As mentioned previously, couples routinely become more hopeful after we identify their maladaptive circular process as the cause of their distress. They can also gain hope when we show them how this systemic malfunction can be reversed by better meeting each other's fundamental human needs (Shaddock, 2000).

Mirror images. Some desires and needs are essentially mirror images of the fears I have just discussed. Desiring attachment or love, people will fear situations where these are lacking. All of us seek affirmation rather than shame and guilt, and we all prefer a certain amount of autonomy to feeling excessively controlled. More generally, all of us want to feel "safe" and "secure," which amounts to the absence of all the feared danger situations just discussed.

Affirmative co-constructed desires: Dancing together. Some human desires, however, involve pleasures that cannot be understood merely by noting that their absence causes distress. This is especially true of desires for joint, coordinated, or "co-constructed" activity: for dancing together, for sharing and building lives together, for having sex with a beloved partner, for merging resources and efforts, for raising children together, for watching sunsets, and for sharing thoughts. Such wishes contain the crucial ingredient of affect sharing. Rather than simply leading parallel lives, partners hope that their spouses will share their joys and support their successes. These desires cannot be subsumed under needs for "attachment," however, because that need, precisely defined, is about wanting assistance when one is threatened or upset. They are related, but not identical, to self psychology's identification of a (selfobject) need for "twinship," a felt sense of similarity and closeness with a like-minded life companion. They cover the same ground as Weingarten's (1991) enlarged definition of "intimacy" as "the co-creation of meaning."

These sources of pleasure all depend on the presence of a partner, often a particular partner, but they require more than the simple presence of that partner. Even if a partner is physically present, one's desires will remain unsatisfied unless both partners are involved or invested in the joint effort. Ideally, partners must be independent agents, not simply means to our ends—subjects, rather than mere objects (Benjamin, 1995). Appreciating people's frustration in attaining these shared, co-constructed ends helps us empathize with complaints about too little pleasurable time together and with fears of losing a shared life through divorce.

The desire to be known. Most of us want others to know how we feel, what we like, what we hope for, and how we are doing—that is, who we are. Success feels better when it is shared; defeat is less distressing with someone to console us. Our needs for empathy and intimacy include this desire to be known. Being known is also a precondition for partners' being invested in each other's life scripts and dreams, a central component of marital love (Kernberg, 2011).

The desire for empathy when our partner fails to meet our needs. Spouses who frustrate us often remain impassive or unsympathetic to the distress they have caused. This makes the trauma worse, just as when an athlete who disputes a call is assessed an additional penalty for protesting (Ken Newman, personal communication, November, 1987.) This pattern of double disappointment occurs most often when the offending partner tries to escape guilt and shame by refusing to acknowledge the frustration he or she has caused (Ringstrom, 1994). Much of the intensity of client distress during negative interaction cycles can be explained by the failure of such secondary empathic containment, and much of the restorative power of "softening" derives from a partner's providing it.

The desire for unencumbered time alone. Couples frequently ask us to help with their mismatched wishes for time spent together versus time spent apart. Earlier in this chapter, I discussed the distress associated with feeling dominated, controlled, or excessively intruded upon. Here, I can add a more positive understanding of the impulse to be apart, related to inborn motivations for what Robert White (1959) termed "effectance" and that, more recently, was subsumed under "exploration," by Lichtenberg, Lachmann, and Fosshage (2011). Having a more positive and nuanced view of the desire for independence, solitude, or outside activities (e.g., hobbies or "going out with the guys") can help us avoid reflexively siding with the partner who seeks more closeness.

The desire to hurt the partner. Wanting to injure the partner is almost always the downstream result of some injury to the self, or "narcissistic rage." It is also quite real and frequently hidden. Many psychoanalysts emphasize the importance of helping clients own these intentions as a useful prerequisite to maturity, self-awareness, and marital harmony. A woman I treated was well aware of her "attachment insecurity" when her husband was unavailable to her, but her anxious panic subsided only after she came to own the vindictive anger that threatened to erupt at such times. Her hostility was not expressed directly, but came across in her tone of voice, which drove her husband further from her. Helping her to own her "dark side" wish for revenge, not just her need for closeness and companionship, helped her and her marriage.

Such clinical situations are the basis for the couple therapist David Schnarch's (2011) critiques of attachment theory as applied monolithically to couple therapy. He sees this approach as too "Disney-esque" or "nice" when it always assumes that "people are doing the best they can" with only "good intentions," whereas their aim—hidden from the partner, the therapist, and even the self—may be to hurt. Getting this vindictiveness out in the open can also help partners, who can now see that they have not been "over-reacting" when they felt put off, but were responding to a covert attack.

Sometimes, to help normalize wishes for revenge following marital injury, I tell the story of a young man who asked a trusted mentor if he had ever contemplated divorce. "Divorce?" the mentor replied. "Never! But, murder? Often!"

The wish for unconditional love and idealized partners. We have previously discussed the wish for unconditional love from an idealized partner as something that makes marriage difficult. Sometimes, this is simply the desire for a partner who can listen whenever we need it and accept whatever we say. We expect to have to put up with aggravation from our bosses or our children, but not from the person who is supposed to be our best friend and loving supporter. And should our partner fall short, the potential for wounding is high, resembling Caesar's dying lament, "Et tu, Brute?" The wish for a partner with no imperfections or hot buttons will always be frustrated, even as some amount of loving responsiveness can still be expected.

WORKING WITH HIDDEN ISSUES, FEARS, AND DESIRES

I now present suggestions for uncovering and working with the hidden issues, fears, and desires discussed above. These interventions interrupt and calm negative cycles by exposing the engines that power them, allowing us to foster insight and to repair and strengthen the couple bond.

Our goal is for both partners to recognize their own hidden fears and desires *and also* those of their partner. This will help them to meet those needs more effectively and to repair the relationship when those needs are not fully met. They will also develop a better, more detailed, map of their relationship to replace their previous simplistic, maladaptive one. This improved map will help the partners discuss and interrupt their pathological dance, now identified as their shared and *comprehensible* enemy.

Therapists schooled in individual psychoanalytic psychotherapy will be familiar with the methods used for fostering insight: empathic immersion, reducing resistance, accepting ambivalence, interpreting (reframing) behaviors, and exploring the past.

Useful methods for strengthening the couple bond include (a) helping clients voice their hopes and fears more effectively *to each other*, (b) exploring and countering partners' reluctance to "soften" and alter their negative responses, and (c) helping couples use their new insights and enhanced bond to develop a plan for preventing and reining in future negative cycles.

These goals and methods are intimately and complexly related, so that discussing them separately would be excessively complex and redundant. Instead, this section aims to present practical suggestions that, in most cases, will serve multiple functions.

Begin With Empathy and Work to Maintain It

All of the interventions I will be advocating here are grounded in an empathic stance. As therapists, we must make the effort to put ourselves into each partner's shoes. We do so by tapping our imagination and our memory, the latter including similar experiences with the couple in front of us, with other couples, and in our own lives. It will help to pause, from time to time, to consider consciously what it might be like to be each of the partners *and* what it might be like to be married to each of them: Recall that I got in touch with Tina's despair by noticing how uncomfortable I felt listening to the overbearing intensity of Dick's tirade about Christmas.

Interrupt the Negative Process by Focusing on Hidden Issues

In Couple Therapy 1.0, the therapist cools the escalating negative process by getting in the middle of it—sometimes simply by interrupting it verbally, but more commonly by providing empathy, understanding, and alternative explanations for the distressing feelings and actions that the couple are displaying. In the upgraded version we are now discussing, we continue to provide a strong blend of empathy and curiosity, but *we focus our empathic attention more sharply on the motives behind the maladaptive steps of the negative interaction cycle.* We are looking to uncover the specific hidden hopes and fears that will make the maladaptive steps less mysterious and more comprehensible and sympathetic to both partners.

In individual psychoanalytic psychotherapy, exploring the client's defenses brings us to deeper understanding. *Similarly, the critical initial task in couple therapy is to interrupt and explore the process that is interfering with its own examination and with analyzing the deeper hopes and fears of the partners.* This is somewhat of a circular, bootstrap process. It usually begins with massive amounts of empathy, curiosity, and reframing by the therapist. As safety increases and the clients' moods soften, our explorations of individual dynamics can go deeper and will usually, though not invariably, be accompanied by reciprocal sympathetic responses from witnessing partners.

Reframe Defenses and Secondary Emotions

A powerful way to foster empathy and increase insight, safety, and curiosity is by "reframing" or re-narrating the meaning of clients' behavior. Therapists reframe (interpret) the latent, underlying motivations for otherwise distasteful or defensive behavior by describing them more sympathetically. Reframing allows partners to "cognitively reappraise" what they have previously been evaluating so negatively (Fishbane, 2013). When it is effective, "hard" emotions and behavior (self-righteous anger, rigid coldness) often shift to "soft" ones (sadness, anxiety) in both partners.

Perhaps the most common reframes in couple therapy are of the "secondary emotions," emotions (and their attendant behaviors) that literally come second and serve to conceal their upstream predecessors (Greenberg & Goldman, 2008). Extreme anger can be redefined as emanating from "hurt feelings" or from a pressing need to be understood. Anger that manifests as yelling, nagging, or swearing can be reframed as originating in hopelessness when engaging a partner who seems functionally deaf, emotionally abandoning, or unbending in an attack on one's pride. Insults that sting can be reframed as understandable (secondary) efforts to obtain revenge so as to "even the score" after one has been wounded. The goal here is not to banish legitimate expressions of anger or frustration, but to help injured partners "report" their feelings, rather than disqualifying themselves and their complaints by presenting them in ways that their partners experience as excessive.

Another way to look at this is simply to say that one emotion can both conceal and point to a deeper one that is closer to the client's true feelings, but is assessed as more dangerous. Clients commonly report feeling "anxious" when some other, more distressing emotion threatens to emerge (Freud, 1926). And just as the defense of intellectualization serves to conceal and dampen underlying emotions, so "emotionalization" uses one emotion to conceal another. Many such substitutions are possible: anger as a cover for hurt pride, or guilt as a defense against anger.

Secondary emotions do not just defensively conceal other emotions, they are frequently the almost instantaneous *reactions to some earlier, primary emotion*—as when some people become angry when asked to join a conversation they fear will make them feel inadequate. In another common sequence—noted by Fruzzetti (2006) and Johnson (2008)—a person who experiences a softer, primary emotion ("I miss him.") may then experience an intense reaction to that feeling or thought that obscures the initial emotion ("I'm stupid to be in love with him! I'm such a poor excuse for a woman! I feel so worthless!" or "He's such a jerk. It really makes me mad that he never gives me what I want! He's so selfish!").

Stonewalling and failing to respond sympathetically to a spouse's tears or agitation can be reframed not as the behavior of a self-centered, unconcerned spouse, but as the external appearance of someone too flooded with emotion to talk. It may then be helpful to cite Gottman et al.'s (1998) finding that seemingly unmoved partners often have elevated heart rates and great subjective distress.

Overall, we want to help clients appreciate that the aim of their secondary emotions and defensive behaviors is to conceal what they fear exposing. People who call their metaphorical troops to battle do not feel safe or hopeful when they are expressing their needs, and people who raise their metaphorical drawbridges do not feel safe responding to such requests. Over time, consistent with the goals (Gehrie, 2011) and results (Perry & Bond, 2012) we find in individual psychodynamic therapy, we can anticipate decreased defensiveness in both partners.

Reframe Unrealistic Wishes

Just as we can reframe secondary emotions and defenses, we can renarrate unrealistic wishes. Demanding or entitled people with seemingly unrealistic wishes—say, that the other be able to intuit their needs—should always be viewed as behaving in ways they believe are essential and sensible. I previously made this point from the perspective of systems theory, suggesting that angry, entitled, "least likeable" partners resemble drowning swimmers with unresponsive partners, but this is also a tenet of modern psychoanalytic thought, as summarized by Wile (1981):

> [T]roubled individuals, traditionally viewed as gratifying infantile impulses, are actually deprived of what in many cases are ordinary adult satisfactions . . . Irrational reactions, viewed by some therapists as purely destructive, are seen as providing important information about the relationship. The irritability, sulking, and romanticized longings of partners are often the only available indicators of an alienation and dissatisfaction from which both may be suffering. The appropriate therapeutic task, accordingly, is to expose these underlying issues.
>
> *(pp. 2–3)*

Rather than explaining that it is unrealistic to expect one's spouse to read one's mind—which Wile terms "turning insight into coercion" (p. 55)—it is more empathic and productive to dig deeper, to wonder why the client thinks this is the only option. By doing so, we will often discover what constrains more open communication.

Ask Some Good Questions

Some questions are particularly helpful in uncovering deeper concerns. I use these pretty much every day:

- "What nerve just got touched?"
- "Can you help us understand the intensity of your feelings?"
- "If your tears could talk, what would they say?"
- "Can you talk from your fear?"
- "What were you hoping for when . . .?"
- "How did it make you feel when John just said . . .?"
- "Did you know that was how Sarah feels?"
- "Have you felt strongly like this before?"
- "Did something like this happen when you were growing up?"

Shift the Focus Back and Forth Between the Partners

All the tactics known to individual therapists for fostering insight are useful in couple therapy. With the partner present, however, one must block counterproductive partner reactions ("I've always known you were insecure about that!") that can impede continued safe exploration. One way to do this is by shifting back and forth between the partners, alternating the project of analyzing each person's hidden issues.

Do a Better Job Than Your Clients in Making Their Case (i.e., Articulating Their Hopes and Fears)

Contemporary couple therapists often work to help clients make a better case for what they want: "to find their voice" or to make "differentiated" "relational claims" on their partners (Fishbane, 2010; Greenberg & Goldman, 2008; Real, 2007; Wile, 1981). Because client communications are often ambivalent, poorly reasoned, or packaged in rage, tears, or guilt-tripping, partners routinely dismiss them as illogical, crazy, or excessive. *Therapists can help clients express their deeper concerns more clearly and more thoroughly, so that they can be heard by their partners.*

With this goal in mind, Wile (1981) uses a technique he calls "doubling" to re-state clients' positions better than they themselves have been doing. He speaks for them, often moving himself next to them and speaking directly to their partners. He begins respectfully, conveying that this is a first draft, "Let's see if I can state Andy's case in a way that makes sense to you, Sally . . ." and continuously checks to see if he is fairly representing his client's position. This intervention conveys empathy, as the partner the therapist speaks for feels validated and understood. But it does more than that. The main reason to speak for clients in this manner is that they are generally not doing a good job of it themselves. Not only are they being interrupted by their partners, but—lacking a sophisticated understanding of themselves and often highly conflicted about voicing their thoughts—they get muddled in trying to explain themselves succinctly. Just as I have been discussing "hidden" issues, Wile (1981) identifies "left out" issues, and explains:

> People who discuss their feelings in obscure ways appear to be caught between a wish to express them and a fear of what might happen if they did. Their solution, conscious or otherwise, is to lay out controversial thoughts in a semidisguised manner and to leave it to others to acknowledge them or not. These individuals may be partially hoping that what they are saying will go unnoticed; they also appear to be wishing it might be picked up.
>
> *(p. 114)*

Such clients unconsciously hide their needs not only from their partners, but from themselves. For instance, when Beth railed at Fred for not doing some household task, she did so conflictedly, fearing that she was, as he so often told her, "an unreasonable bitch." At such times, she was unaware that her complaints usually arose just as Fred was about to leave for an extended business trip. As I pointed out these issues, both Fred and Beth softened and moved closer to each other. Therapists who are more aware of their clients' conflicted desires than they are, who are less afraid of their clients' partners, and who know the benefits of straight talk are better positioned to state their clients' cases than they are. And when we speak for a client, that client also hears what we are saying and benefits from our clarification. More than in Couple Therapy 1.0, where our goal was to help partners listen to each other, here we are also working to help them listen better to themselves.

In summary, *making a client's case better than he or she can is a powerful, multifaceted tool that interrupts negative cycles, provides validation, interprets and reframes behavior, and places previously hidden hopes and concerns clearly on the table.*

Make Explanatory Interpretations

Interpretations are interventions containing a "because" that attempt to foster improved self-understanding by explaining why things are occurring and how they are connected. They can look like this: "Despite very much wanting to have sex last night, you didn't bring it up because you believe that doing so is unromantic. You tell yourself that asking for sex is unromantic, which it is somewhat, because you are afraid that asking directly will lead to rejection, and then not only will you not have sex, but you will feel unloved and embarrassed." Other interpretations will be far shorter: "Because so many conversations with George have gone south, it's natural that you try to avoid them."

Les Greenberg (personal communication, 2013) has suggested a useful formula for making interpretations in couple therapy: the "no wonder" intervention. For example: "No wonder you're so down. You had your hopes up that you could spend the evening together and your plans fell through." Here, "because" is conveyed by the more sympathetic "no wonder." Greenberg's wording has the advantage of conveying the therapist's comforting concern and validation, along with the causal explanation.

Interpretations can also be more speculative and framed as questions: "Could so much rage come from feeling so alone for so long?" This format not only allows clients to modify the details, but encourages them to join in the task of interpretation.

Work to Understand and Reduce Resistance

Most interpretations offer opportunities to convey empathy, including when explaining defensiveness, as in, "It makes you feel more in control to be righteously angry when you express your hurt or loneliness than to do it in a gentler, more vulnerable way." Providing empathic explanation is a powerful way to lessen constraints clients place on their own self-awareness.

Another way to work with defensiveness is to call attention to shifts in involvement as they occur. Similar to the "close process monitoring" of psychoanalyst Paul Gray (1994), we can work to help clients maximize self-awareness by highlighting moments when they constrain their thoughts and limit themselves. For example, a therapist might say, "Tom, you changed the subject just now when your wife brought up her concerns about your upcoming trip to visit her parents. Did that stir you up?"

Encourage Intensity by Repetition and Evocative Metaphor

Another way to help patients access their deeper concerns is by having them repeat emotionally charged statements more than once, as in, "When you're away, I feel so alone. When you're away, I feel so alone. When you're away, I feel so alone." A therapist can also encourage intensified feeling by using evocative, metaphorical language and visual images: "When she criticizes you, you feel under attack like a man caught in a hurricane. You feel so scared, small, and angry that you have a hard time thinking, while you mostly just want to run away to safety."

Allow Clients to Be Multifaceted

To help clients expose their hidden issues, it helps to acknowledge their ambivalence and complexity. Uncovering and voicing ambivalence not only gives a more accurate representation of what is going on inside, but works to make clients more sympathetic to their partners and to themselves. In the various named interventions below, Wile (2012) describes how he enables clients to be multifaceted in the service of gaining self-awareness:

> **The how-much, how-much intervention**. I'd ask, "Okay Karen, how much are you saying, 'Yeah, yeah, yeah, tell the truth, Barry, that's not what you really feel' and how much are you saying, 'What worries me the most is that you don't really care about me'?" This question allows me to tease apart Karen's angry reaction and her underlying vulnerable feelings. I'm inviting her to elaborate on these feelings while leaving her room, if she prefers, to reassert her angry reaction.
> **The fraction-of-a-second intervention**. Speaking for Karen, I'd say, "Barry, for a fraction of a second I thought maybe what the therapist just said about your feelings is true. But then I said to myself, 'Nah! I don't want to get my hopes up just to be disappointed.' Though it would be wonderful if I were wrong."

Wile also describes *asking multiple-choice questions* to allow clients to select from a range of options or, when appropriate, to pick "none of the above" or "all of the above." For example, "Do you feel (a) upset with María for bringing this up, (b) embarrassed by her bringing it up, (c) relieved that it's now out in the open, or (d) something else entirely?" As with his other interventions, Wile's multiple-choice questioning allows clients to be ambivalent. Those who might freeze up when asked to tell us how they feel may also be greatly relieved by this format. Even if a client rejects all of the possibilities we offer, we have primed the pump.

Recognizing that our clients are complex and multifaceted also makes room for their ambivalence about us and about the therapy: "What are you taking away from this session that's useful, if anything, and what hasn't been so good about it?"

Explore the Past

Significant trouble with inhibited or intensified desires and with excessive interpersonal fears almost always begins prior to the current relationship, so exploring experiences with parents and with the parental marriage, as well as with prior marriages and other long-term relationships, is fertile territory. Hidden issues may also be better understood by discussing the couple's experiences when they spend time with their parents in the present, including during family holidays, vacations, or reunions.

Heal and Restructure the Interpersonal Bond

Beyond clarifying the motives, hopes, and fears that drive negative interaction cycles, we can use this information to help us heal and restructure the damaged bond between the partners. Such healing is more likely when the partners become aware, and then accepting, of their spouse's underlying issues. This is a clear benefit of conjoint therapy, as couples soften and move emotionally toward each other. This softening and increased closeness, in turn, not only counter and calm the vulnerability cycle, but offer corrective emotional experiences.

Greenberg and Goldman (2008) have outlined the steps that need to occur:

1. Partner A reveals a core experience.
2. Partner B perceives A's underlying experience and now perceives A in a new way.
3. This changes B's response to A.
4. A perceives B's new response and this supports new organization in A.

This is only half of the corrective process, since most therapies will uncover unmet needs and vulnerabilities in both partners. Enabling partners to perceive and experience each other in new ways promotes change in both their external interactions and their internal experiences.

Partners who are "drawn in" and become warmer and more intimate are very different from distancers who have been "hounded" to pay attention by pursuers who have had to beg for closeness or, for that matter, from clients whom therapists have instructed to come together through instruction in relationship skills.

Such "moments of meeting" (Lyons-Ruth, 1999) and intimacy, when the partners are vulnerable, are never simply an intellectual event, but hold the potential for a profound transformation in the couple's experience of each other. Over time and many sessions—not all of them as dramatic as made-for-TV therapy scenes—genuine changes in trust and connection evolve out of this therapeutic process as it uncovers hidden issues and reframes hurtful behaviors. This is the positive picture of success, the goal line of EFT and EFT-C therapy, when couples soften and attach intimately. It is the "solved moment" in Wile's Collaborative Couple Therapy one that is also foregrounded as "witnessing" in Michael White's (2009) more structured variety of narrative couple therapy.

Encourage Further Intimate Contact (Sometimes)

As couples move toward greater empathy, trust, and connection, it becomes both possible and beneficial to ask them to talk even more intimately to each other. When the moment is right, therapists can say such things as:

- "Beth, can you tell Fred what you need from him when you feel that way?"
- "Tina can you look at Dick and tell him just how much you miss him?"
- "Tom, can you look Jennifer in the eye and tell her how overwhelmed you feel when she is sad?"
- "Sarah, can you tell Susan how afraid you get that she will leave you?"
- "Roger, can you at look Ted and express the love and concern you seem to be feeling as you've listened to what he's been saying?"

Other times, therapists should simply step out of the way and let the couple do the talking—or hugging.

Back Off to Cool Things Down (Sometimes)

But there is potential danger here, as well. Sometimes, as one uncovers deep hurt, the partners may get even more lost in the emotion schemas that evoke pain—regret, anger, revenge, distrust—such that they have a hard time "returning to their senses" and feel worse at the close of sessions. At such times, therapists will want to slow things down using the tactics discussed before for cooling the emotional room temperature and ones we will discuss later, under psychoeducation and emotion regulation.

Address Constraints on Partner Empathy

In some scenarios that will require more therapeutic work, spouses open up, express their needs, and make themselves vulnerable, but their partners fail to be moved. Therapists inviting clients to be supportive with the phrase, "Can you tell her/him that it's OK to be scared [or sad, or weak]?" may find the partner unwilling or unable to comply. Worse, some partners will appear vindictively triumphant, stating that the uncovered issues confirm what they have been saying for years—that their partners are neurotic and that this has nothing to do with them! Others will respond defensively to authentic reports of anger and frustration.

When partners fail to be drawn in or to empathize, the therapy should then examine the constraints that block this softening. This is another obvious advantage of couple therapy over individual therapy, in which the personal growth of the partner in therapy may be insufficient to improve the relationship because of rigidity in the absent spouse.

Perhaps the most frequent deterrent to partners becoming empathic is their fear of becoming vulnerable; letting the other off the hook just feels too dangerous. Many spouses also fear that empathizing is tantamount to absolving the partner of guilt for distressing behavior, and that being understanding and supportive will only lead to more of the same problem in the future. And some clients who were socialized to be caretakers for others—more often the wife, but sometimes the husband—may believe that expressing empathy will inevitably lead to loss of self and bondage to the needs of the other (Scheinkman & Fishbane, 2004).

Other partners back away from empathizing out of fear of "catching" the painful feelings their partner is expressing. The challenge for the listener is to manage the feelings he has taken on as a result of showing empathy to his partner. Therapists faced with spouses who seem unable to manage such feelings should explore the specific impediments to their doing so.

Partners can also fail to provide empathic connection when they rush in too quickly with advice. These are most often men, who tend to underestimate the benefits of showing that they understand and are concerned about their partner's hurt feelings. Such spouses often feel unduly injured when their attempts to problem-solve are rebuffed. When they experience failure in their efforts to help, they may become detached, thinking that "nothing will help," while conveying a rejecting attitude that is the antithesis of empathy.

Or spouses may fail to empathize because their own needs for empathy at that moment are too pressing. When this happens, therapists may have to pull back and meet the distressed partner's needs for attention and succor, as a prerequisite, before that partner will be able to provide empathy to his or her spouse.

A final, common obstacle to empathy derives from combinations of moralistic thinking and failed imagination, as when partners maintain that their spouses should not be so upset by a particular event because they brought it on themselves, or because the event appears (to them) to be insufficient to cause such distress. These failures of empathy occur more frequently in overly logical partners who have trouble accessing their own emotional lives. In the former situation, the therapist can point out that just because a person contributed to his own pain does not mean there is no pain to empathize with; indeed, the pain may be *greater* due to shame or guilt. In the second case, the therapist can help the partner to recall a similar, if not identical, painful event in his or her life as a way to foster empathy.

Develop a Plan for Preventing/Interrupting Negative Cycles

After working hard to increase couple insight and bonding, therapists can plan with them how they might use their new, improved "instruction manuals" for themselves and each other to prevent future unhappiness. Therapists can ask questions like: "Can you tell her how she might act so as to be less threatening to you?" "Knowing that your husband is so afraid of your criticism, how might you make it safer for him to listen to you?" "What can you do to feel less uncomfortable when your wife starts telling you she is upset about her job?"

Sally and George: Working with Underlying Issues

The following case illustrates some of the key points made in this chapter.

Even after his depression lifted—about eight months into our conjoint therapy—George remained relatively passive in his marriage. His high-energy wife, Sally, who confidently ran the show at her large factory outlet store, not only wanted George to do more, but wanted him to initiate things. This wish was especially strong when it came to her desire that he approach her for sex.

At her most exasperated, at the beginning of therapy, Sally had alternated between forlornly crying and bitterly attacking George as uncaring and unloving—something that only made matters worse as George retreated into wounded immobility. Sally had been close to divorcing George for this persistent problem, which dated to the early days of their marriage. At the same time, Sally was grateful for all the support George had given her during their marriage: encouraging and financing her college education in her 30s and minding the fort when she was working long hours. But despite this gratitude (which stimulated some guilt), Sally had been at the end of her rope. Couple therapy was her last hope to change George and make him more to her liking.

For his part, George was terrified of losing Sally, who was so central to his life and whom he so admired, especially for her executive functions in the marriage. Sally and George seemed to me a pretty typical, increasingly entrenched, pursuer–distancer couple who cared deeply for each other, but who felt stymied by their inability to satisfy each other's desires.

In the early stages of treatment, I worked with George to understand his reluctance to take the initiative. As it turned out, he had difficulty asking directly for what he wanted, and his lifelong, self-protective strategy had been to avoid frustration via passivity. We uncovered an important key to this issue when he described his many disappointments when he was young and had repeatedly tried, unsuccessfully, to get his depressed, exhausted-from-work father to play catch and otherwise engage with him. It also helped us to link his childhood experiences of rejection with his current, similar, realistic fears of rejection as he looked for work after having been laid off (i.e., rejected) by the corporation where he had worked for many years. Understanding her husband better helped Sally to soften, and being validated helped George to stretch himself in his job search. Eventually, he found a new job, for which we were all relieved and happy.

George's depression lifted, and some of the heat went out of the couple's financial anxieties, especially their concern about how they would pay for college for their four children. As a result, there was less generalized squabbling of the type that distracts from more basic concerns. This initial therapeutic work had consisted largely of Sally's witnessing what was basically my individual therapy with George, a supportive/insight-oriented process focused on uncovering his hopes and fears. Sally's being there to hear about them, now reframed in more sympathetic terms, greatly reduced her demeaning attacks on George as "irresponsible" and "unloving."

Inside the marriage, the couple dance changed, as George became more involved and less passive-aggressive (an aspect of their pursuer–distancer cycle). In the past, when Sally had asked him to perform certain tasks around the house, he had often procrastinated, secretly not intending to do things quite as she had asked and certainly not as soon as she would have liked. Now, because he experienced her as less shaming, he was more responsive and willing to "accept influence." As he became less angry and accommodating, he was also able to admit his prior secret satisfaction in irritating and getting back at Sally— an example of insight and greater maturity following behavioral change in both partners.

Many wives would now have been delighted to have a husband who was so easy-going, so adaptable (he was happy to go out to whatever movie or restaurant she chose), and so pleased to be married to her. However, Sally was still unhappy with George's passivity about initiating joint activities. Her unhappiness showed in her generalized mood of dissatisfaction with him and her preference for spending time with their children. A clear benefit of this "witnessed" individual therapy was that I could observe Sally's reluctance to become fully empathic and present, even after George's considerable progress.

With this in mind, the therapy moved to an exploration of the marriage from Sally's end.

I first recognized and empathized out loud with her wish that George be more proactive. This was made easier because of some individual sessions with him during which I also felt burdened by having to initiate topics and keep the conversation flowing. I told her that I could easily imagine a husband who would be more willing to keep things going, although I also remarked on the disadvantages of marriage to a dominating spouse (someone like Dick, who was described at the beginning of this chapter).

My having validated Sally's wish for things to be still better made her more amenable to exploring why it was so painful for her to accept what she had. As it turned out, her wish that George initiate actions—rather than just sharing activities they both enjoyed, like camping or sex—was based on the half-conscious belief that his originating and planning such activities would signify that he "*really* loved her," valued her intensely, and had her "ever on his mind." This was a lifelong wish of Sally's from childhood. Her parents had provided attachment assistance when she had been distressed, but had never given her the sort of strong affirmation she was hoping for from George. Sally yearned to be "desired" as someone who was "captivating" and "really special."

On hearing Sally state these underlying desires more softly and clearly, George was able to empathize and to do somewhat better. He started giving Sally some of the hugs she so wanted and, without asking, took over some of the tasks related to their daughter's college search. His greater responsiveness also grew out of our uncovering an unrealistic wish of his: that his can-do wife would be self-sufficient, unlike the family dog, who needed "a hug a day." This insight lightened things up with some humor, and Sally started to approach George with a playful, "Woof, woof!"

Their sex life also improved, as we learned that Sally's preference that George get things started derived not only from her wish to be desired, but from lingering guilt over sexuality—guilt that lessened some as we talked about it openly and as George also admitted to some guilt and insecurity in the bedroom.

Many husbands ("the standard-issue" ones that populated Sally's mind) might have become still more proactive after learning the strength of their wives' desire, but not George. He continued to be phlegmatic, slow and hesitant to initiate sex and most other joint activities, though always happy and content to follow Sally's lead. What it came down to at the end of this successful couple therapy was helping Sally accept that, while her wish that her husband be still more proactive might be normal and reasonable—even with its roots in her lingering doubts about her desirability—it was something she would have to let go of and mourn. This took some time to accomplish, as her wishes kept resurfacing, but acceptance was facilitated by our empathy for her disappointment, which replaced George's prior invalidation. As she mourned her loss, Sally was assisted by, and became more aware of, the considerable pleasures they did share, and of how she, like George, did not want to lose her life partner.

Therapy Requires More Than Uncovering

Experience shows that change is unlikely if we fail to get at underlying issues, but it is not always true that simply accessing deeper concerns leads to change for the better. Some more "assembly" may still be required. In the following chapters, we explore some additional psychoanalytically informed upgrades, all of which depend on first exposing hidden issues, fears, and desires.

Notes

1 The most important of these include Bergler (1949), Dicks (1967), Donovan (2003), Gerson (2010), Hazlett (2010), Leone (2008), Livingston (1995), Ringstrom (1994, 2014), Sager (1994), Scharff and Scharff (2008), Shaddock (1998, 2000), Siegel (1992, 2010), Zeitner (2012), as well as therapists who are not psychoanalysts and do not identify themselves as writing from this perspective, but who have, nonetheless, made important contributions to a depth psychological perspective: Greenberg (Greenberg & Johnson, 1988; Greenberg & Goldman, 2008), Johnson (Greenberg & Johnson, 1988; Johnson, 1996, 2008), Real (2007), Scheinkman and Fishbane (2004), and Wile (1981, 1993, 2002, 2013a).
2 The psychoanalyst Edmund Bergler (1949) was probably the first to emphasize that such "malevolence over trifles" indicates that deeper unconscious issues have become engaged, noting that "the trifle is only the hitching-post for a deeper unconscious conflict" (p. 66).
3 Modern behavior therapists have reached a similar conclusion: that something bigger than isolated behavioral complaints drives negative cycles. They call these "themes" and provide examples of ones that involve core issues of love, respect, and conflicts over closeness (Jacobson & Christensen, 1996).
4 For those unfamiliar with psychoanalytic self psychology, Heinz Kohut (1971, 1977, 1984) and others (e.g., Stolorow, Brandshaft, & Atwood, 1987) have stressed the formative and lifelong human (selfobject) needs for affirmative connection with others—for interactions that provide empathy, companionship, idealization, and protection. The term selfobject refers to an "object" (a person) who performs functions necessary for stabilizing and invigorating the self. Applying this psychological understanding to marital partnerships, self psychologists stress that people search for positive (selfobject) support from their partners, and that when this support is lacking, emotional symptoms—including entitlement, (narcissistic) rage, devitalization, and overall mental collapse (fragmentation)—may follow.

7
FOCUSING ON DIVERGENT SUBJECTIVE EXPERIENCES

> Couples in dysfunctional relationships are often caught up in conflicts about *"the truth"*: "That's not what *really* happened . . .," and similar statements are frequent. In competent marriages, there appears to be a well-developed and shared ability to recognize the less frequent occasions in which *the truth* is important ("The tax deadline is tomorrow. We've got to get the form to the mailbox.") and those more frequent occasions when subjective reality is far more important than the truth.
>
> J. Lewis, summarizing results from the Timberlawn family studies (1997, p. 76)

In the last chapter, we explored the value of uncovering hidden issues, especially fears and desires that power negative interaction cycles and cause marital unhappiness. This often allows us to discover idiosyncratic or person-specific meanings of events that evoke conflict between the partners, as we saw with Dick and Tina, who became deadlocked over celebrating Christmas because the holiday had different meanings for each of them. The meanings things have for us are often incompletely known to us (because they are unconscious, disavowed, or "unformulated") or are assumed to be universal (because they were learned in childhood, because they are embedded in cultural givens, or because we have never met anyone who thought differently) and, therefore, frequently cause puzzling discord between partners. In this chapter, we look at this problem of divergent subjective experiences more closely.

The opening quote from the Timberlawn family studies suggests just how important this topic is to couple happiness: Across many couples and many conflicts, Lewis and colleagues found that "competent" couples were distinguished by their ability to respect each other's differing subjective experiences. Such couples only rarely fought over "the truth." Looked at from the opposite direction, Gottman's extensive observational studies (2011) found that the vast majority of couple arguments—times when couple competence had broken down—began with differences in the "perception" of events. Even when partners concede that they have different perspectives, they frequently argue (pointlessly) that there is only one *correct* perspective. When this occurs, neither partner stops to listen to the other and polarization continues until the (usually obvious) truth on each side is acknowledged.

The Rob Reiner film, *The Story of Us* (2000), shows a couple on the verge of marital separation as they rush to get their kids to the camp bus. Their drive slows down when they are caught behind the unlikely impediment of a house being towed. The mother reacts anxiously, seeing the house as an obstacle they must not allow to deter them from their mission; the father, who is driving, instead finds it a source of amusement and family bonding (noting how its zip code keeps changing and wondering what would happen if someone flushed a toilet). Both are right: The house is both an obstacle *and* a source of amusement. Both parents are hurt and deflated into silence, however, when their individual perspective is not acknowledged. This particular polarity—the wife all work and the husband all fun—plagued them in other situations, too, and was central to their marital troubles.

The Foundational Significance of Human Subjectivity

In addition to the *specific* resonances and meanings of events, some disputes engage the fundamental human desire each of us has to be recognized as an independent person, what psychoanalyst Jessica Benjamin (1995) terms a "subject." This subject has the right to independent action (agency) and thought (subjectivity), as contrasted with an "object," who is merely a character in another person's play. In healthy relationships, we allow others to operate as subjects, who are therefore "usable" (meaningful/valuable) as independent actors providing us honest reactions to our behavior (Winnicott, 1960; Newman, 1996; Ringstrom, 2014).

Because such relating is risky, *people often attempt to control their partners, including by attempting to rule out the existence of alternate realities.* In our consulting rooms, this manifests as one partner telling the other, "Only an idiot would want to do it that way!" When this happens, partners correctly sense that something more is at stake than the particular topic being discussed. They feel a threat to their right to "subject" status, and may react powerfully to that threat, by either counterattack or resignation.

Mentalization Deficits and Psychic Equivalence

While some clients defensively disallow the psychic reality of their partners mostly in the heat of battle, others do so more pervasively, due to their psychological deficits. As noted by psychoanalyst Peter Fonagy (2000) and his collaborators, some clients are especially deficient in their capacity to "mentalize," that is, to comprehend the minds of others and—relevant to this discussion—to appreciate the possibility of alternate realities. Some of this empathic deficit is due to their failure to accept the possible difference between what they are experiencing and what "is." Such "psychic equivalence" is common in people with severe personality disorders and seriously interferes with their ability to relate to their partners and to work with us as we explore alternative accounts of marital events (Ringstrom, 2014).

The "You're Both Right" Intervention

My experience with couples in conflict over divergent subjective experiences inspired what I came to call the "You're both right" intervention: The therapist points out that while the partners seem to believe that there is only one correct way to see a situation, in fact, both can be simultaneously correct. When making this postmodern point, I point out how two people can react very differently to the same movie, often because they have focused on different scenes or characters. A more memorable way to make this point is by showing couples the Rubin vase (Figure 7.1), which can be seen *simultaneously* as both a vase *and* as two faces in profile.[1]

The "Life Doesn't Come With Labels" Intervention

Sometimes I call the challenge of differing subjective experiences the "Life Doesn't Come With Labels" problem. More than most people realize, our daily lives are a continuous Rorschach inkblot test, where our perceptions and

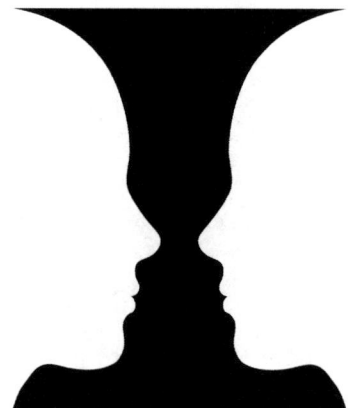

FIGURE 7.1 The Rubin Vase

Photo Credit: pio3/Shutterstock.com. Used with permission.

judgments are mental events reflecting internal concerns and templates. The newspaper headline, "Teen Sex on the Rise!" may cause alarm to parents, but might be a cause for rejoicing in teenage boys. Many arguments between couples are prolonged needlessly by semantic wrangles that can never be resolved objectively. Whether Fred's working late makes him a "good provider" or a "neglectful husband" cannot be determined by looking at the clock when he arrives home. Fred and Beth have to work out their differing preferences without reference to absolutes.

Another example: A client of mine, Sarah, who had suffered greatly in the wake of delivering a stillborn son two years previously, got into prolonged, heated arguments with her mother-in-law over whether her new infant daughter should be referred to as her second child, as Sarah preferred to think of her, or as her first, as advocated by her mother-in-law. Since there was no objective way to settle this semantic dispute, I interpreted it as a proxy battle over whether the mother-in-law could validate Sarah's painful memories or whether Sarah was required to present herself, falsely, as exclusively delighted because she now had a living baby. As might be expected, this dispute reminded Sarah of other times when she had felt similarly forced to put on a fraudulent happy face.

Some Common Arguments Over Labels

Many ongoing arguments can be seen as battles over definitions or labels, which often stem from dissimilar cultural experiences and values. Couple therapists frequently see arguments over the correct definitions of "neatness," "responsibility," "fun," "love," and "punctuality." Peter Fraenkel (2011) adds several more relating to time: the correct tempo for making love, the correct speed to drive, and whether fun time should precede or follow time spent working. Many arguments over whether something was "thoughtful" or "insensitive" hinge on divergent subjective definitions. As described by Brent Atkinson (2005):

> Relationships begin spiraling downward when, rather than seeing their partner's behavior as arising from legitimately different priorities or ways of maintaining emotional stability, each partner interprets the other's behavior from within their own framework. From their own way of looking at things, the other person appears as insensitive, selfish, misguided, irresponsible, lazy, controlling, etc. (e.g., "I would never treat him the way he treats me!"; "I would never get upset over such a little thing!").
>
> (p. 227)

Once a couple acknowledges that many events do not come with objective or ethically absolute labels attached, they can stop being quite so judgmental and, instead, explore their specific reactions to their differently experienced life events and discuss how to work together to deal with their differences.[2]

Fraenkel's Three R's

When working with couple differences, I find it useful to follow Fraenkel's (2011) easily-remembered sequence, his "Three R's": *Reveal* (uncover the difference), *Revalue* (notice that there is value or truth on both sides—similar to my "You're both right" intervention), and *Revise* (work out a compromise).

When Events Themselves Become Debatable

Although the subjective meanings of events are not determined by external realities, that does not mean that there are no external, objective facts, and sometimes couples fight fiercely over "the facts" concerning what each believes has occurred. One common argument concerns whether one partner did or did not communicate something to the other, as in "I told you to do that!" followed endlessly by "No, you didn't!" and "Yes, I did!" Having listened to this back-and-forth many times, I now interrupt it by suggesting two possibilities: (a) that speakers who are certain they told their spouses something may have been distracted at the moment of telling and are now remembering *their intention* to tell, and/or (b) that listeners who were indeed physically present may have been distracted and never registered the communication.

Sometimes, however, the therapist gets the impression that one partner is clearly misrepresenting facts that any neutral person would consider consensual reality. In such cases, to quote a remark generally attributed to Senator Daniel Patrick Moynihan: "You're entitled to your own opinions. You're not entitled to your own facts." When one partner makes little distinction between consensual facts and his or her wishes—and does this repeatedly in an arbitrary, histrionic, or rigid manner, usually as a transparent effort at self-protection—his or her partner may, understandably, get angry and anxious. These feelings intensify when details appear to be up for grabs and there are no solid facts to anchor the discussion.

When working with such couples, I first direct them away from their courtroom debate over what precisely occurred by reframing gross alterations of the facts as an effort either to get an emotional point across or to avoid shame. I acknowledge that one spouse considers this a form of rhetorical cheating, while my reframe tries to show him or her that it's more important to hear the underlying message. My goal is to slow the irate spouse down sufficiently to allow me to work with the person who is exhibiting this urgent need to play fast and loose with the facts.

Sometimes, we also discover spouses particularly allergic to such defenses—usually the result of having had parents who similarly distorted facts, a practice that threatened the child's inner sense of reality. Some of these spouses will seem to be excessive sticklers for the facts, never cutting their partners any slack. As pointed out by Virginia Goldner (2013), like small children, such "gladiators for the truth" will often require and appreciate the validation of facts ("Yes, I saw that, too!") more than unalloyed, empathic soothing ("That really hurt!").

Divergent Attitudes About Emotions

In *Meta-Emotion: How Families Communicate Emotionally* (1996), Gottman, Katz, and Hooven discuss people's overall approach to their emotional lives: Not only do some people have more trouble with *specific* emotions in themselves and their partners (e.g., shame, guilt, sadness), but they can have divergent attitudes about emotions in general. They call these beliefs "meta-emotions," and differentiate two types of people. One type are "emotion distancing," believing that people can control their feelings and should simply use "the power of positive thinking" to "suck it up" when they have powerful emotions. They view intensely emotional people as being out of control. The other type are "emotion-coaching," and believe that emotions are like an internal GPS that can help guide us in our actions. Gottman et al. found, also, that an untreated meta-emotional discrepancy between married partners predicted divorce with 80% accuracy.

While "emotion distancing" may be superior in situations of great stress (e.g., in battle, when one must suppress emotion and do what needs to be done), in most marriages, seeing emotions as "trying to tell us something" is more productive.

A client who asserts that one should "be polite" and "not complain," and "If you can't say something nice, don't say anything at all," poses a particular challenge. The therapist can expect some hard sledding against this entrenched meta-emotional belief system, and will need to help this person uncover the hopes, fears, and cultural beliefs that maintain it.

Divergent Attitudes About Discussing Past Injuries

Closely related to divergent attitudes about exposing versus suppressing emotions are disagreements about the merits of discussing past injuries. Many arguments over past injuries between spouses—from those about last Saturday night's insensitive remark to those about extramarital affairs—take this form: *The injury really did occur and cannot be forgotten, and the injurious event is really past and so might be forgiven so that we can move on into the future.* We will return to this subject in the chapter on forgiveness. For now, I note that this common type of argument, like others discussed earlier, cannot be settled simply by referring to some absolute principle. Clearly, there can be value in venting and reviewing painful events, but it can also be beneficial to let them go and focus on recovering and enjoying life. Both approaches have merit. In specific instances, couples will have to work out when to review and when to move on.

MIKE AND CINDY: DIVERGENT EXPERIENCES

Mike had come to me, sheepishly and guiltily, referred for therapy by his wife, Cindy, after she discovered some erotic emails he had been sending to another woman. I quickly restructured the therapy to include Cindy. After the first of their four children was born, Cindy had left her career to devote herself to being a full-time mom, and Mike had become increasingly involved in his demanding job. As Cindy's sexual interest dropped off, Mike was silently resentful, but accommodated. Their family soon came to resemble many diagrammed in Minuchin's (1974) Structural Family Therapy: a cross-generational alliance between mother and children, with father left out in the cold. The "quasi-affair" via erotic emails was, I thought, Mike's attempted home remedy for the intimacy-deprived state to which he had become resigned. As I worked to help Mike both to apologize for the damage he had done and to explain his deeply felt loneliness, sexual frustration, and insignificance, Cindy softened. The long-term structural problem improved, and Cindy's insecurity-driven guilt-tripping lessened. Nonetheless, one day they came to therapy after an event that Cindy said had nearly taken them back to Square One.

What had happened? Mike had arrived home—battle-weary from work—and seen Cindy playing happily with the family sheep dog, Bertie. Cindy had then said to Mike, "I know you didn't want a dog, but you've got to admit Bertie is just the cutest dog!" to which Mike had nonchalantly joked, "Oh, you need a dog to love you!" . . . and they were off to the races. As will become clear, this vignette illustrates how the same event (a wife enjoying the family dog) evoked divergent meanings for these partners and how uncovering the details got them back on track.

Part of what hurt was that Cindy really did love Bertie and loved the way Bertie loved and responded to her. Both she and Mike had noticed this before. Reflecting on the event, she told us that, in her financially strapped, emotionally arid family of origin, she had always known that she could never ask for a dog. More generally, on many occasions when she had been enthusiastic about something, her mother had failed to mirror that enthusiasm. Later, although uncertain about whether she would ever be able to love her children and somewhat afraid of dogs, Cindy had committed herself to creating a warm, loving household for her children that included the dog she had never believed she would have. Both the children and Bertie responded to her love and enthusiasm in kind.

What she was selectively blind to was how she was unconsciously replaying her mother's behavior by depriving Mike of the love and enthusiasm he also needed. After Mike's "affair," Cindy had been unconsciously evening the score by remaining (defensively) aloof from Mike and lavishing her love on her children and their dog. She could be seen as the one taking an extramarital lover or, at least, that was how it looked to Mike. Interpreting the event for Mike, who would have preferred to dismiss it, I explained that for him, the scene resembled a husband seeing his wife falling all over a former boyfriend. They both laughed in agreement, though Cindy remained wounded.

We continued to explore Mike's insensitive remark, something he wanted to attribute mostly to having been tired. I reminded them of how we had previously discussed times when Mike had felt on the periphery of family activities, and Mike agreed that this counted as yet another one. Hearing this during this intimate "moment of meeting" in the session reduced Cindy's retaliatory anger at Mike. It also challenged her assumption that Mike's snotty remark was a calculated effort to hurt her feelings and helped her to reinterpret other situations where Mike "just blew up for no reason." These incidents had been another important reason that Cindy had sent Mike for therapy, as she assumed that Mike simply "had a bad temper and needed anger management training." Instead, analysis of their divergent experiences of several situations like this one helped her see an alternative: that Mike's outbursts were often triggered by some disappointment in their relationship. Mike, in turn, came out from behind his superficial defensiveness ("I was just tired") and became more aware of his frustrated needs for love and affection.

In the next chapter, we examine couple psychodynamics from the vantage point of transference, an additional way to understand and work with divergent couple experiences.

Notes

1 The Danish psychologist Edgar Rubin did not invent this illusion that carries his name, but he made it famous in his studies of perspective.
2 Considerable research has shown that couples who are more similar than different across many variables do better (Hamburg, 2000; Pines, 2005). One obvious explanation is that such couples are far less likely to disagree due to radically different reactions to their shared experiences.

8
FOCUSING ON TRANSFERENCE

Another way to dig deeper into the psychology of a couple's negative interaction cycle is to examine their transferences to each other. The basis for the concept of transference in psychoanalytic theory is the observation that people often distort events so that they experience them not as they objectively are or as they would be experienced by a hypothetical transference-free person, but as modified by their current (frequently unconscious) wishes and fears. These wishes and fears, in turn, derive from a combination of inborn motivations, past experiences, and current emotional needs (Cooper, 1987; Greenson, 1967). Past experiences with childhood caretakers, with siblings,[1] with peers (especially in adolescence), and with prior intimate partners are all important sources.[2]

Transference Wishes and Fears

Transferences can usefully be divided into the subtypes of transference fears (or negative transferences) and transference wishes (positive transferences). Referring simply to "transference" or "the transference" erroneously omits this distinction and should be avoided. A "negative paternal transference," for example, refers to a feared situation related to a person's father.

Transference wishes and fears correspond to the relationship desires and fears we have discussed previously. The point I am adding here is that, while everyone has powerful desires and fears concerning relationships, each of us has some desires that are more pressing and some fears that are more unsettling. Explanations for this variation may be found in a person's history, just as the histories of nations can illuminate their current distinctive concerns. Differences in intensity also result from temperament (some of us are born more easygoing or "agreeable") and biological state (hunger, sleep deprivation, and depression commonly contribute to stronger negative reactions).

Since transference wishes frequently derive from unmet needs and are thus linked to memories of their disappointment, transference wishes often arrive in the company of transference fears (Stern, 1994; Weiss & Sampson, 1986).

Varieties of Distortion

As with projective tests, some transferences rely less on a simple distortion of facts and more on selective focus (Goldklank, 2009), which, to be sure, then distorts or narrows the overall picture ("I focus on my partner's failings, because I fear being fully aware of how dependent I might otherwise feel" or "I focus on my partner's strengths and ignore glaring problems in the relationship in order to feel safe and protected"). And some transferences result not simply from generalizations about past experiences ("I was disappointed when I asked my mother for help, so I'm almost certain my partner will disappoint me, too"), but from a *current need to distort current events* ("I see my spouse as blameworthy, because I can't stand to feel guilty" or "I see my boyfriend as perfect to diminish my doubts about marrying him"). Consequently, *many transferences serve as self-protective defenses*. Finally, transferences always imply some view of the self in relation to another person, and this view of the self is also subject to potential distortion ("To protect myself from a feeling of helplessness, I (unfairly) blamed myself for my parents' divorce. As a result, seeing myself as unworthy, I feel unable ask them for a loan to help me purchase a house.").

Transferences Evoked by Marriage

Transference reactions are generally prompted by stimuli that have some plausibility (Gill, 1982). The current couple relationship (a husband and wife; a father and mother) and home environment (a house, a kitchen, children) easily evoke transference hopes and fears based in childhood experiences in the family home. Recall my client, Dick, who so feared a replay of his traumatic experiences of Christmas that he wanted to protect his new family from them via a Grinch-like ban.

Home and family life will often evoke transference wishes for an unconditionally loving, supportive spouse (parent) and transference fears of control or criticism. A husband may return home at day's end with highly ambivalent feelings: dreading the childhood mother who controls and who may unreliably provide what is needed, while hoping for freedom from the taskmasters (parents) at work and for the comfort foods (grilled cheese sandwiches or Mom's apple pie) that instantiate dependency-gratifying, unconditional love.

Transferences as Expectations

Transferences—seen as desirable or feared expectations—can be placed in the larger framework of people's general expectations about themselves, others, and their environment. In general, our expectations are automatic and semi-conscious, if not totally unconscious, which frees us from reinventing the wheel when we encounter familiar situations. Some of our expectations will be reasonable, while others will be unrealistic, often overgeneralized from idiosyncratic prior experiences.

Not only about people. Some negative transferences may not be so much a feared reprise of an interpersonal situation (excessive criticism or abandonment by a parent), but fear of a return to an earlier traumatic situation in which the child felt overmatched and helpless. Such feared situations can include traumatic exposure to poverty, to illness or death, to war or natural disasters, or—perhaps the most common trauma haunting the clients I see—to the experience of parental discord and divorce. Any of these feared situations can reverberate through the marriage and drag it down, especially if the feared situations remain unconscious.

Self-fulfilling expectations. One important source of trouble is that our expectations tend to be conservative and, thus, self-fulfilling: "The more I believe it, the more I see it, the more I believe it." Many social psychological studies corroborate clinical experience showing that our expectations of how others will treat us also affect how we act and, subsequently, how others treat us, frequently in ways that confirm our initial expectations (Bradbury & Karney, 2010). If we believe the world is flat, we won't sail west from Europe, and we won't discover America! Kelly, Fincham, and Beach (2003) cite studies showing that "distressed couples expected fewer positive and more negative behaviors from their spouses than nondistressed couples" in both low- and high-conflict tasks; and that "marital satisfaction was significantly correlated with positive and negative *expectancies*" (p. 728, italics added). More recently, a prospective study of 767 married couples found that expectancies from childhood related to attachment security correlated with expectancies toward spouses, which predicted subsequent marital satisfaction (Kimmes, Durtschi, Clifford, Knapp, & Fincham, 2015).

Such self-fulfilling expectations help explain deterioration over time in attitudes between marital partners. During courtship, we see excessive idealization (positive transference wishes for an ideal partner) and dismissal of negative qualities in the service of forming this picture-perfect bond. Spouses may continue to view each other as globally positive for a while, attributing anything negative to external circumstances (the partner was late due to traffic), but if things start to go downhill, they may come to see even objectively positive behavior through a negative lens ("He only gave me a birthday present because he knew I'd be upset if he didn't"). Such corrosive narrations will impede efforts by partners on the receiving end to disconfirm these negative expectations (transferences).³

Attachment security as transference expectations. Attachment security is a crucial subset of guiding beliefs, the healthy (secure) version of which comprises, according to Mikulincer, Florian, Cowan, and Cowan (2002):

> a set of expectations about others' availability and responsiveness in times of stress, which are organized around a basic prototype or script. This script seems to include the following if–then propositions: "If I encounter an obstacle and/or become distressed, I can approach a significant other for help; I am a person worthy of receiving help; he or she is likely to be available and supportive; I will experience relief and comfort as a result of proximity to this person; I can then return to other activities."
>
> (p. 406)

Insecure attachment can be viewed as negative transference expectations concerning the same variables. Mikulincer et al., who are pre-eminent in the field of attachment research, report that some client "working models" of relationships are not simple generalizations from prior relationships, but are "relationship-specific," that is, based on actual experiences with the current partner. In this regard, they cite "suggestive evidence that marital quality correlates better with the latter [the "relationship-specific" working model] than with the general form" (p. 412). This finding should give us hope when working with couples, since even if partners' transferences are grounded in childhood, their current form may be less entrenched than we might have thought and, thus, more amenable to modification in therapy.

How We Discover Transferences

The main way we formulate hypotheses about the internal mental structures we call transferences is by looking for redundancies across "relationship episodes," a method made explicit by the psychoanalytic researcher Lester Luborsky (1990). Relationship episodes will involve people from the client's formative years, their present life, and their current therapy (their therapist and, in couple therapy, their partner).

Dimidjian, Martell, and Christensen (2008), in their summary of Integrative Behavioral Couple Therapy (IBCT) similarly advocate searching for important relationship "themes" across incidents that have gained power from painful sensitization in the past. The example that follows shows how they do this and serves to further illustrate the points I have made so far:

> Eve may complain that Dillon spends too much time watching television, but she may also become angry when he goes hiking with friends . . .

> The IBCT therapist is able to see the themes of abandonment and responsibility in Eve's complaints. Actions by Dillon that abandon her and leave her shouldering family responsibility are distressing ... These behaviors of Dillon's are reminiscent of her past, when she was often left by her working parents to care for her younger siblings, and rouse similar feelings of abandonment and unfairness in her.
>
> *(p. 81)*

In formulating transference hypotheses, therapists will be assisted not only by repetitions and redundancies across episodes, but by singular childhood events, usefully termed "model scenes" (Lichtenberg, Lachmann, & Fosshage, 2011). For instance, a client related a painful disappointment from when he was six. He had approached his mother cautiously, with a request for a fishing rod, so he could go fishing with his friends. His mother angrily quashed his hopes, telling him he was "unworthy" and couldn't have fishing equipment until he earned the money for it himself, an absurd requirement for a six-year-old. This painful model scene helped explain this man's pervasive sense of unworthiness, his delight when anyone mirrored his enthusiasm, and his inability to say "no" when his wife (a shopaholic) eagerly asked him to fund a new purchase.

Another way to access transference wishes and fears—advocated by Hendrix (1988) and elaborated by Singer and Skerrett (2014)—is to ask each partner directly to reflect on his or her childhood, and then talk about, "what I wanted, but didn't get" (stability, affirmation, financial security, fun) and then "what I got, but didn't want" (chaos, coldness, anger, excessive control).

Permutations of Transference Roles

Because transferences are structured internally as *patterns of self and other in interaction*, once we know the pattern, we can use it in some not-so-obvious ways. Clients may play out the role of self or other or both, sometimes with different partners and sometimes alternating roles with the same partner. We also see people striving not to repeat painful roles from their past. The man who didn't get the coveted fishing rod from his mother had trouble saying "no" to his wife's requests for jewelry, but was excessively fierce in denying his employees raises they deserved. Mostly, though, he found himself conflictedly obsessing over these choices, shifting internally between the roles of gratifying others (as he wished he had been) and turning them down as "unworthy" (as his mother had done to him).

Another practical point: How people treat each other (well or badly) is a useful indicator of how they treat themselves. Our internal relationships with ourselves are shaped by, and similar to, our external relations with important others. As summarized by Hazlett (2010):

[I]n established couples, how people treat their partners is directly related to how they treat themselves on the inside. So if Mike is relentlessly self-critical and demanding with himself, he will eventually treat Lisa that way. And if Lisa uses denial and avoidance to shut down her own feelings, she will also use them to shut out her partner.

(p. 31)

Transference Allergies, Core Negative Images, and Default Settings

When discussing transference fears with clients, I find it helpful to call these "psychological allergies" or "transference allergies." Just as a person with a prior exposure to bee stings or peanuts may later have an excessive reaction to them, so a person who experienced early abandonment by parents may have excessive emotional reactions to a spouse's business trips. With transference allergies, people smell psychological smoke and assume they will soon experience an emotional fire. Susan Johnson (1996) refers to these as "raw spots"; in common parlance, they are "hot buttons"; and in technical psychoanalytic language, they are "negative transferences." With our human inclination to think, "Better safe than sorry," prior traumatic experiences understandably put us on high alert, making our "smoke detectors" go off too easily (Stosny, 2006). Our job as therapists is to help clients tell the difference between their hair-trigger warning systems and genuine looming catastrophes.

Terrance Real's (2007) "core negative image" (CNI) is another good way to put the negative transference concept into lay language. As he defines it, the CNI is:

> that vision of him or her that you feel most hopeless and frightened about. You say to yourself, in those furious, or resigned, or terrified moments, "Oh my god! What if he or she really *is* a vicious person? . . . a cold-hearted witch? . . . a betrayer? an incompetent? Constricted? Selfish?" Your CNI is your worst nightmare. It is who your partner becomes in those most difficult, irrational, least-loving moments.
>
> *(p. 83)*

To communicate the idea that transference fears and dispositions operate unconsciously in the background, I compare them to default settings on a computer. Most people know that their computers arrive with options or preferences preset at the factory (the "default settings") and that until we look for them, we may not even know we have choices concerning how our applications will function. In a similar way, adults have "preferences" or "settings" that operate in the background, were not consciously chosen, and are often not experienced as options but, rather, as the only way to deal with the world.

These settings include not only views of the self and others interacting in traumatic scenarios, but also beliefs about whether anything can be done about them. This last element helps explain why we so fear our CNIs: because of an attendant belief (setting) that we are helpless to do much about them.

"Double" or "Failed Assistance" Transference Allergies

People in the throes of a negative transference reaction or transference allergy enter a minor state of panic where—overtaken by their worst nightmare CNI—they feel overwhelmed and hopeless. They have trouble thinking and expressing themselves clearly. Usually, they are conflicted and confused. To fully empathize with such states, one must understand that *traumatic situations are not solely about the initial adverse event, but also about what happens next*, including how others react. The most serious childhood traumas are "uncomforted traumas," those in which attachment figures have not only caused or failed to protect the child from the initial ordeal, but have also failed to be empathic and helpful after it occurred. Handling distress is a skill one learns with help from (and modeling by) others. Thus, the uncomforted child may not learn how to comfort and soothe him or herself following frustration. When similar situations occur later in life—whatever the specific initial CNI—persons entering this state are likely to (a) feel helpless to calm themselves; (b) doubt that they will obtain help from others; (c) experience conflict and confusion about who is responsible; (d) need considerable empathy and assistance from their partners; and (e) react (allergically) with still more disappointment and negativity should partners fail, as early caretakers did, to provide that needed assistance.

These last two steps, both independent of the specific CNI that evoked them, explain the special utility of attachment theory and psychoanalytic self psychology for understanding and treating marital impasses. Both theories stress the role of supportive partners or therapists (attachment figures; selfobjects) in assisting people in need by providing support, empathy, validation, and soothing. Put another way, *what we commonly see in couple negative interaction cycles is a "double transference allergy"—the first to the feared CNI, and the second to partners who resemble caretakers who failed to assist their traumatized child-self*. I call the second a "failed assistance transference" or a "failed assistance allergy." While this can be hard to tease apart from the inciting transference allergy (say, to an initial experience of abandonment or failed empathy), much of the panic that follows a CNI concerns this second allergy to failed assistance—to the current partner who fails to repair the situation via care, empathy, or apology.

Interlocking Negative Transferences

Failed attachment assistance commonly results from concurrent or "interlocking" negative transferences. When a couple seeks therapy, it is almost universally true that *both* partners are *simultaneously* experiencing transference allergies, so that neither can soothe nor empathize with the other during episodes of emotional distress. This pathological situation contrasts with Kohut's (1984) comment that "a good marriage is one in which one partner or the other rises to the challenge of providing the selfobject function that the other's temporarily impaired sense of self needs at a particular moment" (p. 22). Not only do partners become functionally unavailable to provide support, but *their defensive reactions make matters worse by further confirming the validity of their individual transference fears*. This confirmation helps explain the ensuing tenacity and escalation of the cycle. I use the term "interlocking transferences" to portray this simultaneous fitting together of each spouse's transference fears with confirming behavior from his or her partner. When such confirmation occurs, the couple system moves further toward meltdown, with increasing levels of anxiety and maladaptive defensive behavior.[4]

Contemporary psychoanalysts stress that transference beliefs and neurotic symptoms, like the bones in our bodies, though apparently stable and unchanging, are actually in a constant state of self-creation and remodeling (Cooper, 1987; Schlessinger, 1995; Wachtel & Wachtel, 1986; Wachtel, 2014). To be maintained, ingrained negative transferences require confirmation of their adverse expectations. With this in mind, we can see reasons for both hope and despair. Hope emerges because the cycles required to maintain couple transference expectations are so palpably present in our offices; if we can block these cycles and provide disconfirming alternatives, we can expect to remodel our clients' negative expectations and turn things around. Indeed, this is just what we see in our successful cases and in research on changing attachment models in marriage (Mikulincer et al., 2002).

The bad news, however, is that we can anticipate an uphill battle as, after each additional cycle of CNI confirmation, partners grow increasingly entrenched in their negative transference expectations. In most cases, these negative expectations have been solidifying for many years before the couple comes to us for treatment. Worse, as we work to alter the couple's negative cycles, the partners may, despite our efforts, continue to confirm each other's worst relationship nightmares—even in our offices, where they had hoped to feel better and revive their love for each other. So, when couple therapists ask the question, "Has this negativity gone on so long that this marriage cannot be saved?" we are usually asking whether our weekly sessions can reverse many years of CNI-confirming cycles of interlocking negative transferences.

Positive Transference Issues

When clients present for couple therapy, it is rare to see them distorting their views of each other in a *positive* direction, as couples so often do during courtship. Nonetheless, we often see positive transferences manifesting as one or both clients expressing intense, importunate, or entitled desires for reassurance, affection, support, or empathy. Their spouses often react badly to these wishes, viewing them as excessive, burdensome, or childish. As therapists, however, we should view them as powerful statements of precisely what our clients need most. These intense transference desires result from some combination of current and formative experiences, specifically, from their not being met in childhood or in the present relationship. A wife who must constantly be told that she is lovable may never have received the kind of loving support as a child that would have allowed her to internalize a solid sense of self-worth. Or, she may actually be receiving too little current affection from her husband, which might make anyone cry out for more. In either case, we will want to uncover the wishes, explain them sympathetically, and work to help clients become better at both getting their needs met and living with inevitable disappointments.

WORKING THERAPEUTICALLY WITH TRANSFERENCES

The basic approach to uncovering and working with transference wishes and fears was laid out in the chapter on hidden issues. Here, I will mention some nuances not previously discussed.

Individual Psychodynamic Therapy in the Presence of the Partner

One logical consequence of the realization that past sensitivities are critical to the pathological dance is to shift the focus from the here-and-now couple interaction (Couple Therapy 1.0) and explore, instead, the historical origins of those sensitivities. This obvious modification (upgrade) amounts to doing individual therapy in the presence of the spouse, and is a common practice for most psychodynamically oriented couple therapists. Recall the case of George and Sally in Chapter 6 where, for brief periods, each became the therapeutic focus while the other sat and listened.

Because such a shift in focus away from the couple's dance to the historical roots of transference sensitivities frequently involves discussions of childhood caretakers, it is often termed "family of origin work" by couple therapists. This format is probably better labeled "individual psychodynamic psychotherapy in the presence of the partner," since it can employ all the interventions available in individual psychodynamic psychotherapy.

I choose to proceed this way—to work as an individual therapist with one of the partners—not simply to cool the process down (as in the TTEO model), but because I know how to do this psychotherapeutic work. Nonetheless, I sometimes enlist the listening partner to help with the exploration, and I often encourage partners to think along with me about possible psychodynamics. Sometimes, partners serving as co-therapists provide useful information that has been repressed or downplayed by their spouses.

Taking time to gather basic historical information in my initial diagnostic evaluation of the couple allows me to make preliminary guesses about where their sensitivities lie and what further exploration might help. Sometimes, however, the relevant historical material surfaces while we are examining the couple's pathological process. When the material emerges this way, the historical events uncovered are often more compellingly linked to current problems and are regarded, ever after, as their sensitizing causes.

Some couple therapists will find it useful to pursue historical issues more systematically by constructing formal genograms (McGoldrick & Gerson, 1985; Wachtel & Wachtel, 1986). My personal preference is to gather model scenes and memories of the past as they emerge in the context of discussing a particular CNI. While working as I do has the advantage of increasing my confidence in the transference formulations, it has the disadvantage of missing some patterns that may only surface when one is more systematic.[5]

Working with Long-Past Incidents: Mike and Cindy, Continued

Recall Mike and Cindy, who reacted so differently to his arriving home while she was playing happily with their dog, Bertie. I will now describe some subsequent events from that same therapy session that illustrate individual therapy in the presence of the partner, work with the listening spouse, and a failed assistance allergy. This example also demonstrates how to work when partners bring up hurtful incidents from the past that their spouses think are long gone, should be forgiven, or are now beside the point.

As we discussed Mike and Cindy's divergent reactions to the dog incident, I saw it as a scene in which Cindy's wish to share her enthusiasm had been thwarted, so I asked her how it had been when, as a child, she had been excited about something and had wanted to tell her parents. Unable to recall a single incident when they had been happy for her, she instead remembered how her "proper" mother required her to keep her hair short throughout childhood, despite Cindy's protests and the fact that her friends' mothers allowed their daughters to wear their hair long. Her mother had not only continued to cut Cindy's hair short herself, but had been unsympathetic when Cindy had cried about it (which set up a later failed assistance allergy). Cindy then told us of her great pleasure in now having long (beautiful) hair, similar to her pleasure in having the dog her mother wouldn't let her have. What emerged from this inquiry was the picture of a girl whose severe, fundamentalist-religious family tamped down pleasure and dismissed dissent.

Cindy described the same pattern with respect to her clothes. Her mother disapproved of pretty or fashionable clothes, whereas Cindy was now able to have a wardrobe that gave her considerable pleasure. She then recalled a painful marital fight from five years before. She had purchased a new dress and was eager to show it to Mike, but instead of the enthusiastic response she had hoped for, he seemed lukewarm and asked about the price. As she thought about it now, his reaction *still* made her angry.

In the session, as at home during the dog incident, Mike felt unfairly attacked. Not really getting it, he told Cindy that the dress episode was long past and was no big deal anyway. Didn't he work hard to give her a beautiful home and clothes, not to mention their dog! When she continued to criticize him, he shut down sullenly.

The long-past episode of the dress, together with Mike's current lack of empathy, provided more evidence confirming my formulation about Cindy's transference desire for enthusiastic support when she was happy and for empathy when she was disappointed. Hoping to make the components of her double allergy clear to both of them, I said, "Mike, I think the reason Cindy is thinking of the time you weren't excited by her new outfit five years ago is that it's like what she's talking about now: how she wanted you to be enthusiastic about her enjoying Bertie. These events touched the same nerve. Without intending to, you set off her CNI, her despair about getting a strong, affirmative response from you, something she so wanted in childhood, but so rarely got from her parents."

"Worse than that," I continued, "the reason she got so angry right now is that she's despairing that you will ever understand how your response let her down. She's worried that her need to reach out to you when she's upset will *also* be rejected."

Having made this lengthy intervention, I hastened to Mike's rescue, saying something like, "But of course, while she was reacting to *her* allergies, you were also in a traumatic state—wounded by the scene with her and the dog that felt like the many times when she's been so animated and happy with the kids, but not so enthusiastic about being with you, her hard-working husband." The therapy continued to work successfully with both partners' transferences, which could be seen as painfully interlocking and reinforcing.

Begin by Recognizing the Reality Trigger

After I have formulated a hypothesis about a transference pattern, I share it with the couple. I begin by identifying and validating that the client is, indeed, reacting to something real. With Mike and Cindy, we began with the scene with Bertie and with the individual meanings they ascribed to that scene. That scene triggered strong, but different, emotional reactions, which I helped them explore as transference allergies and desires. In psychoanalysis, the importance of validating the reality of the triggering stimulus has been emphasized by Gill (1982) and Kohut (1977, 1984), among others, and in couple therapy, it is also the best place to start (Goldklank, 2009). When the therapist interprets one partner's transference CNI, the other partner will usually feel validated, since the therapist is also confirming the spouse's overreaction or misperception. For this reason, good transference interpretations in couple therapy tend to be "You're both right" interventions.

Make Transferences Acceptable, Rather Than Shameful

When interpreting transference wishes and fears, we don't want to sound judgmental, as in, "You pretend not to feel such and such, but you really do!" Rather, we want to help clients experience the previously unacceptable/ disowned material as a legitimate part of themselves that is being warded off for understandable reasons, saying things like "You seem rather harsh with yourself when you sense any hint of sexual feelings," or "You seem to expect something terrible to happen to you if you have any wish to be taken care of," or "I have the sense you're angry at your mother but think it's awful of you to feel that" (examples from Wachtel & Wachtel, 1986, pp. 125–126).

Corrective Experiences via the Listening Partner

A key benefit of doing individual work in a couple format is that partners witness the exploration and can become more aware of whom they married. We have previously discussed the value of achieving greater compassion and increased closeness as a way to heal the damaged couple bond. *We can now see couple therapy through the lens of transference as an opportunity to correct negative transference expectations.*

In interlocking transference cycles, partners tend to confirm each other's worst fears. When things go well, however, it is precisely the opposite. As in psychoanalysis, possibly the most mutative moments in couple treatment occur when a transference need is expressed or "tested," and the partner responds not as feared, but with sympathy and loving concern. This process fits Greenberg and Goldman's (2008) research finding that what most changes a maladaptive emotional (transference) pattern is the "substitution of one emotion for another," not simply the uncovering of the painful emotion. In couple therapy, such moments of corrective emotional experience can be quite intimate and can remind us that similar episodes of intimacy—where partners risk sharing their deepest fears and desires—are central to the experience of romantic love (Goldbart & Wallin, 1994; Kernberg, 2011). As such, these moments of intimacy can provide glue for repair and fuel for reawakening love between partners.

The Challenge of Disconfirmation

But what can we do when partners fail to soften and continue to confirm negative expectations? Although the psychology of transference is valuable to both the couple therapist and the individual therapist, couple therapy involves an important complication not present in individual therapy. In psychoanalysis or psychoanalytic individual psychotherapy, the empathic, relatively anonymous, professional therapist—lacking a real-life stake in clients' decisions—finds it relatively easy to provide corrective emotional antidotes to clients' negative transference expectations (Greenson, 1967; Strachey, 1934; Weiss & Sampson, 1986). The presence of interlocking transferences, however, makes it more likely that partners will confirm their CNI nightmares, even in the therapist's office.

Much of the art and difficulty of couple therapy lies in convincing spouses that their negative expectations are unrealistic, selective, or exaggerated, since they repeatedly experience these transferences as accurately predicting future couple scenarios. Disconfirmation will take more effort with a couple than with an individual and usually involves (a) reframing the speaker's concerns to make them more sympathetic and less likely to provoke confirmation; (b) reframing the listening spouse's negative-transference-confirming responses as understandable, rather than malevolent (Fred withdraws not because he doesn't care about Beth's suffering, but because he fears being overwhelmed by it); and (c) helping both spouses overcome their reluctance to play the scene differently (encouraging Beth to trust that opening up to Fred will prove comforting; challenging Fred to hang in even when his wife is angry and in tears).

Working with Listeners Toward Disconfirmation

When a partner is revealed *not* to be sympathetic or capable of listening, the first step is to reframe or re-narrate the speaker's concerns, so as to make them more sympathetic and less provocative. Should this fail, we then shift to discussing possible dynamic reasons for the insensitivity of the listener. We want to make clear that the listener's unsympathetic response is not inevitable, but flows, instead, from the listener's psychology and history. Since we have discussed this problem of listeners not "softening" before, I will limit myself here to additional suggestions related to the listener's transferences.

Feared identification. Listeners may sometimes be unsympathetic—paradoxically, it turns out—because listening to another's painful events reminds them of analogous events in their own lives and stirs their own transference concerns. Spouses often turn out to have very similar issues and sensitivities, although they may be perceived as more prominent in one spouse than the other. Exposing them more clearly in one partner may cause distress and subsequent defensive distancing in the other. If, however, we succeed in reaching through this distancing to its source in partner identification, the spouses may experience deep connection, as they learn that their partners "have been there, too."

Transference fears of emotional incapacity. Many listeners fear that they will be overwhelmed by the emotional or caretaking responsibilities that would follow should they fully register what their partners are saying. This was true of Fred, who not only felt sorry for his depressed mother (they both suffered because of his father's absence), but also felt guilty and inadequate when he realized he couldn't make things better. This can almost always be interpreted as an erroneous transference belief, since our clients are far more able to help and comfort now than they were as children.

Transference fears of unfair demands. Negativity and inattentiveness will also be more intense if the listener was once "a parentified child," "a well sibling," or a child who was in other ways overly or unfairly burdened by family circumstances. These clients have emotional allergies to being asked, yet again, to do more than seems fair.

Blocking the "I'm Not Your Mother!" Response

Once spouses have acknowledged being sensitive in a particular area, their partners may try to use this against them. The spouse who says, "Stop worrying that I'm not going to pay the bills. I'm not your mother!" implies that the complaint that preceded this remark has been rendered invalid by the experience of having an irresponsible parent. "Now that we know that you're terrified of being poor because your father lost his job when you were a kid, there's no reason we can't buy that plasma TV I want!" Uncovering one partner's neurotic fear should not give unrestrained license to the partner less afflicted by emotional scars.[6]

Blocking the "You Know I'm That Way!" Response

Conversely, spouses with a now-uncovered, validated-in-therapy sensitivity may label their partners insensitive and heartless if they press their agenda, as in, "You know I was sexually abused by my uncle. I think sex once every few months is about all you should expect." The main goal of uncovering transference meanings and sensitivities is to increase the partners' compassion. That doesn't compel capitulation to the person with the transference allergy. Ideally, newly insightful spouses will work to reduce their sensitivity and minimize its impact on others.

Encouraging Joint Problem Solving

Awareness of transference allergies and desires does not end the discussion, but raises the question of what to do next. *The challenge for spouses who now know about scars, allergies, and latent desires is to use this knowledge fairly in resolving conflicts.* As found in follow-up studies of psychoanalysis (Schlessinger & Robbins, 1983) and couple therapy (Seedall & Wampler, 2013), ingrained patterns of relating do not disappear due to therapy. Rather, once they are recognized, they are more accessible to modulation. Seedall and Wampler provide a summary of how therapists can help:

> Rather than focusing on fundamentally changing longstanding models of attachment, therapists could conceptualize their work as helping clients enhance the security of their interactions by (a) becoming more aware of their relationship patterns, including their propensities and automatic responses; (b) more consciously responding to their partner's distress; and (c) learning to signal and express their needs more appropriately during their own distress.
>
> *(p. 434)*

Working Toward Mourning and Adaptation

What should the therapist say when a client asks, "OK, I get it that Beth is sensitive to criticism because of how she was treated by her parents, but why should I have to deal with this? Isn't this unfair?" My answer is "yes and no." I begin by telling couples that it is adaptive and rational to know their partners' emotional weaknesses and sensitivities. Surely, if their friend had a shoulder injury, they wouldn't slap him on the shoulder when greeting him. One way to move forward is simply to ask the couple, "What are you going to do about this? How are you going to contain this problem?" This admonition to adapt to your partner's vulnerabilities is an effort to counter the unconscious transference wish that we all have that our partners have no weaknesses that might interfere with their optimally being with and caring for us.

I then ask how they would respond if their spouse needed a wheelchair: Is there a difference between a physical disability and an emotional one? How much responsibility can one expect from a person with a disability? And how much accommodation and assistance can the disabled person expect from his or her partner?

What ultimately helps is accepting that one partner has warts and scars (actually *both* partners do, of course) and that, for the sake of the couple, they must figure out how they are going to handle this situation. Their discussion, managed well, can make the couple stronger, as they each accept that the other will not be "everything they had in mind" when they married. Some mourning and adapting will be required.

Transferences to the Therapist

Clients have transference fears, assumptions, and desires toward therapists when they are in couple therapy, just as they do in individual therapy or psychoanalysis. This is a complex and important topic. Because it overlaps standard discussions of psychoanalytically oriented individual therapy

(Basch, 1988; Greenson, 1967; Malan, 1979; Summers, 1999), I will limit myself to a few remarks specific to couple work.

First, a certain amount of therapeutic leverage comes from allowing clients to idealize the therapist—to allow, in Freud's language "an unobjectionable positive transference" or, in the language of self psychology, "an idealizing selfobject transference"—to see him or her as a source of expertise, hope, and succor. In the early going, I mention my relevant credentials and try not to interfere with idealizing transferences. Hopefully, I will be able to deliver on some, though not all, of my clients' expectations.

At the same time, I try not to let either partner idealize me as a far better spouse than the one he or she has. Mostly, I accomplish this by being aware of the danger and, when appropriate, by injecting a certain amount of personal humility into the therapeutic mix.

In addition to titrating idealization, I try to address incipient negative transferences early, before they can do too much damage. Negative transferences to me frequently concern my presumed lack of neutrality or my excessive criticism. I try to welcome discussion of these, since they can jeopardize the therapeutic alliance and the treatment itself. At my best, I am able to link client fears to historical events, to show how transferences to me resemble those to the spouse, and to help clients make productive use of this knowledge.

Countertransference

When assessing clients' transferences, it is essential that I monitor my own countertransferences, since these often facilitate guesses about the complementary role expectations in play (Catherall, 1992; Racker, 1968; Tansey & Burke, 1989). As mentioned before, I experiment internally with thoughts of what it would be like to be married to each of the partners, and I wonder to myself whether I would experience the same sorts of frustrations and disappointments they are describing. If it seems likely that I would have the same problems, I feel more confident that those problems are worthy of attention. If I see different problems not yet mentioned, I may wonder why a spouse is willing to be so complacent and uncomplaining. If I am not much bothered by the problems mentioned, I am more likely to wonder whether the complaining spouse is having allergic reactions. Of course, all of these musings depend on my having a working knowledge of my own personal biases, emotional allergies, and current concerns.

It is particularly important for therapists to work internally with negative countertransferences to clients. Sometimes these are purely personal—actually, better identified as our *own* transferences, rather than countertransferences—and are elicited by clients' similarities to people who have disturbed us in the past. Knowing yourself will help you to disentangle how much of your discomfort is your own responsibility and how much is what I call "usable countertransference," which can inform you about how most other people would respond to your client.

When you find a client particularly repellant, you should first consider the possibility that he or she is not doing a good enough job representing his or her position or needs. If you can do this, then using interventions that reframe, uncover, and give coherent voice to the repellant client's concerns should help. In addition, you might want to re-read the discussion in Chapter 2 on the benefits of siding first with the less-likeable client.

The other option is to share that you, too, would be distressed by a particular behavior—say, by his or her repetitively breaking promises. Confronting clients like this evolves from an "other listening perspective," as contrasted with attempts to see the world empathically through their eyes. This will momentarily put you squarely on the side of the complaining partner, while making it clear that you are not afraid to direct the conversation toward maladaptive behavior. Timing and tact are critical. As noted by Ringstrom (2014), "the evasion of such material risks reinforcing the patient's solipsism and undermining an increased capacity for relationality through mutual recognition" (p. 58). When done judiciously and sensitively, such interventions can lead to exploration of the hidden motives behind the disturbing behavior.

Disclosing Humility

I am far more likely to share relevant personal experiences with my clients now than I was when I was younger. While there is always the possibility that this will backfire or become problematic (say, by undermining the client's professional idealization or trust in me), self-disclosure can convey humility in the face of life's daunting challenges.

I confess to couples that I can lose it and act in many of the counterproductive ways I suggest they avoid. By acknowledging my flaws, I can undermine the (transference) belief/wish—so often portrayed in movies—that it is easy to be married. I want my clients to know that I have applied what I am teaching them to my own life. Taking the position of someone who has "been there," I am freer to discuss the specific emotional challenges to behaving maturely. Such self-disclosure, in moderate doses, strengthens the therapeutic alliance by promoting the solidarity of a team whose members accept, without shame, that change is not easy and that success in relationships requires effort.

In the next chapter, I will build on the ideas presented here as I discuss projective identification, a defense that begins with a transference to the partner.

Notes

1 Sibling transferences are often overlooked in couple therapy. However, because married partners are often close in age, they can easily serve as reminders of past problems with

siblings. If you look, you may find husbands' and wives' transferences to brothers or sisters that signal old resentments about parental favoritism or mistreatment by siblings.
2 In psychoanalysis, the concept of structuralized expectancies, desires, and maps of others and the world is carried by transference. Very similar psychological territory is covered by "working models" or "schemas" in EFT; by "themes" in behavioral couple therapy (Dimidjian, Martell, & Christensen, 2008); by "filters" in PREP (Markman, Stanley, & Blumberg, 2001); and by "attributions," "expectations," "perceptions," and "schemas" elsewhere in psychology (Durtschi, Fincham, Cui et al., 2011). In psychoanalysis, they are also described by "states of mind" (Horowitz, 1979), RIGS (Representations of Interactions that have been Generalized) (Stern, 1985), core conflictual relationship themes (Luborsky, 1990), and "organizing patterns" and "expectancies" (Lichtenberg, Lachmann, & Fosshage, 2011).
3 The destructive, self-perpetuating impact of increasingly entrenched negative transferences has also been noted by non-psychoanalytic researchers, who use different terminology. Markman, Stanley, and Blumberg (2001) called this "negative interpretation," while Gottman (2011) called it "negative sentiment override." For more discussion and research on the movement from idealization to impervious negativity, see the articles reviewed in Niehuis et al. (2011), especially those by Neff and Karney (e.g., 2004).
4 This mutual maintenance and interconnection of partners' transference fears and defensive reactions has been called the "marital neurosis" by Graller et al. (2001), "mutual influences of self-protection" by Berkowitz (1999), "mutual projective and introjective identifications" by Scharff and Scharff (2008), and "interlocking sensitivities" by Wile (1981); and is central to the operation of the "vulnerability cycle" of Scheinkman and Fishbane (2004) and the "cyclical psychodynamics" of Wachtel (1986, 2014).
5 I am currently rethinking my position on this. One significant impediment to gathering systematic historical data is that clients are usually in a rush to deal with more pressing matters. As convincingly argued by Wachtel and Wachtel (1986), however, unless therapists inquire about grandparents, brothers and sisters, and aunts and uncles, many clients will not think that information about these people is relevant. Moreover, constructing genograms actively enlists clients in historical detective work and often allows them to see their parents more sympathetically, thus loosening the grip of childhood assumptions. Finally, sometimes this historical work is assisted by conjoint meetings with family members (Framo, 1976). I have done this relatively rarely— usually when a family member is part of a systemic problem—but when I have, it has almost universally proved helpful.
6 Therapists, who are trained to perceive such sensitivities, and who have the professional standing to back up their perceptions, are sometimes the worst offenders in misusing such insights against their partners. Beware!

9
FOCUSING ON PROJECTIVE IDENTIFICATION

Another way to examine marital conflict and unhappiness from a psychoanalytic perspective is through the lens of projective identification (PI).[1] Projective identification was once thought to occur only in people with serious personality disorders, but it is easily observed in healthier individuals as well. As we will soon see, one reason for its theoretical appeal is that projective identification bridges the gap between intrapsychic psychology and interpersonal process.

PI as an Interpersonal Defense

Projective identification is a type of *interpersonal defense* whereby people recruit others to help them tolerate a painful intrapsychic state of mind. This contrasts with purely intrapsychic defenses like repression, where others are not (mis)used in this fashion. In one common form of PI, an internal conflict ("I want to buy a new car, but I think I should be saving money") becomes interpersonalized as a debate between partners ("I want a new car, but my wife thinks we should save our money"). When you are conflicted about an issue, you can sometimes conceal this complexity from yourself and take the easier course by staging an argument with another person. This is because when you know (even vaguely) the truth about your conflictedness and the details of your doubts, it becomes challenging to come to a univocal solution to your dilemma.

In another common form of projective identification, a disturbing self-evaluation is externalized: "I worry that I'm too needy," becomes "He won't give me what I deserve." Debates about one's goodness or lovability are frequently interpersonalized; as one client put it, "I feel better when my husband hates me, than when I hate myself" (Scarf, 1987, p. 180). In these situations, the projector is unable to maintain a complex, conflicted, or "good enough" view of the self, and instead splits things into polar opposites, seeing them in black-and-white, all-or-nothing terms. From this perspective, adversarial couples can be seen as trying to force each other to accept the shameful designation of imperfect person by externalizing it, tossing it back and forth like a hot potato.

While what is most commonly disowned (projected) is some negative character trait, admirable qualities that make the inducer anxious may also be projected ("He's the smart one in our marriage"), so as to provide unconscious psychological advantage ("Since he's the smart one, I don't have to expect too much of myself").

PI as Unconsciously Enacted Scenarios

Most depth psychologies propose that not only do people unconsciously misperceive others based on their past experiences and current needs, but they also unconsciously attempt to actualize or enact specific role relationships based on those experiences and needs (Sandler, 1987; Stern, 1994). To accomplish this, they invite or induce others to play roles in their real-life dramatic creations. While it is well known that children enact their internal concerns in play and that adults often do so in their sex lives, it is less well known that adults also do this, in a more disguised manner, in the course of their everyday transactions. The concept of projective identification will help us understand this scripting of others (e.g., the helpless damsel in distress who enlists a rescuing knight in shining armor).

Component Steps of PI

Projective identification begins with two theoretically separable, but frequently simultaneous, steps: (1) an intrapsychic projection (transference) by the person wishing to expel an unacceptable part, combined with (2) actions by that person (the "inducer") to encourage the partner (the "recipient") to behave in ways consistent with the projection. In subsequent steps, either or both partners may "identify" with what has been projected and may behave accordingly.

To illustrate these steps, consider the following example: A woman who is uncomfortable with some part of herself (say, her social anxiety) first sees this, somewhat unrealistically, as present in her husband ("He never wants to go out and socialize!"). This improves her self-concept, as it locates the problem outside of herself; it may also give her an ego-boost, via felt superiority, and an excuse to skip an upcoming social event. This step amounts to her unconscious use of a transference in the service of defense.

The process of projective identification then moves beyond the transference (the distorted perception) when the recipient is not only misperceived as an unacceptable part of the self, but actually *comes to feel and behave accordingly* (to identify) because of pressure from the inducer to do so. Thus, the husband who is repeatedly told that *he* is the socially anxious one may begin to doubt himself, and this uncertainty may be followed by anxious, socially awkward behavior.

PI as a Costly Defense Mechanism

By forcing partners into polarized roles, projective identification can powerfully interfere with couple intimacy, problem solving, and well-being. In addition, as long as recipients are close at hand, clients attempting to locate problematic states in them face the danger of the projected feelings returning, like a boomerang. A person who has located anger and malevolence in a spouse will have to be on perpetual guard. And one who, in addition, *provokes* that spouse to anger—rather than just imagining him or her as "the angry one"—will be in even worse shape. Attempts to "remote control" some feared state of mind by locating it in another are risky and, even when temporarily successful, may saddle the projector with a partner who is devalued or out-of-commission.

PI Explains Feared Situations Coming True

Therapists frequently observe that partners don't just neurotically (unrealistically) fear or complain about anticipated negative outcomes; they tend to elicit them. We encountered this when discussing the concept of interlocking transferences and saw how each person's fears and defenses can stoke the flames of the other person's fears and defenses in an escalating, maladaptive dance. Projective identification provides an additional explanation for this phenomenon. *As with interlocking transferences, client defenses elicit apparently unpleasant outcomes, but when projective identification is at work, there is an additional unconscious psychological benefit that powers the process.* For instance, while the wife described above may consciously complain that her husband is socially inept, she has had a hand in his behaving that way and has unconsciously benefited from his evoked disability.

PI Explains Failures to Soften

Projective identification similarly gives us another explanation for the failure of some clients to "soften" after their partners have exposed their vulnerabilities. *Failures to empathize can result from precisely the same forces that caused a prior projective identification.* Since their inability to contain a feeling in the first place has led projectors to locate it in their partners, we should not be surprised when they fail to welcome their partners communicating it back to them.

Recipient Containment

Like all defense mechanisms, projective identification is employed unconsciously when people are unable to accept or "contain" some way of feeling or thinking about themselves or their world. We can classify subsequent events by noticing how the projected/induced feelings or personal delineations ("*You're the one who doesn't care!*") are handled by recipients. Since Bion (1962), psychoanalysts have emphasized that if the receiving therapist can "contain" the projection, "metabolize" it, and then feed it back to the projecting client in a more manageable form, the client may become more able to tolerate the projected state of mind (Ogden, 1982; Tansey & Burke, 1989). By containing, metabolizing, and feeding back the transformed projection, the therapist provides "emotional holding," similar to the physical holding that helps soothe children and adults alike.

In the same way, spouses who remain emotionally capable and empathic can assist when their partners have become overwhelmed by inner states of distress. Such assistance can be conceptualized in psychoanalytic psychology as containment and holding (the object relations view, just described), as disconfirming a transference fear (ego psychology), as passing a wishful transference test (control mastery theory), or as providing a selfobject function (self psychology). These amount to different vantage points on the same interpersonal function, which I shall refer to here as "containment."

Providing containment for others when emotions run high is no mean feat and will challenge most spouses. When spouses fail to provide containment, we generally see one of three common patterns:

- The recipient fights to put the projected traits back in the projector ("No, you're the insensitive one!"); these are *adversarial couples*.
- The recipient distances from the situation, leaving the projecting partner dissatisfied after the attempted interpersonal defense has fallen flat; these become *pursuer–distancer couples*.
- The recipient identifies and goes along with the induced role, which creates *identified-patient couples* and other varieties of *polarized couples* (to be discussed later).

In all of these cases, the therapist must work to help *both* partners understand and contain their distressing states of mind. To do this, the therapist must first grasp and personally contain what is being disowned. We do this by turning our attention to tasting the distressing feelings and the attendant pressures to behave badly in response. As Catherall (1992) put it, "It is imperative that therapists not treat the disavowed material as something that they would never feel" (p. 360). The therapist who can acknowledge how challenging it is to remain emotionally present can help normalize the situation: "Mary, it's also very stressful for me to see Joe out of work, week after week. It's tempting to run away from this feeling by blaming Joe, or by focusing on something else that's not so painful."

The Recipient's Predicament

Once containment has failed and you have been pressured into enacting a role in another person's drama, extricating yourself can be particularly challenging. Almost universally, recipients know that their induced self state is "not all of me" and, consequently, they resist one-sided, negative characterizations. They will fight for fairness and a more three-dimensional characterization by citing facts and counterexamples. Nonetheless, the inducer—who is strongly motivated not to listen—will dismiss their objections. The recipient will then feel victimized and trapped in a no-win situation. So it was for the Congressman, who after being dubbed "America's dumbest legislator," called a press conference to deny it. Attempting to refute or deny attributed roles frequently just digs one in deeper. Therapists who have been caught in similar binds when paranoid patients have dismissed all efforts to establish the therapist's good will, including by interpreting negative transferences, will know how this feels.

Inductions: Motivated and Unmotivated

A common question in clinical discussions is whether clients have an *unconscious motive or intention* to elicit the distressing outcomes (depression, anxiety, underperformance) experienced by their spouses . . . or by their therapists. A common criticism of the concept of projective identification is that its proponents too readily and uncritically see clients as unconsciously intending these outcomes. To give these critics their due, and to clarify my position, it helps to distinguish between "unmotivated" inductions and "motivated" inductions, where only the latter qualify as bona fide projective identifications. In unmotivated inductions, careful examination reveals that, while a client's behavior *did* contribute to eliciting distressing behavior in his or her partner, this outcome *produced no emotional gain for the client*. On the contrary, these are the "ironic processes" I referred to when discussing couple dances in Chapter 5, in which clients elicit precisely the *opposite* of what they desire. A husband who badgers his wife about leaving lights on may generate so much resentment that she "forgets" to turn them off more often, and a pursuing wife who is afraid of abandonment may elicit even more distancing. In such cases, when feared scenarios perversely or ironically occur, it is best to assume that the result is not due to projective identification, but to maladaptive behavior that has backfired.

By contrast, some induced outcomes appear to be unconsciously intended. Such outcomes are unconsciously rewarding, even as they are often simultaneously the subject of complaint. *While "unmotivated inductions" describe unwanted scenarios that people generate via flawed assumptions and maladaptive behavior, "projective identification" should be reserved for scenarios that have an unconscious purpose or benefit.*

This distinction, between motivated and unmotivated inductions, is important, not just semantic. When clients repeatedly put themselves into painful situations without intending to, we have work to do, including helping recipients resist their reflexive reactions. Paul Wachtel (2014; Wachtel & Wachtel, 1986) has, for many years, convincingly emphasized the vital role of such unintentional inductions of negative behavior in recipients (who now become "accomplices" to the neurosis) as necessary to maintain a client's pathological beliefs. However, *when clients have an emotional stake in maintaining those situations, we have a still greater challenge: to expose and modify the motivations that impede improvement.*

Inductions via Inaction

Another common criticism of the concept of projective identification is that it can seem mysterious, or even supernatural. How exactly do people "put" or "locate" a part of themselves in another person and get them to identify with that part? How are inductions actually accomplished? PI is not accomplished by telepathy. Rather, *in projective identification, much of the influencing force is non-verbal, "written between the lines," and is accomplished through inaction.* A lack of emotional support tends to make insecurity, loneliness, or narcissistic rage worse. A relative lack of worry in a dangerous situation tends to increase anxiety in others who are present. To convey this idea to clients, I mention how a driver, speeding and nonchalantly oblivious to danger on a dark and winding road, will induce anxiety in a passenger. Indeed, the anxiety of the passenger is a direct function of its absence in the driver, and illustrates what I call "the conservation of anxiety," a concept that instantly resonates with anyone who has been called "overly anxious" in such situations.

Since non-responsiveness, inaction, and psychological blindness are often the mechanisms of induction, inducers characteristically feel falsely accused by recipients (noting, correctly, that they *haven't done anything wrong*) and think they should not be held responsible for their partners' reactions. This allows them to play the blameless victims of their partners' psychopathology. Further, since no one can point to something they did to cause their partners' distress, they grow even more convinced that their partners really are the embodiment of what they fear. Nonetheless, they are committing sins (PI inductions) of omission.

The following case illustrates projective identification with an induction resulting from inaction (inattentiveness, lack of support, and failure to engage contradictions).

Rex and Caitlin: PI to Cope With Grief

Caitlin began a session reporting that she had succeeded in overcoming her reluctance to contact Rex's mother, with the goal of mending their long-standing, emotionally distant relationship. We had discussed this mission in the previous session as something Rex wanted Caitlin to do to cheer up his recently widowed mother. But after Caitlin reported her persistence (her mother-in-law had, as usual, been hard to reach) and modest success toward improving their relationship, Rex had remained unmoved.

Rex and his father had been extremely close, talking on the phone every day. The father had been very supportive of Rex and his family, and everyone now missed him. I viewed his untimely death as the main source of Rex's low-level depression, but had not been able to get Rex to discuss this directly. It now occurred to me that his desire for contact between his wife and his mother was an attempt to partially reverse his loss, with the women standing in for him and his dad. Rex was the playwright in a projective identification drama that enlisted his wife as an actor, yet failed to diminish his pain.

Possibly irritated by Rex's lack of affirmation, Caitlin then brought up what she saw as Rex's double standard concerning spending money. She pointed out that when she spent money on clothes for herself or on special foods for their son, a picky eater, Rex criticized her for being wasteful. At the same time, Rex was now showering toys on their son and purchasing expensive items, including a new luxury car, for himself, without comment. Rex ignored this obvious incongruity and, instead, pointed to the value of the toys he had bought for their son. He then extolled his less-privileged upbringing as superior to Caitlin's family's suburban lifestyle. This tangential response riled Caitlin up further, since not only was he ignoring her point (that not all of the "out-of-control spending" was her doing), but he was also forgetting *her* actual lack of money as a child and, more importantly, her lack of parental attention (now being repeated in their exchange). What I saw was that Rex was inducing in Caitlin the panicky feelings she had felt as a child, when she was so often neglected by her parents, *feelings that matched his own currently disavowed ones,* as he tried hard not to miss his deceased father.

Attempting to help Caitlin "contain" the projections and not make matters worse by returning them, unmetabolized, to Rex, I gave her a supportive, nonverbal look and suggested that we explore Rex's issues more deeply. Trusting me that this would be more productive than continuing her unsuccessful debate, she allowed me to take charge.

I then tried to draw Rex out, starting with the financial worries that I knew were on his mind. He dodged this by voicing concern about having to support Caitlin's parents, who, he believed, lived beyond their means and might run out of money if they lived long lives (an allusion to his father's premature death, I thought), unlike some of *his* relatives, who were older than her parents, but more fiscally responsible (again, I noted the reference to longevity and his effort to place "virtue" in his court).

Rex then described the pressure he felt, working in an industry that was stagnating (another allusion to depression and death), and his fear that Caitlin's spending would require him to work longer in order to make enough money to sustain their retirement. Provoked (induced), again, by his painting her as responsible for his suffering, Caitlin interrupted, pointing out inconsistencies in his descriptions of his anxiety and personal frugality: Their ample portfolio made such anxiety unnecessary and, she railed, "You should shut up about my buying new boots! *You're* the creep who needed the new car and stereo system!"

Noting to myself how Rex's projections had, again, exceeded Caitlin's capacity to contain them, I now cut in with several interpretations:

> Rex, I think the key event here is your father's death. It shows up in your concerns about your mother—who is also suffering greatly from the loss of your father—and your worries about your economic future. Every time we start to talk directly about your having lost your dad, you get upset—understandably—and then you run away. An important way you cope is to locate the loss of your father in your mother and your worries about your financial future in your wife's spending. It is certainly easier to face these issues than to stay with some of your own inner concerns: The loss of your father has reduced your drive and vitality and makes it hard for you to go to work. And the loss of pleasure has made you want to indulge your son and yourself.
>
> The danger here is that since you feel guilty about your spending and, to some extent, your own avoidance of talking to your mother [she was a difficult person and, although he avoided engaging her himself, he was always defending her], you try to address these issues indirectly by blaming Caitlin: You say that *she, not you,* is the one who is trying to feel better by buying things; that *she, not you,* is the one who has a hard time relating to your bereaved mother; that *she, not you,* is the one with "emotional problems." *You sustain these inaccurate, negative beliefs about Caitlin by ignoring when she helps out or when she protests your inconsistencies.*
>
> The problem is not only that you fail to address your own inner distress, but that you also deprive yourself of what would really help you with your grief: for you and Caitlin to comfort each other, feel close, and see yourselves as being in the same boat, not just financially, but emotionally.

This was quite a bit to say all at once, and it was too much for Rex to absorb in one session (and I'm sure I didn't say it quite that eloquently in the heat of the moment). We worked on the components of my intervention for many weeks to come. On that day, Rex listened respectfully and worked a little more on mourning his father.

Over time, Rex gradually allowed me to help him stop scapegoating his wife in order to conceal his feelings from himself. Like many men, he found it easy to see women as weak and sad, but couldn't admit to having those feelings himself. Caitlin had been a convenient repository for Rex's grief, since she readily expressed her profound sadness over his father's death. As I worked with Rex, and as his vulnerability and tears emerged, Caitlin was also listening. She was able to back off from pointless debates with Rex and stay focused on how she and Rex would fill the void left by his father's death. The better they managed that challenge, the less Rex needed Caitlin as someone to represent the feelings that he was unable to contain, and the more he could see her as the supportive partner she actually was.

PI as the Royal Road to Success in Couple Therapy

Projective identification proved a very powerful tool in the case of Rex and Caitlin, as it has with many other couples I have worked with. Indeed, *when I reviewed the files of my most successful couple therapy cases, I found that helping clients own their disowned or projected parts was very often the most dependable route to success.* This was not something I had anticipated. The following is another success story, illustrating how a common and uncomfortable self-experience—shame following a failure—was located in *and* induced in a spouse, and how helping the inducer to reclaim the projected shame led to improvement in the marriage.

Rachel and Matt: PI to Cope With Shame

Soon after her failure to make a private retail store a success, Rachel, a 40-year-old woman, came for marital therapy, complaining, "My husband gives me a sick feeling!" She was ready to leave Matt, whom she considered a disappointing provider and lover. Her foremost complaint was that his earning capacity—though in six figures—had never been what she had hoped for and was less than that of many of her friends' husbands. Although she acknowledged that Matt loved her, that he had helped her deal with her contentious family, that he had been supportive when she had been addicted to drugs, and that he was well-liked by their friends, she was now certain that she should never have married him.

Rachel's contempt for her husband (one of Gottman's dreaded Four Horsemen) was obviously a projection of her own shame and disappointment at the failure of her business. Indeed, this was so easy to see that I had to work hard to contain my initial negative countertransference to her as an insensitive, entitled whiner! Note that the contempt I was working to contain was induced in me by Rachel's failure to acknowledge the patent unfairness of her indictment (a countertransference induction by client inaction).

But Rachel's contempt was not limited to a defensive projection. Her vociferous attacks intensified Matt's anxiety over performance, further undermining his actual performance at work and in bed. Specifically, his growing insecurity led him to avoid trying to solicit new business because he feared rejection, something he was experiencing daily at home. He also avoided approaching his wife for sex, since his erections began to fail him. Rachel's defense against *her* shame and failed performance had succeeded in inducing just those qualities in Matt. Matt hardly moved or spoke in our sessions, and his stooped body language screamed "loser." Matt felt ashamed and was unable to defend himself when Rachel compared him unfavorably to a self-confident military officer who had attracted her interest. As I sat with him, I tried to imagine him soliciting customers; I could neither envision him mustering the courage to make the necessary calls, nor picture any clients trusting him with their business. In all of this, Matt seemed to confirm his wife's (projected and induced) belief that he was "a poor excuse for a man."

The interventions that helped reverse this process of projective identification began with my helping Rachel own and contain her shame about the collapse of the business venture she had hoped would transform her life and increase the family's income. This proved relatively easy to do, in part, because Matt remained supportive when I had Rachel review the store's rise and fall. Soon, Rachel was crying and began connecting her business failure with her inability, as a child, to get her stern, businessman father to pay attention to her. As she felt safer, she told us that she also felt terribly ashamed of her relapse to abusing prescription drugs, a coping mechanism that had now backfired and intensified the distress it was meant to conceal.

Matt's support and his failure to confirm Rachel's expectation that he would shame her for her financial failure or her drug use (as her father had shamed her, for much milder offenses) provided an important corrective experience, further reducing her shame. As Rachel's self-esteem rose, she became more hopeful and pursued a new line of work, one that eventually provided professional camaraderie, self-esteem, and income. These gains, coupled with her regained closeness with Matt, helped her find contentment with her new job, even though it lacked the cachet and earning potential of her failed business.

I also worked to help Rachel feel less ashamed of Matt's real limitations, most of which were the flip side of his considerable strengths. Although Matt was not the conquering, alpha male Rachel thought she would have preferred, he was extremely loving and patient as a husband and father. As Rachel's contempt lessened and her genuine gratitude emerged, Matt's mood brightened and his posture straightened. Feeling more confident, he sought career counseling, which led to greater professional success. Under less (inductive) pressure from Rachel to fail, he became more successful.

As the virtuous circle continued to revolve, Matt's self-confidence grew, which enabled him to provide critical emotional support to Rachel when she would develop doubts about herself: not only about her career or her drug use, but about her physical appearance and her abilities as a mother. Feeling Matt's support, Rachel had less need to externalize her negative self-image. Their sex life also improved, although Rachel had to accept that she would be the one to initiate most of the action. The contemptuous, shame-inducing cycle of projective identification that had brought them to therapy was replaced by a positive, mutually supportive cycle. Where the old cycle had been driven by shame, distrust, and criticism, the new cycle reflected increasing pride, trust, and support, which resulted in greater happiness for both of them.

Fifteen years later, when Rachel consulted me for help in coping with her aging parents, I learned that their therapeutic gains had withstood the test of both time and some significant external challenges. I came to see this couple as one of my greatest successes: moving from contempt and the brink of divorce to profound respect, intimate connection, and genuine appreciation.

Dating or Marrying the Problem

Another common form of projective identification involves what I term "dating or marrying the problem." Here, one partner—having passively experienced a childhood trauma—seeks out relationships and/or engineers events so as to actively restage the trauma with a happier ending, thereby achieving some mastery over it. Partners may be selected to fit the required role or induced into playing it, as one "dates" or "marries" the problem. In either case, the idea is that the childhood role of suffering victim is located outside the self. Someone who was shamed and bullied as a child now shames his or her adult partner. Someone who was abandoned by a parent becomes the abandoner. Others may find or induce a partner to be wounded or injured in some way and then attempt to "cure" them, thus vicariously mastering their own childhood suffering. Sometimes, we see combinations of these two patterns as a partner may first induce a problem and then effect a partial cure, or repeatedly induce the "illness," so as to continue to play the role of (unconscious) victimizer and (more conscious) rescuer.

Dating or Marrying the Cure

Although some clients attempt to cure themselves by dating or marrying their *problem*, others try to date or marry their *cure*, by seeking out partners likely to be induced to provide either missing psychological functions or reassurance about their feared defectiveness. *Such efforts at cure can be viewed as projective identifications, because clients faced with internal distress induce a concordant distress in their intimates and thus pressure those intimates into the role of rescuer.* We examined this situation in some detail in Chapter 3, when we discussed unrealistic hopes for cure.

When the requirements for cure are not too great, one or both spouses may be able to provide the functions missing in the other. These couples present to us when one partner is no longer willing or able to fulfill this supportive role.

Marital Polarities as Examples of PI

Many polarized couples who frequent the literature and our consulting rooms can be understood through the lens of projective identification as (a) one partner who seeks to "marry the cure" and one who seeks to "marry the problem," or (b) two partners simultaneously trying to "marry a cure." Some of the more common and clinically useful polarizations are: the hysterical (feeling/free-spirited) versus the obsessional (thinking/planning); the overadequate (overfunctioning) versus the underadequate (underfunctioning); the angry/entitled versus the stoical/long-suffering; and the "sane" (victimized/enabling) versus the "crazy" (identified-patient). Such couples range along a continuum, from relatively benign "complementary couples" to more pathological "fatal attractions."

Complementary Couples

Some polarizations can be relatively benign and stable over time. These are complementary couples "in collusion" (Willi, 1984) making "projective tradeoffs" (Scarf, 1987) through which partners not only disavow and locate a part of themselves in their partners, but vicariously enjoy seeing that part in action . . . at a distance. In this form, "identification" with the disowned part occurs in both partners and is experienced positively by projectors. A man denying his dependent needs enjoys buying expensive jewelry for his wife or taking over the driving at night when she is anxious. A woman who has disowned her own aggressiveness enjoys seeing her husband assert himself with others. There is usually more to such trade-offs than simple vicarious pleasure. For instance, an "overadequate" spouse may also feel a sense of masterful superiority, while an "underadequate" one may feel relief at not having to face certain life challenges. These benefits further stabilize the pattern.

When the arrangement is working, the spouses are like teammates who have accepted differing roles. Danger lurks to the extent that these polarized partners never quite see eye to eye on the projected traits. They may feel emotionally disconnected from each other, and will have difficulty resolving conflicts in areas of radical difference, such as how much to socialize or how strict to be in parenting. That said, these couples should be distinguished from those who—after a short honeymoon period—experience the projected parts as strongly distasteful, usually for the same reasons that they were projected in the first place. These are the "fatal attraction" couples that Diane Felmlee (1998) found to be common in relationships that do not last.

Fatal Attraction Couples

Many important marital polarities can be discovered if we ask spouses what originally attracted them to each other. Those who select partners typecast for their ability to play a required (usually polarized) role will need to apply less inductive pressure to enact their desired scenarios. Typecast partners will also be less likely to change than ones who have been more actively induced into their roles, with the result that they almost invariably frustrate their spouses' attempts to cure their problem by marrying it. When the qualities of the selected partner come to be seen as more burdensome than rewarding—after having failed to either effect a cure or maintain a disavowal—we have a "fatal attraction." Two examples from Pines (2005):

Attraction
Wife: He was a very persistent pursuer. He made me feel desirable and adored.
Husband: She seemed like a dream come true, almost unapproachable.

Disillusionment
Wife: He doesn't let me breathe. He's always in my face.
Husband: She never lets me feel like she wants me.

Attraction
Wife: He seemed very smart, very capable.
Husband: She respected me. I felt accepted and appreciated.

Disillusionment
Wife: He makes me feel stupid and incompetent.
Husband: She feels bad about herself and blames me.

(p. 223)

Although the term "fatal attraction" suggests that such dyads invariably divorce, some polarities in which partners are recruited and needed in particular roles are long-lasting, and the attendant unhappiness seems endless. These are the couples everyone thinks should split, but who go on and on, bound together in a dance of mutual projective identification.

Amplification of Polarities

Earlier in this chapter, I showed how anxiety could be induced in a partner by a relative absence of it in the inducer: how an oblivious, speeding driver induces terror in a passenger. A more in-depth examination of such "polarities of worry" will help us better understand the amplification and maintenance of these and other marital polarities.

Polarities of worry begin when two people experience different levels of concern/anxiety about a problem (e.g., finances, teenage driving). *Their discordant assessments of danger frequently induce further polarization.* The more worried person experiences the spouse as in denial, unsupportive, and unhelpful, all of which increase the burden and anxiety surrounding the situation. Simultaneously, the person who starts out less anxious may become even *more* blasé. This may happen because the non-worrier (a) feels the worrier is taking care of things (so there is less need for concern); (b) is irritated by being told to worry, and finds it easier to blame his or her discomfort on the nagging than on the external situation; or (c) finding some truth in the worrier's anxieties, feels an increased need for defensive disavowal leading, paradoxically, to still *less* conscious concern and *less* empathy for the partner, who then becomes the defensive repository for even *more* disavowed anxiety.

Just as excessive or insufficient worrying can be mutually inducing or amplifying, almost any initial difference can become increasingly polarized as partners disavow each other's emotional state and induce its opposite. Thus, the spouse who is very angry, sad, or underfunctioning may elicit, respectively, excessive calm, denial, or accomplishment. People who present themselves as totally capable and unflappable may elicit states of depression or lassitude in their intimates. Depression will be induced when the high-performing partner, bent on not "catching" the discouraged state of mind, withdraws from the depressed partner; this distancing further intensifies the depression . . . which induces still more defensive distancing. Laziness and underperformance will be induced when the overfunctioning partner's extraordinary achievements or excessive indulgence (i.e., enabling) decrease the depressed partner's incentive to function competently.

In all of these situations, although the initial conditions have been set by personality predispositions and defensive needs, *the final state of polarization develops also from the systemic interaction between the partners.*

Polarities Centered on Other Emotions and Roles

Just as polarities of worry can begin with one person being less able to tolerate anxiety, other polarities begin and are maintained by difficulties containing other emotional states—the main driving force behind projective identification—including those that commonly attend certain life challenges.

Individuals who are afraid of anger may induce angry outbursts in their spouses and then label their partner "the angry one." Mike and Cindy, from Chapter 8, are an excellent example. While they both agreed that Mike was the one needing "anger management," it was Cindy's constant nagging and sarcastic criticism—expressions of her own chronic and disavowed anger—that usually provoked Mike to counterattack. Further, Cindy's need to block out awareness of anger in herself and others made it difficult for her to see it coming in Mike; consequently, she always experienced Mike's outbursts as coming "out of the blue," which confirmed her belief that Mike was the problem.

Individuals who are afraid of the challenges of adulthood are the "underadequate" spouses who grew up in households where successful mature functioning meant losing parental love, or where unsuccessful efforts were unduly shame-inducing. Such clients appear immature for their age and "afraid to grow up," calling out for assistance to the partners they need, and thus inducing them to serve as their protectors.

Individuals who are afraid of autonomy often pair with ones afraid of dependency. Each partner becomes the spokesperson for the value of his or her end of this spectrum. Once polarized, these couples appear as pursuer–distancer couples, in which "the woman may recruit the man to express her 'bad' needs for independence and the man simultaneously may recruit the woman to express his 'bad' need for dependence" (Middleberg, 2001, p. 343).

Existential Polarities

Some couple polarities amount to existential human dilemmas, in which each partner argues the merits of one way of living, although both sides have value.

Current gratification versus future gratification. These couples debate how much time to devote to work versus play, to housework versus relaxation, to planning versus spontaneity. One may want to spend more money now ("You can't take it with you!"), while the other wants to put more into savings ("You have to save for a rainy day!"). We all face such dilemmas. Both sides are "right," and whatever choices we make will involve some loss.

Letting bygones be bygones versus continuing to process the past. We have discussed this common polarity before and noted, again, there is truth on both sides: The injury really did occur and cannot be forgotten and, simultaneously, the painful event is over and needs to be let go of for the couple to move into the future. Variants of this polarity concern whether to "see the glass as half-empty or half-full," and whether venting about a recent frustration is a good thing or mainly an irritant. In these cases, as with other polarities, therapists should try to help each person concede the merits of the other person's preferred stance and then guide them together toward making a concrete decision that takes both extremes into account.

The polarities just mentioned are common, but therapists may discover others. In the following case, a relatively common polarized debate over how much time a husband should be at home came to be understood via a more customized (idiographic) version of projective identification.

Mary and Joe: An Idiographic Polarity

Mary complained that Joe never wanted to spend time with the family, and Joe defended his need to continue to have "nights out with the boys" and weekends playing sports as he had in his bachelor days. After I helped Mary to accept her disowned wishes for respite from her children, and Joe to accept that his rationalized wishes for time away concealed how inept and superfluous he felt when he was at home with his young children, much of the heat went out of this recurring debate. Although it would have been easy to view this as a typical pursuer–distancer dance, with a polarization between the need for closeness expressed by the wife and the need for autonomy expressed by the husband, the specific hidden desires that were projected and the fears that were defended were quite different, and uncovering them was critical to this couple's progress.

Polarizations: An Individual or a Systemic Problem?

The beauty of projective identification as a concept is that it links individual and systemic dynamics. In many couples who become polarized, one or both partners are having individual difficulty containing unacceptable or overwhelming emotional states (Rex and his grief; Rachel and her shame). They then involve their partners in their interpersonal defense (PI), which often manifests as a polarization. And when such motivated inductions are *mutual*, they will be still more challenging to combat.

In other situations, couple polarizations result from the progressive amplification of initial differences—with each side "waving the flag" for his or her position, and then waving still harder after the other side fails to salute. This results in more extreme behavior (polarization). Such inductions are often less intensely individually motivated, since they derive largely from the failure of each side to acknowledge the valid-but-different position of the other side. Such polarizations are more a property of the system than of individual character pathology, and will generally be easier to reverse.

In both prototypes, individual and systemic properties mesh to maintain the pattern, but to varying degrees. In most cases that present for therapy, we will find both individual and systemic contributions.

Working With PI: Healing Splits and Assisting Containment

Combined with recommendations I've made previously, the following interventions are particularly useful when dealing with projective identification.

Point out the truth on both sides. What usually helps—independent of how entrenched or motivated the difference is—is to help clients accept that there is merit on the other side of the polarity. The more blocked clients are to that possibility, the more difficult our task. Clients who accept that both sides have a point will provoke and induce their partners less. And those partners—like the scapegoats in groups or families after inductive pressure has been reduced—will behave in less extreme, contrary, and polarized ways. Less polarized behavior in one spouse will, in turn, lessen fears that such behavior will be viewed as intolerably dangerous. Finally, helping spouses own their own negative traits (those located previously only in their partners) promotes greater acceptance and less reactivity when partners do, indeed, manifest the feared or distasteful personality trait, as when Rachel became more accepting of Matt, who, in fact, was not the most financially successful husband on the block.

Make genetic interpretations. How one helps clients accept disowned parts of themselves is a complex topic and equally applicable to individual therapy as to couple treatment. I will make only a few suggestions here.

We begin by fostering a safe, empathic, non-shaming environment where curiosity is encouraged. We can then make "genetic" or "family of origin" interpretations, as we reframe problematic disavowal more sympathetically, by appealing to its self-protective genesis. Discussing projective identification, Middleberg (2001) gives paradigmatic examples of ways to explain to clients the origins of a specific constricted personal repertoire:

> Three suggested reasons to disown a feeling or part might be the following: (a) *To protect a person*, for example, "You would have had to disown any needs to be taken care of, because you had to grow up fast and take care of your alcoholic father"; (b) *To protect self*, for example, "You learned not to express your need for autonomy because your mother took it as rejection and punished you with withdrawal"; or (c) *To follow family rules,* for example, "Maybe you had to disown your hurt to follow the family rule about not showing weakness because it gives others an advantage."
>
> (p. 349, italics added)

Make contemporaneous interpretations. Sometimes, we simply make *contemporaneous* interpretations (causal statements) pointing out the current unconscious value of the projective identification process. Recall the extensive interpretation I gave Rex about how he was attempting to conceal various aspects of his distress after his father's death by locating them in his wife, mother, and son.

Point out benefits. Another way to help a person who is complaining loudly of distasteful, disavowed characteristics in his or her partner is to point out that these same characteristics come with benefits, often ones that powered the initial romantic attraction. Here, we are attempting to reverse the usual deteriorating course of "fatal attractions" by showing that when one spouse is the "meticulous one" and the other is the "fun one," between the two of them, they can get the job done and celebrate afterward. This intervention, despite its rather limited power, has proved useful in the final stages of helping clients mourn the hard reality of their remaining differences (recall the case of Rachel and Matt).

Facilitate corrective experiences. Change also depends on opportunities for projectors to expose their disowned, feared states and experience positive, rather than calamitous, effects. Clients who locate dependency, weakness, or inadequacy in their partners gradually improve their tolerance for these feelings as their therapist and their partner listen and provide empathy, understanding, and reassurance. Clients who fear their own aggression do not get over this simply by knowing where their fears came from; they also need to have chances to voice their anger openly and have their complaints responded to constructively. Clients who fear being left alone and attempt to cope by locating this fear in others can become able "to commit" by experiencing beneficial connection in our offices.

In sum, we reduce projective identification by helping clients to own and accept certain previously warded-off aspects of themselves. The next chapter continues to probe this topic of acceptance.

Note

1 The following authors, in historical order, have made important contributions to our understanding of projective identification as applied to couples: Dicks (1967); Willi (1984); Wachtel & Wachtel (1986); Scarf (1987); Slipp (1988); Zinner (1989); Catherall (1992); J. Siegel (1992, 2010); Berkowitz (1999); Middleberg (2001); Donovan (2003); D. B. Stern (2006); Lansky (2007); and Gurman (2008b).

10
FOCUSING ON ACCEPTANCE AND FORGIVENESS

> If love always, and unconsciously, turns into hate, hate does not so effortlessly return to love.
>
> *Muriel Dimen (2003, p. 247)*

The Origins of Acceptance Theory in Couple Therapy

In *Acceptance and Change in Couple Therapy* (1998) and *Reconcilable Differences* (2000), Neil Jacobson and Andrew Christensen, two of the most distinguished developers and researchers of behavioral couple therapy, discussed a major change in their outlook. In those books—the first for therapists, the second for the lay public—they relate how they came to see forgiveness and acceptance as powerful tools to add to their previous emphasis on negotiating compromises, facilitating positive exchanges, and teaching communication and problem-solving skills. Examining outcome research for behavioral couple therapy, they found improvement rates without relapse at two years of about 50%, which was similar to the rate in other forms of couple therapy, and far better than no-treatment control groups. Exploring their data to see why this metaphorical glass was still only half full, the authors discovered that the couples who remained stuck with irreconcilable differences showed less capacity for accommodation, compromise, and collaboration, suggesting that a focus on those variables might be beneficial.

As they studied the problem more closely, Christensen, Jacobson, and their colleagues observed the apparent paradox that when people stopped trying so insistently to get their partners to change, the desired changes often began to occur spontaneously, suggesting that previous foot-dragging had been the passive-aggressive result of constant criticism. They observed other benefits, as well, which I will discuss shortly. Years later, outcomes for what they came to call Integrative Behavioral Couple Therapy were indeed found to be superior to Traditional Behavioral Couple Therapy (Dimidjian, Martell, & Christensen, 2008). More recently, Gurman (2013) called this focus on acceptance the "third wave" in behavioral couple therapy, while Sprenkle, Davis, and Lebow (2009) consider appreciating one's partner's differences a "common finish line" for most current schools of couple therapy. Although it was two behavioral couple therapists who helped put this topic on the couple therapy map, I have placed this chapter in my psychodynamic section because most, though not all, interventions to facilitate acceptance and forgiveness focus on uncovering and altering (frequently unconscious) psychological impediments to letting go and moving on.

Dealing With Unsolvable Problems

Therapists who use interventions based on acceptance and forgiveness help partners to accept or contain differences and chronic problems that may never change, termed *unsolvable* or *perpetual problems* by Gottman and *irreconcilable differences* by Christensen and Jacobson. One important category of ongoing problems concerns past hurtful events that cannot be undone, but might be "forgiven."

Acceptance. Sometimes, helping clients abandon their efforts to change what seems unchangeable leads, paradoxically, to the desired change. Even when changes are *not* forthcoming, however, *acceptance helps diminish what commonly becomes the most toxic characteristic of a couple's marriage: not so much the unchanging problems, but the incessant wrangling over them.* To be sure, this is working toward change, but it is a very different kind of change than clients have usually envisioned.

Conversations about how to *contain* unsolvable problems also offer opportunities for intimacy and bonding. While partners may never totally agree about how much to socialize or on what counts as "being late," they can expect that conversations about these ongoing problems will bring them closer, as they share their struggles and views on their differences.

Forgiveness. The value of forgiveness has captured the interest of psychologists and psychotherapists in recent years (Fehr, Gelfand, & Nag, 2010) and has given birth to new forms of therapy aimed at facilitating forgiveness (Enright & Fitzgibbons, 2000; Luskin, 2002). Important contributions have come from couple therapists attempting to help clients recover from major betrayals, from students of gross human rights violations, from theologians, and from psychoanalysts, all of whom have investigated how to assist people in letting go of consuming states of vengeful preoccupation.

A New Tool

As a therapist whose attention had centered on helping couples manage conflict, I found interventions aimed at facilitating acceptance and forgiveness to be welcome additions to my therapeutic toolbox. Of course, I had engaged these issues when they came up, but I had not really thought about them conceptually. In what follows, I present selected practical ideas that I have found helpful when working toward acceptance and forgiveness. I differentiate between them somewhat arbitrarily, based on the severity of the offense: *acceptance* applying to common, everyday frictions, and *forgiveness* to more serious acts of betrayal and injury.

ACCEPTANCE

Three Choices and the Serenity Prayer

When faced with adversity, one should first assess the situation honestly to determine one's desires, the relevant obstacles, and the likely outcomes of possible actions. After this initial assessment, one has three choices: Attempt to change the situation, leave it, or accept it. These options call to mind *The Serenity Prayer* (often attributed to the theologian, Reinhold Niebuhr, and promulgated by Alcoholics Anonymous): "God grant me the serenity to accept the things I cannot change, the courage to change the things I can, and the wisdom to know the difference."

The decisions couples make—what to change, what to accept, or whether to abandon ship—are, of course, theirs to make. What "acceptance theory" makes clear is that when our couples become caught in that vague, unformulated experience of wanting change, while realizing that efforts to achieve it seem only to make matters worse, we can propose a third option: working toward serenity and acceptance.

Not Everything

Of course, we should never advocate accepting the truly unacceptable: physical violence, substance abuse, ongoing extramarital affairs, persistent mistreatment, or deep lack of concern. These are serious violations of the basic couple contract.

Some less severe violations are also unacceptable. An individual client of mine, at the recommendation of a previous couple therapist, had achieved considerable success in accepting his wife's chaotic behavior (e.g., leaving clothes strewn all over the house), but quelling the warfare between them about this particular issue had not addressed the core of their marital problems. Their central problem was *not* a polarization over orderliness, but her pervasive inability to acknowledge his "independent subjectivity" (Pizer & Pizer, 2006). The result of my client's pseudo-acceptance was that he remained devitalized and irritable, and mystified about why. After his wife summarily went off to pursue her career in another city—while expecting him to pay her bills and to comfort her during the transition—he realized what continuing this marriage would mean, and left it. The lesson? In working toward "acceptance," therapists must aim for something better than grudging resignation or doleful surrender to a miserable status quo.

Common Unsolvable Problems

Some unsolvable problems or debates are unique to a couple (how much time to spend with Aunt Sophie), but the most frequent ones turn on temperamental, stylistic, or personality differences. They concern disagreements over how close, orderly, spontaneous, frugal, or timely one should be. They include the differences we have discussed previously about how to behave during conflict: the value of discussing the past, voicing complaints, and communicating emotions. Such disparities frequently interfere with partners' ability to understand each other, leading them to think that their partners are misinformed, were poorly brought up, or may be mentally ill. But since virtually all marriages contain some incompatibilities, and since they are unlikely to yield to pressure tactics to change, couples often do better trying to contain, manage, and otherwise accept them.

Costs and Benefits: Cole and Jennifer

The costs of not accepting differences include: *dysphoric moods and reduced energy*—depression, anger, anxiety, insomnia, and lost mental resources due to obsessing about a grievance; *counter-reactions of hostility and passive-aggressive non-compliance* that follow one partner's coercive attempts to change the other partner via nagging, guilt-tripping, or vilification; *hostility contaminating other marital interactions*; and, most important, *estrangement of the partners and erosion of the marital bond*.[1]

Marriages benefit, however, when partners accept what is less than perfect and appreciate each other's sacrifices and compromises. "Taking a hit for the team" is easier when it is recognized by one's partner and harder when it is not, as illustrated in a case presented by Dimidjian and colleagues (2008, pp. 96–101): Although Cole and Jennifer had previously agreed that she would return to work after their second child was born, when the time came, Jennifer developed doubts and wanted to remain home as a full-time mother. This angered Cole, who wanted her to continue to be the family's major breadwinner. Cole's lack of empathy made it harder for Jennifer to mourn her wish to be a full-time mom and hindered her ability to move forward and "do the hard thing." This is a common situation, where one spouse's change of heart or ambivalence stirs anxiety in the other, which throws the couple off track.

Unpleasant actions are much more likely to be performed when requesting spouses empathize with their partners' predicament. Saying "I know how hard it is for you to return to work when you would prefer to stay home" would have gone a long way toward helping Jennifer do what was difficult. *Accommodating (accepting) spouses also gain the benefit of narrating their actions as sacrifices made in the service of their partners and the partnership, rather than as grudging capitulations to their partners' desires.*

Things may get even better if the requesting spouse, now free of anxiety about the outcome, is able to voice some guilt or doubt about having pushed his or her agenda. Rather than hiding behind "We had an agreement." or "You know it's the right thing to do," Cole could acknowledge that what Jennifer is doing is more to his liking than to hers. He might even offer that he "owes her one." And whenever one partner makes an accommodation—by changing or by accepting their spouse as is—it is more likely that the spouse will be similarly accommodating around some other issue.

Working Toward Acceptance: Applying What We've Covered Before

A partner who gives up trying to change a spouse and bows to his or her requests, as Jennifer did, will achieve acceptance only after mourning what might have been. A number of factors we have already discussed can help move spouses toward serenity and acceptance.

Maturity. The components of maturity (self-awareness, self-esteem, responsibility, etc.) that foster success in marriage do so, in part, by helping people to accept ongoing problems and periodic disappointments. Facilitating the development of these capacities will often allow partners to accept each other better.

Acceptance of self. Letting go of excessive idealizations of romantic love and allowing both oneself and one's partner to be imperfect is a form of acceptance. Accepting one's imperfections—"containing" them, rather than resorting to projective identification—contributes to the ability to forgive one's partner and accept his or her failings. And the capacity to accept oneself, warts and all, is a prerequisite for making a sincere apology.

Acceptance of imperfect interactions. Clients who can accept less-than-perfect marital interactions will also do better. Those from severely dysfunctional families of origin—who never experienced the less-than-perfect reality of life in a healthy, "good enough" family—can be helped by being gently disabused of the illusion that perfect interaction is possible.

Empathy, sacrifice, and commitment. Since putting ourselves in our partners' shoes is foundational to accepting them, it is no surprise that empathic ability has been shown to correlate with the capacity for forgiveness (Fehr et al., 2010). The related capacities of commitment and sacrifice (Stanley, Rhodes, & Whitton, 2010) and "accepting influence" during conflict (Gottman & Levenson, 1999) have also been shown to correlate with success in relationships, and indicate a mature willingness to let go of one's personal agenda—a form of acceptance—in the service of one's partner and the partnership.

Transference. Clients aware of psychological hot buttons (transference fears) in themselves and their partners will be more accepting of themselves and their partners. Spouses who acknowledge their own psychological allergies will take personal responsibility for their internal states, rather than blaming their partners. Insightful partners will try not to trigger their spouses' allergies and will be less surprised and more compassionate when they do.

Interpersonal process. Throughout the chapters on psychodynamics, my emphasis has been on facilitating intimacy, bonding, and conflict resolution by helping clients give voice to their deeper hopes and fears. As this occurs, negative interaction cycles give way to cycles that are more supportive and collaborative. When this happens, the resulting *improved interpersonal connection (selfobject bonding) helps couples to mourn their wishes about their partners that may never be met.* Recall Sally and George, the pursuer–distancer couple discussed in Chapter 6. This couple is typical of many pursuer–distancer couples whose improved process allows both partners to accept less than perfect—specifically, their remaining, often lifelong, differing preferences for closeness versus distance. Pursuers who begin to get more intimate connection come to accept less than they had hoped for, partly because they no longer take their partners' distancing so personally. Distancers, having learned how to be better listeners, become more willing to engage in conversation, even at times when they would prefer not to.

Working Toward Acceptance: Additional Options

Uncover reasons for reluctance. My primary approach to facilitating acceptance is to work with the reluctant partner to find out what is getting in the way. There are many possibilities, including issues of fairness, cultural norms, or specific anxieties about what might happen if things don't change. As I explore obstacles to acceptance in one partner, I try to help the other one present his or her needs in a more sympathetic way. Often, I alternate with the partners, ideally helping them meet somewhere in the middle.

Point out benefits. In trying to address a client's aversion to acceptance, I often mention the advantages of letting go, in particular, ending the wrangling over timeworn problems.

Point out that defects are also assets, and that no one's perfect. Sometimes, following Jacobson and Christensen's (1998) recommendation, I gently point out that many actions that hurt also provide benefits: The hard-working husband who disappoints by coming home late is also the husband who helps fund college tuition. The wife who seems too persnickety about how to parent the children is the same mother who identifies and gets the best teachers for them. The challenge is to accept that a character trait may simultaneously have both plusses and minuses and, equally important, that every partner has plusses and minuses.

Discuss compromises. Helping couples work out behavioral compromises, as in the aphorism, "It's better to light a candle than to curse the darkness," can help end repetitive squabbling. Couple therapists can encourage discussion of workable compromises and the challenges they entail, as will be discussed in Chapter 13. A painful fact of life is that any true compromise means that all parties must accept less than they wanted.

Encourage alternatives. Another way to deal with marital disappointment is to find alternative ways to satisfy the frustrated needs. Partners (more commonly women) who try, in vain, to have intimate conversations with their distancing spouses can meet part of their need by talking to like-minded friends or relatives.

Encourage positive couple interactions. Much research (Gottman, 2011; Pines, 1996) has shown that increased frequency of positive couple interaction correlates not only with marital happiness and success, but also with willingness to compromise and sacrifice. We will discuss this more in Chapter 14.

Assign acceptance experiments. Fruzzetti (2006) assigns the following homework task to help clients move toward acceptance:

> Identify what you keep doing to get your partner to change (e.g., nagging, critical looks). Observe how often you do it. Then stop! Next notice the upsetting feelings you get, including judgments of yourself and your partner and the discomfort of not getting what you want. See if you can handle this. Take care of yourself in other ways to make up for it; help yourself through the mourning process. Become aware of the costs to you of continuing your efforts to change your partner. This may involve not only reflecting on the frustration, but actually feeling it happen if you continue trying to get your partner to change.
>
> *(pp. 160–161)*

This exercise helps clients become more aware of the costs and benefits of giving up trying to change their partners. When I use this exercise, I focus on the discomfort it evokes and use this to facilitate understanding obstacles to letting go.

Encourage and teach repair conversations. Overarching acceptance of one's partner and one's marriage is greatly facilitated by efforts to repair emotional damage soon after it has occurred. Absent this, clients will increasingly view their partners as sources of aggravation, the very opposite of acceptance.

Teaching clients how to have repair conversations—including those that occur in our offices—is an important means of fostering acceptance.

Once the couple has cooled down, the repair conversation is used to review and repair the recent damage and, optimally, to plan how to do better in the future. Repair conversations implicitly encourage couples to accept the painful truth that their life together includes episodes of mutual injury that require repair.

People try many things to repair their relationship after a fight: apologizing, doing something extra nice, promising to do better, agreeing to forgive and forget, offering a hug. They all work sometimes, but they all fail when the partner is not receptive. None guarantees that the problem will not recur. Couples are more likely to find a long-lasting solution if they examine what happened, acknowledge responsibility, appreciate the reasonableness of each other's behavior, and plan how to do things better in the future.

One problem with a simple apology like "I'm sorry I was so insensitive" is that it may be perceived as an attempt to sweep the issue under the rug, rather than as a sincere attempt to understand what caused the fight and to heal the partner's injury. Even if they are not experienced as insincere, such apologies are incomplete. Partners who "kiss and make up," while tacitly colluding to shut down further discussion, may achieve near-term marital harmony, but they are likely to repeat the unpleasant scenario. For these reasons, couples will need to do more than make a quick apology.

Repair conversations should aim for an atmosphere of "unified detachment" (Lawrence & Brock, 2010), in which the couple convenes on a "platform" above the fray (Wile, 2013a) to review painful events, perhaps with a little levity. When helping couples with repair conversations, I offer my own acceptance and encouragement. I tell them that marital health does not mean *never* hurting each other, and that their marriage can be improved if they can learn to work together *after* their fights. I teach this explicitly and compliment couples on their ability to process their distress after the fact so as to head off lingering resentment. I remind them of the folk wisdom to never go to bed angry (though I disagree that repair must always precede sleep).

The basic principles of repair conversations essentially echo recommendations for "fighting fair" in the first place. I will discuss these more explicitly in Chapters 11 and 13, but for now, the main point is to encourage spouses to try to put themselves in each other's shoes and to prioritize good listening over self-justification.

A couple should be in a moderately receptive, calm mood, before embarking on repair. If they set the process in motion in order to "have it out now," they are likely to make matters worse. I advise clients not to expect instant reciprocation and understanding from their partners. Indeed, it is very likely that the early stages of repair conversations will be marked by the same painful experience they are trying to fix. Steeling oneself to this possibility may prevent what Wile (1993) calls "nice-guy backlash," the desire to counterattack and resume the fight after one's nice-guy attempts at repair have failed to elicit similar conciliatory behavior.

The fundamental emotional challenge in repair conversations is to make a detailed apology—specifying precisely what you did that caused your partner distress. Once one person does this, the other is usually more able to admit his or her contributions. Wile calls this an "admitting–admitting" couple state. Thus, in addition to observing the general rules for fighting fair, we advise clients that *the first rule of recovery conversations is to talk only about your own contributions to the fight* (Wile, 1993). This is critical, as any mention of your partner's contributions will invalidate your apology, making it appear as an insincere rhetorical device positioning you for the next round of debate.

It is difficult to follow this rule when everyone is still feeling injured and adversarial, but if one person can make the first tentative move, a virtuous cycle can begin, in which each partner's admission of responsibility stimulates the other's. Both partners then gradually feel, and sound, more authentic and conciliatory, as they see that their apologies are not met with ridicule or scorn. If the conversation stays positive, the couple bond will be strengthened, and negative transference expectations will be weakened. Repeated experiences of successful repair will further strengthen partners' trust in the process and in each other by allowing them to acknowledge wrongdoing and forgive each other. Having accomplished sufficient repair, couples can proceed to discuss how to prevent future fights.

We turn now to the related, but more challenging, situation, in which one partner is clearly more culpable and the offense more reprehensible.

FORGIVENESS

Major Betrayals

I distinguish offenses requiring "forgiveness" from those requiring "acceptance" by their severity, with most of the former experienced as major betrayals. Increased severity raises new questions about whether and how to forgive. Examples are shown in Table 10.1.

These offenses have in common a substantial violation of the implicit marital contract to care deeply about the partner, to put his or her needs ahead of those of others outside the relationship, to extend oneself in a crisis, and to be honest about activities that might impact the partner. These breaches threaten the foundations of the relationship, shaking one's confidence in one's partner's honesty, trustworthiness, and loyalty.

Although such transgressions can surface in the course of ongoing couple therapy, they are commonly presenting problems. In my experience and that of others in the field (Baucom, Snyder, & Gordon, 2009; Enright &

Table 10.1 Serious Couple Offenses

- Physical violence.
- Extramarital affairs.
- Online porn, chat rooms, or strip clubs, when viewed by a partner as equivalent to affairs.
- Secret injurious financial activity: gambling, risky investments gone bad, undisclosed pre-marital debt, concealed expensive purchases.
- Other important deceptions that impact the partner: criminal behavior, drug abuse, concealing the loss of a job.
- Breaking an important promise.
- Divulging confidential information.
- Failing to provide support during childbirth, a major illness, or the illness of a parent or other close relative.
- Not taking a partner's needs into consideration during a major life event: unduly pressuring a partner to have an abortion, accepting a job offer without discussion.
- Ignoring or disparaging a partner's major life achievement.
- Seriously embarrassing a partner in public.
- Seriously offending important friends, family members, or colleagues.
- Not taking the partner's side in important disputes with others, especially family members.

Fitzgibbons, 2000; Greenberg, Warwar, & Malcolm, 2008, 2010), *such couples require a distinctive approach, especially in the early stages of therapy,* because—unlike other couples seeking therapy—one partner is sharply defining the other as the offender. What the injured party demands of the perpetrator is an apology and reassurance that the offense will not repeat. Another defining feature of such couples is that injured partners are preoccupied with the betrayal and cannot seem to let go of their anger and distress. Unsurprisingly, forgiveness is often decisive in enabling these couples to recover and has been found to "increase marital satisfaction, psychological closeness, relationship investment, and to rebalance the couple's power distribution" (Greenberg et al., 2010, p. 29).

The Psychology of Forgiveness

Forgiveness is often poorly or simplistically understood by both clients and clinicians. Many clients begin by thinking that they "should" forgive, but after noticing that they "just can't," they give up on the idea. Both therapists and clients must understand that forgiveness is a complex psychological experience, which—if it is to occur—requires time and work. They must also realize that the goal is not to "forgive and forget." Forgetting is simply not possible. Rather, forgiveness requires one to let go of a grievance about a still-remembered event. Such letting go is often frightening, as it can threaten the injured partner's conceptions of equity, safety, trust, and identity. Forgiving is actually far less like forgetting, and more like giving up one's right to call in a debt. By bestowing forgiveness, one absolves the perpetrator from living under the cloud of his or her transgression. Forgiveness can also be a gift the forgiver gives him or herself, choosing personal happiness going forward over remaining mired in a state of injured self-righteousness.

Forgiveness always includes letting go of the grievance, but there are different levels of achieved empathy, reconciliation, and restored trust. Some clients may eventually agree that, had the roles been reversed, they might have acted as their partners had. An example: A wife came to acknowledge that she might have kept secret that she was sending money to an ex-spouse—the offense her husband had committed that had so enraged her—for fear that he would suspect it was not a purely charitable gesture. For most partners, however, forgiving rarely includes coming to condone the hurtful action.

Forgiveness does not universally lead to healing the relationship or to reconciliation. Some partners will do well to acknowledge the irreparable damage and then divorce. Others will develop empathy for the wrong-doer and continue the relationship. Whether to let one's guard down and allow trust to return will be a central question for couples who wish to get past the offense. After reviewing the writings of experts in the field and comparing it with my own clinical experience, I find it useful to distinguish the following possible eventual states of mind for offended partners, with each adding an element missing from the one prior: unforgiveness, acceptance (adding letting go of the grievance), forgiveness (adding empathy and understanding), and forgiveness with reconciliation (adding the continuation of the relationship).[2]

Unforgiveness

Unforgiveness of a betrayal is a painful state characterized by rumination on the offense, agitation, sleeplessness, and grave doubts about the partner, oneself, and life in general. The wronged partner is consumed with questions: "How could this happen?" "How could I not have seen this coming?" "How long has this been going on?" "What kind of person could do this to me?" "What kind of person am I to have let this happen to me?" "Who else knew about this, and why didn't they tell me?"

Victims feel intensely angry, often more angry than they have ever felt before. This anger is hard to contain and includes generalized irritability and occasional attacks on innocent bystanders (co-workers, children, friends, therapists) standing in for the perpetrator. There are wishes for revenge, apologies, and validation from others, and thoughts of permanent flight from the perpetrator. These painful states of mind cycle unpredictably. Victims find it hard to concentrate on anything else as their minds are colonized by thoughts related to the injury. Grave doubts about honesty, fairness, love, and one's fundamental safety can emerge and lead to hopelessness and despair. All students of forgiveness describe this painful state of obsessive distress and disillusionment in which victims are emotionally stuck and unable to get on with their lives.

The state of obsessive unforgiveness exists in relation to various complementary states in the perpetrator-spouse. These range from deep regret to defensive denial and include varying amounts of shame, guilt, suppressed anger, fears for the relationship, strong wishes that the partner move on, and doubts that the transgression will ever be forgiven.

Helping couples move past these states of distress is not easy. Some remain stuck for years; some never recover. In describing what can help, I will first discuss the situation from the perspective of the injured spouse in isolation; this is similar to mourning other traumatic life events and involves clearing away constraints that prevent the person from moving on. I will then consider the role and psychology of the perpetrator in inhibiting or facilitating that movement. After that, I will make some additional therapeutic recommendations.

Constraints Interfering With Mourning

Some injured partners forgive too easily for fear of losing the relationship or facing their own deep hurt, or because of characterological doubts about their personal value (Akhtar, 2002; Spring, 2004; Summers, 1999). This amounts to defensively sweeping the damage under the rug. The drawbacks of this survival strategy are that the offense may recur, that the defense will prove inadequate to suppress painful feelings, or that the relationship will continue to weaken. These injured partners may come for therapy years after the offense, either when their marital bond feels strong enough to allow discussion or when the hurt has grown unbearable.

More commonly, the process of getting beyond the injury has become stuck in an openly unforgiving, ruminative state. As with other traumas in life (a tornado destroying a home, a reckless driver killing a child), the traumas of marriage (a husband hitting his wife, a wife cheating on her husband) will have both universal and idiographic characteristics and significance for the victim. The therapist's task will be to facilitate discussion of the trauma while conveying empathy for the obvious losses involved, curiosity about idiosyncratic meanings, skepticism concerning simplistic accounts, and hope in the face of the client's pessimism about recovery.

Grievance Stories and Unenforceable Rules

Fred Luskin (2002), a major contributor to our understanding of how people move on from unforgiveness, has worked successfully with people who have suffered many types of hard-to-forgive offenses. In addition to the marital injuries listed above, Luskin has worked with people jilted at the altar, fired unfairly from lifelong jobs, abused physically and sexually by their parents, disabled in auto accidents caused by others, and (in some of his most noteworthy research) mothers of children murdered in sectarian violence in Northern Ireland. Like other experts, Luskin focuses on the obsessive post-traumatic state and how that can compound other problems resulting from the trauma.

Luskin begins by helping people become aware of how they have often created what he calls "grievance stories," excessively one-sided, self-serving narrations of their injuries. Clients create accounts to explain what happened; to gain sympathy; or to defend against shame, guilt, and uncertainty about what to do next. Luskin shows people how the *way* they narrate their lives—positively or negatively—can open or block their road to recovery. This is not to say that clients have not been truly victimized, but to note that magnifying victimhood leads to *additional* problems.

Grievance stories progressively lock clients into the victim role, preventing them from taking constructive steps to move on. In part, this is because blaming others blinds people to their own contributions and to options for improvement. Friends and family who were initially sympathetic become worn out and alienated by these self-serving stories, and less available to provide support and guidance.

Luskin illustrates with a client of his, Alan, who was devastated when he discovered that Elaine, his wife of six years, was having an affair. The grievance story Alan created after their divorce was long on blame and short on self-awareness: He was good at listing Elaine's flaws, but overlooked what she had done to try to resolve their conflicts. In his telling, he was uniquely injured among men, and Elaine was the cause of all of his misery: his professional difficulties, his inability to find a new relationship, and his friends' abandonment (as his festering anger exhausted their support and good will). By the time Alan sought therapy, the consuming rage he felt toward Elaine—solidified by his narrative—was hurting only him.

Luskin helps clients notice when they are telling grievance stories—when they tell the stories repeatedly to themselves and others without much effort to provide balance or to check the accuracy of their facts—and advises them to enlist a friend or family member to alert them when they fall into re-telling them. Whether by this or other means of pointing out the existence of grievance stories, couple therapists should then go further: After validating that a real injury has occurred, we should work to uncover the underlying fears and presumed benefits that encourage clients to cling to their self-defeating narratives.

Just as grievance stories block recovery from traumatic experiences, so do what Luskin calls "unenforceable rules." These are strict, usually unconscious, beliefs about how the world ought to be: parents should be loving, spouses should be faithful, business partners should be honest, and teenagers should return home before curfew. All are certainly desirable from the injured party's perspective, but they are not "enforceable."

It is understandable that people become upset when moral expectations are violated, but, Luskin points out, they can make matters worse by *demanding* that others be fair, honest, and loving, and by perseverating on the injustice when others fail them. Luskin stops his argument there, but I would add that a central reason people become stuck ranting at violations of unenforceable rules ("That crazy driver shouldn't have cut me off!") is that such violations reveal that the world is much less safe and fair than we are comfortable believing.

Luskin also thinks we take our traumas too personally. Using the example of a woman who was devastated when her best friend ran off with her boyfriend, he notes that it is simplistic for her to think that the only relevant issues are unfairness and her attractiveness. Who knows what went on in the minds of the two who ran off? While Luskin can sometimes sound too logical and hardhearted, I would say that it is the work of therapy or "mourning" to uncover the overly-personalized meanings and overly-idealistic expectations that make our justifiable hurt both more painful and more long-lasting—in the case above, for instance, the woman's lifelong doubts about her attractiveness or about her ability to identify trustworthy friends.

Luskin reminds us that bad and unethical things happen all the time, and that we should stop being amazed and complaining about them and consider, instead, how to alter our behavior going forward to make a difference. The "victim story" can then shift to a "hero story," in which one works hard to overcome adversity and refuses to be defeated by difficult life events. To help people move on, Luskin reminds them that others have suffered similar or worse disasters and triumphed over them, and he encourages them to seek such people out in support groups or to read about them in literature. Like a good CBT therapist, he challenges overly pessimistic beliefs, such as "I will never be able to trust anyone again," "His hurting me means I'm unattractive or flawed or that I deserved it," or "The new situation will be unlivable."

Luskin also draws attention to the injured person's deepest goals, ones that may appear to have been rendered unreachable by the trauma. He then tries to show the client how he or she has become too narrowly concrete when thinking about those goals. For instance, a woman's husband may have run off, but that need not mean she will never find intimacy again. Focusing on one's deepest goals and imagining attaining them can help one escape tunnel vision.

Shame and Revenge

In his article, "Unbearable shame, splitting, and forgiveness in the resolution of vengefulness," the psychoanalyst Melvin Lansky (2007) argues convincingly that unacceptable shame defended by hostile wishes to "get even" explains much of the stuckness of the unforgiving state of mind. Just as Luskin pointed to the self-defeating impact of grievance stories, so Lansky notes how clients injure themselves and are held captive by their efforts to save face. As he sees it,

> [Vengeful states] offer intrapsychic defensive advantages—moral justification, firmness of purpose, and unquestioned certainty—when they effect reversals of disorganized, humiliated, and uncertain states of mind . . . These defensive advantages, however, are costly ones. The certainty that is crystallized in the sense of being aggrieved, of being the recipient of injustice, being damaged by that injustice, and being entitled to justice seems in the mind of the vengeful person to override the practical, legal, and ethical considerations of doing harm, not just to the presumed offender or betrayer, but to the larger community and its standards.
>
> (pp. 573–574)

The therapist's task here should be clear: Free clients from their largely unconscious beliefs that they have been irretrievably shamed by their spouses, so that they can let go of their defensive reversals, including their desire for vengeance.

A Little Bit of Vengeance Helps the Grievance Go Down

Salman Akhtar (2002) suggests that clients are assisted in moving from vengefulness to forgiveness by mild versions of enacted revenge during the recovery phase, as perpetrators are called out for what they have done. Quoting Heinrich Heine who in 1848 said, "One must, it is true, forgive one's enemies—but not before they have been hanged!", Akhtar notes that by experiencing the guilty pleasure of revenge, even in fantasy, victims can move off their holier-than-thou stance and lay the groundwork for future empathy with the perpetrator.

Are We Blaming the Victim?

A problem arises. Both Luskin's and Lansky's approaches appear radically different from those that assert that forgiveness therapy must begin with all parties—the offending spouse, the offended spouse, and the therapist (in the case of couple therapy)—agreeing unequivocally that the perpetrator has committed a morally reprehensible, injurious act (e.g., Enright & Fitzgibbons, 2000). Shouldn't we worry that focusing on the victim's shame or grievance story comes close to "blaming the victim" for his or her (continued) suffering? How do we reconcile these two views?

Consider the case of a husband hitting his wife in the heat of a verbal battle. This is clearly an unacceptable offense and must be understood as such. When we look more deeply, however, we may find that for the wife to forgive, she will have to admit that it was not so much the physical injury, but the shame she felt about her husband treating her so badly that was most traumatic—that the damage inflicted was to her core sense of lovability, more than to her body. As we shall see shortly, this attack on her self-esteem should also be the subject of her husband's heartfelt apology, if he later becomes capable of giving one. Unless we access this woman's shame, we may remain stuck alongside her in her morally accurate, but psychologically superficial account of events. In this and other situations, underlying shame is hidden from view, "drowned out by the blaring fanfare of the avenger's innocent victimhood" (Rosen, 2007, p. 603), but it must be accessed to allow mourning and authentic forgiveness to occur.

This necessity was confirmed in a recent study of EFT couple therapy in situations requiring forgiveness (Zuccarini, Johnson, Dalgleish, & Makinen, 2013) which found that, for couples to move past the angry surface of expressed hurt and defensive withdrawal, victims had to uncover and express the deeper personal meanings of the injury, often ones involving attachment insecurity. Therapists must then take a complementary or dialectical view of the situation—that a serious "marital crime" has been committed *and* that we have to look into the psychology of the victim—if clients are to move toward acceptance and, possibly, forgiveness, Should we need more evidence that shame lurks, unmetabolized, at the bottom of much unmourned trauma, consider that much bullying consists of actions precisely intended to shame the victim and compel him or her to feel inferior, weak, ugly, or impotent. Recovery from such bullying will, of necessity, require a reworking of that shame.

Therapists treating clients who have been betrayed will need to help them expose the shame the betrayal evoked and see that the shame is not fatal. Forgiveness will include, perhaps surprisingly, a measure of forgiveness of the self. As Lansky (2007) puts this, "Forgiveness in the depth-psychological sense here employed centers around the notion that the underlying shame, felt previously to be unbearable, has been unconsciously reassessed and is now felt to have become bearable" (p. 591).

Complexity and Responsibility

Both Luskin and Lansky see much of the therapy of the unforgiving state as helping clients rewrite the story of their injury as a less simplistic, less one-sided, account. Once their undue shame is exposed, victims may become free to look for still more complexity in the narrative. This "reconsideration of the story" (Akhtar, 2002) is central to most conceptions of how people recover from trauma: Although victims cannot change the past, they can change how they view it in the present. In the new version, victim and perpetrator are more three-dimensional characters, their actions not so obviously black and white, outcomes not so demoralizingly disastrous, and victims more willing to separate the actor from the act. Now free of undue shame, they are able to accept greater responsibility for the events leading to their injury (e.g., the wife who has been hit may admit that her unrestrained verbal attack on her husband's manhood had touched a nerve). Victims may become less self-righteous and more empathic toward offenders, a shift shown to correlate with later reconciliation in the relationship (studies cited in Greenberg et al., 2008).

Empathy for the offender will often involve a re-owning of projected negative self-states, so that the other is no longer seen as so despicably "not-me," the person undeserving of being considered human or worthy of understanding and forgiveness. Usually, injured clients come to some awareness of their own aggressiveness or hurtfulness, which allows them to accept it in offending partners. They may also recall times when they sought to be forgiven. Forgiveness will likewise be facilitated when the victim recalls the good qualities and actions of the perpetrator, actions that can come more into view as the vengeful, obsessive state loosens its grip on the injured person's mind.

In some re-narrations, however, offenders will be seen as *more* responsible than previously. Victims may then blame themselves less and find it easier to reach out to friends and family. Some will become less inclined to reconcile with their offenders.

Trust and the Power of the One-up Position

The loss of trust is frequently the most momentous casualty of interpersonal betrayals. What was previously assumed to be safe—a spouse working late or going on a business trip—arouses fears of a repeat offense. This is true not only of offenses involving lying and secrecy, but also of sins of omission, when a spouse failed to "be there for me." In both situations, the trustworthiness and loving concern of the partner can no longer be taken for granted. And if the offender had previously accused the victim of being unduly suspicious or insecure, it will be still harder for victims to let down their guard.

To become unstuck, victims will have to confront this loss of trust. Ideally, they will do this in the presence of the offending partner, who will validate their concerns and act to reduce them. Sometimes, it will help for the victim to hear the "whole story" from the perpetrator, so that he or she is not left to imagine that the offense was worse than it was or to anticipate additional damaging revelations in the future. Reviewing the transgression may also enable the therapist to uncover mitigating circumstances that had not been mentioned previously. That said, victims may want to rein in their desire to hear every last detail, if these may become triggers that evoke the trauma later on. It may be sufficient for a spouse to know the affair lasted three months, without knowing which hotels and restaurants were frequented.

Trust is never restored in one fell swoop, even with highly repentant offenders. It will take time, and usually behavioral evidence, for trust to return to pre-offense levels, and in many cases it will never return completely. But until trust improves, victims may cling to the moral superiority of unforgiveness that gives them control over a partner, now placed in the humbled, one-down role of supplicant on probation. Indeed, the main benefit of continuing to define oneself as victimized is having (or imagining one has) greater power over the previously out-of-control offender in domains related to the offense.

Victims may reap other benefits, as well—such as control over decisions and resources—that may be hard to give up and may inhibit movement toward forgiveness. In my experience, the most important of these is the increased attentiveness of the partner who was previously preoccupied outside the relationship. As long as the offense is still on the table and court is in session, the offender must sit attentively, on good behavior, in the dock. The art of therapy includes helping victimized clients see that this can become counterproductive by generating resentment in their spouses. Simultaneously, therapists can help clients trust and observe that offenders remain attentive even after being freed from the holding cell of the offense.

Sometimes victims remain stuck in the victim role due to misconceptions about what they would be giving up if they were to become more forgiving. It can help to point out explicitly that forgiveness does not require that the victim come to see things (only) from the perspective of the perpetrator, nor does it mean forgetting or condoning the injurious act, nor does it obligate one to forgo justice from the courts or restitution from the perpetrator (when the offense merits it), nor does it determine whether one reconciles and continues the relationship. All of these depend, also, on the subsequent behavior of the offender. Absent the offender's expression of remorse and promise to reform, the best that can be expected of the victim is an "acceptance" of the offense and a decision to separate from the offender and move on.

As with other behaviors influenced by circular causation, the capacity of victims to rewrite their grievance stories and let go of the moral high ground will depend powerfully on the offender's narrative and behavior, our next topic.

Forgiveness as Transaction: The Importance of Witnessing

Genuine forgiveness that progresses beyond acceptance toward reconciliation is co-created and requires an interpersonal process in which the past is discussed and trust is restored. Forgiveness and renewed trust must be earned. Janice Spring (2004) gives an example of a wife who explained this to her husband:

> Shortly after he admitted his affair, he told her, "I'll never do it again, and I don't want to talk about it—or your grievances—anymore. It's

ancient history." Jane's response cut to her bottom line: "If you don't want to hear my pain, I can't get close to you. I'm not trying to punish or manipulate you. I'm just telling you what I need to forgive you."

(p. 123)

While some victims may be able to forgive their offenders unilaterally and leave, partners who are going to continue to interact will have to listen carefully to each other's stories. The same goes for members of previously warring religious or ethnic groups inhabiting the same country. Gobodo-Madikizela (2008) comes at these issues from her experience with South Africa's Truth and Reconciliation Commission. Like other students of forgiveness, she is interested in how to heal "wounds that cry out," which remain open and consuming, often returning in flashbacks and dreams. Her most significant finding is that both victims and perpetrators can benefit from witnessing each other retelling their stories:

> In bearing witness, confronting their depravity and coming face-to-face with the pain and suffering they have caused victims, perpetrators are re-humanizing not only the victims whose lives were shattered by their actions, but through their remorse they are also reclaiming their own sense of humanity, a humanity shattered by the atrocities they committed. The first step of dehumanization, of rendering the other invisible, is silencing the voice of conscience. The dehumanization of the self is the beginning of that slippery slope into a life of destruction against others who are considered to be enemies. When remorse is triggered in the moment of witnessing, however, the perpetrator recognizes the other as a fellow human being. At the same time, the victim, too, recognizes the face of the perpetrator not as that of a "monster" who committed terrible deeds, but as the face with enough humanity to feel remorse. This does not deny the horrific deeds or set them aside as such; by showing remorse the perpetrator is showing his human side. This becomes an opportunity to integrate these human elements of someone who was perceived as other so that the perpetrator becomes less threatening, and more attuned with the victim's human identity ... It is the recognition of the victim's pain that awakens remorse in the perpetrator, and it is remorse that lays the ground for the emergence of empathic sensibilities expressed on the part of the victim towards the perpetrator.
>
> (pp. 176–177)

For healing to begin, perpetrators must validate victims' experience by hearing them tell their story. As Frommer (2005) puts it,

> Somehow, their recognition of the ways in which they have altered us feels crucial to our being able to do the intrapsychic work that might

lead to our forgiving them ... Under this relational conception of forgiveness, it is an error to conceive of the capacity to forgive in exclusively intrapsychic terms.

(pp. 36–37)

Perpetrators then tell *their* stories, making an effort to explain how they lost their moral bearings.

Note that some therapists (see, especially, Michael White, 2009) make witnessing central to all their couple therapy, not just to therapy following major betrayals. Much of the healing power of the work of Dan Wile, Sue Johnson, and others also derives from the impact of partners truly witnessing their spouses' stories.

Finally, Virginia Goldner (2004) adds another reason to think of forgiveness as requiring a dyadic transaction: "Many authors in the abuse field have pointed out that a victim's healing requires holding the perpetrator accountable *if the victim is to be freed from her confusion about her culpability*" (p. 371, italics added).

Apologies

It is reasonable to expect that, after listening to the victim's account of the offense, the perpetrator will express remorse and convincingly promise to do better. This is a prerequisite to the injured partner's canceling the debt and regaining trust. Indeed, sincere apologies have been shown to make forgiveness more likely (studies cited in Bradbury & Karney, 2010; Greenberg, Warwar, & Malcolm, 2010; Lewis, Parra, & Cohen, 2015; McCullough, Pargament, & Thorsen, 2000; Worthington & Wade, 1999). This research, clinical wisdom, and my personal experience suggest that optimal apologies should include the following elements:

- *Offenders must take responsibility for the damage and must say, "This is what I did to you."*
- *In the early stages, offenders must not qualify their statements by attributing responsibility to the victim* ("You hurt me, too!" or "You get hurt too easily!"). (Recall Wile's similar rule for the first stage of repair conversations.)
- *Offenders must demonstrate a detailed awareness of what damage was done, including damage to trust* ("I made you distrust me and our marriage") *and self-worth* ("I made you doubt your value, not only to me, but to anyone").
- *Offenders must go beyond a simple confession* ("I admit that I did this to you") *or a pro forma script* (like those of public figures doing damage control). *They must include convincing expressions of real concern and "empathic distress" over their actions.*
- *Offenders must convey shame and guilt (personal self-criticism) about the offense.*[3]
- *Offenders must be patient and may have to repeat their apologies many times.*

- *Offenders must take an interest in understanding themselves, including how they came to wrong their partners and how they justified their actions to themselves.*
- *Offenders must promise to do better in the future.*
- *Offenders must "ask" rather than "demand" forgiveness.* "Pressure to forgive" has been shown to impede forgiveness and reconciliation (Greenberg et al., 2010).

Repair Beyond Apologies

Students of forgiveness have identified additional actions that offenders can perform to facilitate forgiveness, including:

- ***Acts of atonement.*** While heartfelt apologies are crucial, concrete actions also help to undo damage, such as apologizing to family members who have been affected or devoting extra time to projects that have been neglected. While some misdeeds immediately suggest appropriate corrective actions, offenders can promote repair by soliciting suggestions: "What can I do that will help you heal?"
- ***Acts that reassure the partner that the offense will not recur.*** In the case of an affair, the offender might change his or her phone number, formally end the relationship (perhaps in the presence of the partner), or change jobs so as not to be around the former lover. When the offense involved alcohol or drug abuse, getting treatment is essential.
- ***Acts that protect the partner from post-traumatic experiences.*** Because the injured partner lives in a post-traumatic state, vulnerable to hurt and doubt, a truly remorseful offender should be aware of potential triggers and take responsibility for keeping them to a minimum. Examples include checking in more frequently without complaint, storing credit card and cell phone records in an accessible place, and generally looking out for the other protectively, in what Spring (2004) calls a "transfer of vigilance."

Helping the Offender

Therapists can assist (willing) offenders by encouraging actions that are both morally virtuous and pragmatically efficacious—witnessing, sincere apologies, and performing acts of atonement and care—but often, more will be required. Just as victims require assistance to move from unforgiveness to acceptance and possible forgiveness, so offenders will usually need our help before they can act unconflictedly to repair their relationships. It is easy to say this, but accomplishing it in a setting where one person has, undeniably, been victimized is more challenging, as outlined by Goldner (2004) in the following quote from her landmark article on intimate partner violence:

> In these treatments, both partners must be defined as clients, yet one is a perpetrator and the other a victim. The two are not on equal footing, and the relationship they are trying to salvage is unjust, unsafe, and unequal . . . To succeed in this work, the therapist must create a context in which the woman [victim] can speak the truth about her life under siege and her partner and the therapist can suffer that truth in the act of listening. At the same time, *the man [offender] must also be recognized in his full subjectivity, not only in terms of his shameful identity as an offender.* In many cases, abusive men carry inside them a child-victim who also has a story that must be told. *Making room for everyone, past and present, is critical for creating the intersubjective conditions necessary for the shift from abusiveness and victimization to mutual recognition and the healing action of the depressive position.*
>
> (p. 347, italics added)

We also should not assume that offenders are 100% on board with the repair agenda: Some will become so, some will apologize but will not wish to reconcile, and some will remain unrepentant. Their authentic choice will usually become clear only after their psychological concerns, including what they imagine forgiving to entail, are explored.

Shame and guilt. Somewhat paradoxically, often the shame and guilt that offenders feel about their hurtful actions are stumbling blocks thwarting their acts of contrition. We commonly see offenders sitting almost frozen, apparently unremorseful, as they listen to their spouses berating them for their actions. Often they look like children waiting for their reprimand to end, rather than like adults genuinely sorry for the hurt they have caused. Just as some clients are unable to tolerate sexual or aggressive feelings, many clients strive mightily to suppress or deny what, for them, is the extreme pain of self-criticism evoked by the criticism of loved ones. Terrified of feeling their own badness or defectiveness, such clients may defensively flee or bizarrely assert their innocence. Often, this need to conceal shameful secrets and the inability to acknowledge problems is what got them into trouble in the first place (e.g., financial errors that, left unchecked, became financial disasters).

One client's wife discovered his infidelity with a prostitute after she developed a sexually transmitted illness. They came to therapy to deal with this betrayal and the many lies that had enabled him to hide it from her. Anticipating that therapy would involve being shamed, and that this was the price he had to pay to avoid divorce, the husband would begin most sessions with his head bowed, sheepishly soliciting punishment, actually saying, "OK, let's get this over with. Let me have it!" His wife often doubted the sincerity of his remorse—thinking him simply a narcissist who had been caught and herself the patsy listening to more of his lies (now, about his contrition)—but it turned out that this rush to penance was an attempt to avoid facing his crushing shame and guilt. A shame-prone person all of his life, he dreaded the prospect of his wife berating him for the behavior that he, himself, saw as unforgiveable. Gradually, in the safety of my office, he became less preoccupied with his shame and guilt long enough to use those feelings to express his genuine regret that he had wounded his wife and risked destroying the family he treasured.

In other cases, offending spouses initially imply that their only mistake was getting caught, maintaining that their partner is overly critical and that no significant damage was done. As was found in the South Africa Reconciliation hearings, such perpetrators have often been able to commit their offenses by shielding themselves from identifying with their victims. As therapists help offenders to listen empathically, this defensive denial may collapse and allow real guilt and shame to emerge.

Clients who fear shame and guilt will be helped by therapists who reassure them that they are not the first to have sinned in this way, and by therapists who help them uncover mitigating circumstances and unmet needs that allow a softening of their moralistic self-reproach. These people will be helped to overcome their beliefs that they do not deserve to be forgiven, that there is no way to heal the pain they have caused, and that their reprehensible actions make them unremittingly bad.

While many clients will come to feel genuine remorse, there are non-sociopathic perpetrators for whom split-off transgressive actions (stealing, exhibitionism, serial affairs) remain egosyntonic. Some of these clients—those with what have been termed "narcissistic behavior disorders"—can benefit from intensive individual psychotherapy aimed at helping them understand the unconscious payoffs of their secret pleasures (Goldberg, 1999).

Fear of being one-down. Many offenders fear accepting responsibility for their transgressions because they believe that they will then be accepting a perpetual one-down position in their relationship. As they see it, if they admit to the full measure of their crimes in the courtroom of couple therapy, their punishment will be forever living in a marital doghouse, handing their partner a "morality trump card" that can be used against them indefinitely (Ringstrom, 2014). Others fear that by giving "sentencing" power to their injured spouses, they will end up undermining their valued marriages. Actually, the opposite is more often the case: Contrition will get offenders *out* of the marital doghouse and allow their marriages to continue, Offenders who are unable to let their guard down, however, will be unable to reassure their partners that they are truly sorry and that the offense will not recur; these latter relationships may never get back on track.

Childhood experiences with forgiveness and apology. Sometimes, we can better understand clients' difficulties with apologizing by asking them about earlier experiences. Some common experiences that impede the beneficial process we are hoping to facilitate include: (a) never having witnessed sincere apologies and forgiveness, so that they are unfamiliar with the process and the benefits; (b) having witnessed incessant fighting over who was to blame, so that admitting responsibility or letting go of offenses seems to invite disaster; (c) having witnessed repeated, hollow, insincere apologies ("I promise I'll never hit you again"), so that apologies appear meaningless; (d) having been compelled to offer bogus apologies or grant false forgiveness ("Tell your sister you're sorry," or "You have to forgive me, because I won't be able to stop crying unless you do"), so that apologizing seems traumatically inauthentic.

Mutual and complex causation. A final, important impediment to sincere expressions of remorse is offenders' believing that forgiveness means accepting all the blame for their actions and agreeing that their transgression is the only problem in the marriage. Apologizing for wrongdoing is made more difficult because, as research and clinical practice show, "victims often fail to acknowledge mitigating circumstances and their own contributions to the problem" (Baumeister, Exline, & Sommer, 1998, p. 85). The same research confirms the parallel observation that "offenders tend to minimize the adverse effects of their actions" (p. 85). In this situation, as noted by Bradbury and Karney (2010), "The process of forgiveness requires the victim to cancel a debt that is larger than the one the perpetrator acknowledges" (p. 304). Similarly, optimal apologies require that perpetrators confess to crimes larger than they believe they have committed. Much of the art and difficulty of working toward forgiveness revolves around this core conundrum.

Therapists, who usually see the offense less moralistically and as more complexly determined than victims do, will be challenged to hold these more complex views in check, in order to allow the full extent of the victim's suffering and trauma to be aired. Trained to look for circular causation, we can easily see how a wife uninterested in sex or preoccupied with her children might have been a factor in her husband's affair, but therapy will not go well if we move too quickly to point that out.

Offenders must similarly be helped to hold in abeyance their own more complex, partially exonerating stories in the service of fully attending to their injured partner's version of events. Even when offenders continue to believe that their offense was not as egregious as portrayed, they can be helped to admit that the injured partner is the sole arbiter of the amount of damage incurred.

Only after the offender has sincerely apologized, and the offended partner has moved toward forgiveness can the therapy begin to address the more complex question of what led up to the offense and what behaviors of the victim, if any, may have contributed. This will be an important step—confirmed by research to be beneficial (Greenberg, Warwar, & Malcolm, 2010)—but it cannot be rushed.

As with lesser offenses requiring repair, as partners approach each other and soften, each may be better able to acknowledge his or her contributions, in a process that becomes progressively more honest and revealing, and this may serve as a basis for making important changes in the marriage. Ultimately, some victims will acknowledge that they have been accomplices to the crime and then, continuing this metaphor, the partners can work together toward crime prevention.

Homework Letters

In their treatment study, Greenberg and colleagues (2010) had partners write letters to each other that seemed to facilitate healing. Offenders wrote letters of apology that were to include: (a) *regret:* saying what they regretted and detailing their understanding of how they had hurt their partners; (b) *responsibility:* taking ownership of their role in the injury by specifying what they were taking responsibility for; and (c) *remedy:* articulating what they would do to help their partner heal from the hurt.

Injured partners wrote letters describing where they were in the process of resolving, forgiving, and letting go of the hurt and anger toward their partners. They were to describe what they did not forgive or were not able to let go of, why it was difficult for them to resolve the injury, and what they needed from their partners to help them relinquish the hurt and anger so they could forgive. If they had already let go of the hurt and anger or had forgiven their partner, they were to write about whether they felt they were able to reconcile.

Steven Stosny (2005, 2006), one of the most experienced clinicians working with abusive men, also has offenders write letters stating what they have done and detailing awareness of the damage this has caused to their partners and to themselves. This assignment encourages partners to take their marriage seriously, to look at themselves honestly, and to take an active, responsible stance toward central relationships issues.

Never Over and Done

Therapists and clients must not hold overly idealized views of the forgiveness/recovery process, especially the belief that healing can take place once and for all. Serious betrayals will never be forgotten. The best we can hope for is that they will be remembered in less painful, more complex ways. As Frommer (2005) points out:

> The state of forgiveness that we long for—free from residual anger, resentment, or ambivalence—is an ideal. In real life, forgiving often coexists with resurgences of doubt, bitterness, hurt, and the painful feeling that the relationship has been inextricably altered by what has happened. We forgive as best we can, which is to say, imperfectly.
>
> *(p. 44)*

As Greenberg's research has confirmed, even when there is considerable movement toward forgiveness, trust returns more slowly. In this regard, therapists should try to normalize this reality and attempt to immunize clients against undue disappointment when things do not progress as quickly as they hope.

Therapists should also be on guard for couples who appear to have resolved their hurt, but are just avoiding reopening the wound. We must use our judgment to decide when to revisit the subject and when to allow respite from the intensity of reviewing the betrayal. I have erred in both directions. Sometimes I have pressed too hard in this work when a rest and discussion of other subjects might have been more productive and sometimes, when I thought we were done and on the verge of ending a successful therapy, I have been surprised by a sudden resurgence of anger and defensiveness showing that the old wounds were still raw and needed more attention.

Therapy Beyond Forgiveness

Couples who move past the forgiveness phase of therapy may continue in conjoint therapy, now focusing on repetitive negative interaction cycles or other specific areas of conflict. Where there has been recovery from an extramarital affair, therapists and spouses will need to pay special attention to the couple's sex life. And some partners may benefit from individual therapy aimed at helping with their propensities to act out.

Many couples who present with a serious betrayal turn out to have been emotionally distant from each other prior to the signal event, leading parallel lives. This distance is often what encouraged the acting out and what allowed it to remain secret. In helping these couples work toward greater happiness, trust, and stability, we must encourage them to increase the number of shared positive activities. These experiences will help carry the couple beyond witnessing and apologizing to further healing and strengthening of the couple bond. Greater closeness will also neutralize the distrust that can intensify when couples are apart too much. Couples should be encouraged to get out and about together, to cultivate shared hobbies, friends, and community activities in the service of restoring a sense of companionship and togetherness.

Finally, while most of this chapter has been about helping couples to forgive, apologize, and reconcile, this may not always be possible or desirable. Some spouses will be so deeply wounded that they will be unwilling to continue the relationship. Others will decide that they should not risk further traumatization by staying together. Some partners will reveal themselves unable or unwilling to give up their hurtful behaviors. In all of these cases, therapists need to shift gears and help the couple to disengage and accept the dissolution of their union. Sometimes, the partners will be able to maintain amicable contact, especially if they have children, but in other cases, hostility will remain. In these cases, even though full forgiveness and reconnection will not be achieved, it is still useful to work toward the lesser goal of acceptance.

Notes

1 Vilification describes a process whereby acknowledged differences between partners are declared to be evidence of personal deficiency, moral weakness, or emotional illness (Jacobson & Christensen, 1998; Dimidjian et al., 2008).
2 Adding to the complexity of the subject, experts use different terms to differentiate these levels of coming to terms with the event and the perpetrator. Confirming the work of Worthington's group (Worthington & Wade, 1999 Worthington et al., 2000), Greenberg et al. (2008) found that the state of "unforgiveness" can diminish, without increasing "forgiveness," where forgiveness is defined as going beyond acceptance and letting go of the grievance to also include "an increase in positive emotions such as compassion, empathy, or understanding felt toward the injurer" (p. 187). By contrast, Luskin (2002) employs the term forgiveness to describe simply the shift out of the obsessive unforgiveness state to that of acceptance, which he correctly notes does not require empathy with, or reparation from, the perpetrator, although empathy and repair can facilitate that shift. Spring (2004) refers to letting go of the grievance, as I do, as acceptance. When the victim adds empathic understanding—as per Worthington and Greenberg above—sometimes coupled with reconciliation with the offender, Spring terms this "genuine forgiveness."
3 Greenberg et al. (2010) found that offenders who acknowledged shame (that their action violated an internal norm) were more positively received than those who acknowledged guilt (that their action injured the other). In my clinical experience, victims vary with respect to what reassures them most. Some feel that if their partners are truly ashamed, they will be less likely to repeat the behavior. Others are more interested in hearing their partners talk about caring about them and are less reassured when offenders dwell on their internal struggles and values.

PART IV
Behavioral/Educational Upgrades

11
TEACHING SPEAKING AND LISTENING SKILLS

The methods I have described so far didn't always work for me. Some couples never seemed to achieve the ability to talk safely and productively. This was true notwithstanding our accessing underlying issues and interlocking transferences, and my interpreting instances of projective identification. There would be moments of softening and closeness, but these would alternate with ones filled with angry recriminations or cold aloofness. Sometimes, I felt like I was writing on sand: Week after week, I would repeat the same interventions, uncover the same patterns, reframe the same issues, and provide the same holding and structure, but I would never turn the corner to find the partners able to perform these functions by themselves.

Frustrated when change was elusive, I began to teach clients explicitly how to have safe conversations when powerful feelings emerge during what Stone, Patton, and Heen (2010) have called "difficult conversations." Teaching these skills had long been central to behavioral couple therapy and had become familiar to me when I began to teach them to college students in my *Marriage 101* class. The communication skills we will be discussing have been developed and popularized by behavior therapists, cognitive behavior therapists, therapists focused on "emotion regulation," and experts in negotiation. In the next three chapters, I will describe them and offer guidance in how to teach them to couples.[1]

Rationale for Skills Training

As noted before, extensive research has found that marital health and longevity are promoted by skillful, healthy communicating (e.g., Gottman, Gottman, Coan, Carrera, & Swanson, 1998). In addition, research has shown that teaching communication skills helps both distressed (Dimidjian, Martell, & Christensen, 2008) and premarital (Carroll & Doherty, 2003) couples. This makes sense for a number of reasons. The most obvious is that marriage is a risky endeavor, and individuals involved in risky endeavors (performing surgery, starting a business) do better when they know which actions promote success and which are tempting but dangerous.

I sometimes illustrate this need for education by describing how my high school wrestling instructor replaced our fuzzy ideas about wrestling (two people grabbing each other and rolling around on the ground) with a slightly more sophisticated understanding, by teaching us named offensive and defensive moves. Clients in couple therapy, too, lack the models and vocabulary they need when they start wrestling with each other in negative cycles. We can help them by teaching them some "named moves."

Another rationale for skills training comes from a different direction—not that clients have yet to learn how to communicate in mature, productive ways, but that because *group* behavior is so often predictably dysfunctional, having rules for safe conduct helps. Whether it is a PTA meeting or a Congressional hearing, it is important to assure that everyone has a chance to speak, that participants listen to one another, and that there are procedures for joint decision-making. Rules, whether Robert's Rules of Order or a national constitution, help make this happen. Couples are well served if they observe rules that assure that both have a chance to talk, that both are committed to listening, and that both know how to work toward resolution of differences. *Some of the "skills" we teach amount to helping couples commit to following specific rules for speaking and listening.*

Although rules in games, sports, and politics are usually written down and explicitly agreed to by participants, the rules we use most tend to be internalized and automatic. Like the conventions deemed "good manners," many of the recommendations for handling difficult conversations, once learned, will operate in the background, to be brought to awareness only when things go awry.

From the perspective of communication rules, we can now understand why some couple therapies are interminable. In many cases, therapists have been serving as keepers of the rules—out of the awareness of the couple, though usually with their tacit consent. In order to bring the therapy to a positive close, we must make these implicit functions explicit and transfer responsibility for their maintenance to the couple.

The Performance Debate

Some clinicians have expressed skepticism about the value of teaching communication skills. They observe that many people "communicate" and behave well with strangers or with colleagues, so it can't be that they just lose this learned behavior in their marriages. These critics, including noted therapists Wile (2013b), and Greenberg and Goldman (2008), submit that the marital problem is not a lack of knowledge, but the challenge of *applying* that knowledge when distressed or angry. And Gottman and Levenson (1999) add the observation that when healthy couples fight, they don't resemble couples using structured empathic listening (as in the speaker–listener technique). These critics question the value of simplistic relationship education and stress the "performance problem" of clients who know better, but behave badly. There are a number of compelling counterarguments to these observations.

People are actually not skillful everywhere else. As well demonstrated by the work of the Harvard Program on Negotiation (Fisher, Ury, & Patton, 2011; Stone et al., 2010), we consistently observe that people in other settings (politics, labor relations, business deals) do *not* know the rules or the relevant vocabulary that might help them when the conversational going gets tough. Contrary to the argument that people only regress at home, we frequently observe similar skill deficits in other conflict situations. We also find business booming for consultants who advise clients on how to manage nonmarital conflicts.

Pressure always exaggerates deficits. Skill deficits will be more obvious when clients are more emotionally distraught. As anyone who has competed in sports knows, it is the fundamentally weak aspects of a person's game that break down under pressure. While it may appear that people are competent in some settings, their skill deficits may appear only during more rigorous testing.

People can be trained to be more skillful under pressure. That performance declines under pressure does not mean that people should not or cannot learn how to function better when stressed. Every athlete with a game on the line will be nervous, every speaker giving an important speech will feel his or her heart pumping, and every person with wounded pride will be upset. Learning how to combat unruly feelings can help people to hit the first fairway, engage the audience confidently, and stick to productive communication strategies when negotiating a deal or arguing with a spouse.

Skill deficits lead to avoidance and interfere with learning to do better. People who have experienced themselves as unable to manage their emotions will avoid them. As noted by Wachtel (2014):

> Learning to express our affects in ways that are socially appropriate, emotionally satisfying, and consonant with our larger life goals is a task that is, in fact, ongoing throughout life . . . When we become afraid of those affects, however, we are deprived of the opportunity to hone our skills in expressing and containing them; and, ironically, we then have more reason to be afraid of them. This creates a self-perpetuating circle in which avoidance creates reason to avoid and hence still more avoidance ad infinitum.
>
> *(pp. 91–92)*

Knowing predictable mistakes helps. We cannot eliminate maladaptive accusations and defensiveness through didactic teaching or moral prescription, but we can give names to various mistakes, point out their costs, and work to help couples resist the temptation to yield to their siren songs.

Skills need not be "natural." Most couples do not use well-defined communication rules spontaneously, but the same can be said for many behaviors and technological advances that, once adopted, have proved beneficial, such as antisepsis during surgery. Across many areas of life, arguing that what is "natural" should be the gold standard makes little sense and, if applied generally to humans, would have us still living in caves and foraging for food. Naturalistic studies of couples might find them rarely using optimal methods of relating, but this may be because they have never learned how to do better.[2]

Skills may be implicit or semiconscious. Many naturalistic studies show more-satisfied couples behaving quite differently from less-satisfied couples. Although we should not hold what is "natural" as our gold standard, studying healthy couples can show us what makes things run smoothly, just as one might study the biomechanics of champion athletes. Indeed, Gottman's most recent research (2011) shows that his more adept couples—his "masters of relationships"—"attune," "turn toward each other," and follow many other constructive communication strategies far more than do his dysfunctional couples. Often, skills training amounts to teaching dysfunctional couples to consciously employ communication strategies that healthier couples follow semiconsciously.

It's not just semantics. While some of this debate over skills training may be semantic—such as how much of what we call psychotherapy is also relationship education—my experience has been that many couple therapists (including my former self) fail to appreciate the value of explicitly teaching couples such things as the benefits of slowing down and following certain conversational rules when the going gets tough.

Having made the case for adding skills training to the therapeutic toolbox, I now proceed to the nuts and bolts of relationship education.

GUIDELINES FOR TEACHING RELATIONSHIP SKILLS

Provide Lessons, Practice, and Homework

Like all teachers giving private lessons, we must individualize our instruction based on each couple's specific strengths and weaknesses; we won't be teaching everything to everyone. Most of the skills we will be teaching do not come naturally or easily. We will often need to repeat our instructions and then ask clients to repeat them back to us. And we can expect couples to relapse and revert to bad habits when they are under pressure (Carlson, Guttierez, Daire, & Hall, 2014; Cornelius & Alessi, 2007). Because new moves will not be learned once and for all, I recommend that clients practice skills between sessions. I also reinforce my message by assigning self-help books pertinent to the skills I am advocating.

Model the Skills

Because many clients have never seen some of the tactics I promote, I often model what one of them might say to the other, and after demonstrating an approach, explain its rationale. This is similar to a dance instructor, piano teacher, or tennis pro demonstrating desirable behavior. Often, this picture is worth a thousand words. Clients who believed that nothing could calm their spouses down are often impressed when they see me accomplish this, and may then become curious about how I did it.

Don't Start Too Soon

Most couples will do better if we allow them to get into the therapy before we start teaching them communication fundamentals. If we start too soon, they may think we don't understand their pain or can't handle the intensity of their feelings.

Don't Wait Too Long

These tools will facilitate our work on process and psychodynamics. A common mistake, especially with volatile couples, is waiting too long to introduce rules for safe communication.

Explain That Rules Promote Helpful Restraint

Most communication rules serve as restraints on maladaptive, spontaneous behaviors, on our proclivity to do what *feels right* when that is precisely the *wrong* thing to do. (Recall how escaping from Chinese finger traps requires us to resist our natural inclinations.) In order to illustrate the utility of communication rules, I use a metaphor from Markman et al. (2001) that compares a nuclear reactor to a couple conversation. In both cases, the key to creating productive energy rather than a destructive meltdown is the internal temperature of the system. And just as the temperature inside the reactor is contained by control rods, so couples' conversational temperature can be controlled by communication rules.

This conceptualization of communication rules as emotional control rods should remind us of Couple Therapy 1.0, in which the therapist was tasked with maintaining an emotional room temperature that was neither too hot nor too cold. We now upgrade that earlier model by teaching couples rules that will allow them to maintain a safe temperature on their own.

Explain Emotional Challenges and Examine Resistances

We should anticipate and discuss the difficulties couples may have following our advice. We will want to offer not only a map of how to act, but also a map of the emotional difficulties clients will encounter when trying to follow our suggestions. Absent such awareness, clients may see our suggestions for skillful couple behavior as simplistic moral platitudes resembling, "Say please and thank you." The failure to attend to these emotional challenges may also explain the limited and sometimes disappointing results of some relationship education programs (Johnson & Bradbury, 2015).

What makes this coaching easier is that most clients will experience our suggestions as sensible and achievable. They will respond favorably to communication skills training because it fits with their (superficial) belief that their problems are, indeed, caused only by "poor communication." They will also like that skills training is backed up by formal research and that the teaching process is more controlled than the free-for-all they've most likely been experiencing.

Nonetheless, some clients will balk from the start, wanting to get on with what seems to them to be more important, and others will seem to go along but will be desultory in complying with our suggestions. Many will find it harder than they had expected. As with other interventions that meet resistance, we should stop and explore the reasons. This will be easier to do after we have clearly described what optimal communication can look like.

Don't Let Your Boredom Discourage You

Teaching communication skills can be boring. I sometimes find myself wanting to skip this slow process and move on to more interesting and emotionally engaging material, but I have learned the value of resisting this urge. I am also sometimes discouraged by empathic embarrassment, as I witness just how much trouble some clients have simply paraphrasing what their partners have just said. But while it may not be emotionally gripping and it is sometimes painful to witness, explicit instruction coupled with supervised practice soon pays off.

Present Yourself as an Expert, a Satisfied Customer, and a fellow Human Being Struggling to Follow the Rules

I tell couples, "I am not only a therapist who has studied couples for many years and seen how successful these skills can be, but I am also a husband who uses them. And even though I teach these skills, I know from experience that following them isn't as easy as it sounds. You should see these recommendations as targets to aim for, but you shouldn't expect to hit them every time."

WHAT TO TEACH

Identify Moves That Are Counterproductive

I usually begin to teach communication skills, organically, by giving names to maladaptive conversational approaches my clients are actually using—ones they think should work, but that are actually making matters worse. I encourage clients to adopt these labels (or create labels of their own) for these tempting-but-maladaptive moves. These forms of fight and flight are familiar to you from earlier chapters. Three labels that regularly get us off to a good start when I identify them in action are: *Disputing the Facts*, as a way to counter a partner's criticisms; *Cross-Complaining*, in order to distract from one's culpability by pointing to one's partner's; and *Getting More Votes*, by pointing out that others agree with one's position.

Remember the Three C's

After noting some particular mistakes that a couple makes, I encourage them, instead, to try to maintain three attitudes that are foundational to all communication rules: When the going gets tough, try to be *calm, curious, and caring*. I encourage my clients to memorize these *Three C's* and take them to heart.

Remaining calm supports the other attitudes and, so, comes first. Curiosity about oneself and one's partner may forestall reflexive, critical judgments. It goes hand in hand with caring as, among other things, it allows people to give their partners the benefit of the doubt. Clients will do better if they preface statements with, "I could be wrong, but the way I remember it is . . ." Caring protects the relationship from the damage that can be done by focusing narrowly on self-interest. Caring fits with a central question partners should ask: not "What's best for me?" but "What will be best for our relationship?" Ideally, *we want clients to ask their partners, "How can I help?"*[3] *As we encourage clients to be calm, curious, and caring, we can remind ourselves that teaching specific rules will simultaneously help them to maintain these attitudes.*[4]

At a Fork in the Road, Stop and Think

I next stress what is arguably the most important relationship skill: to slow down and recognize that what you do next, at this metaphorical fork in the road, can impact your relationship for good or for ill.[5] Just as you slow down when driving conditions become perilous, you need to slow down to avoid an "accident" with your spouse. Terry Real (2007) uses the same metaphor, and a touch of humor, in capturing this idea:

> When immature parts of your personality become triggered—either the wounded, overwhelmed part of you or the defensive, entitled part—in

your mind's eye, take that child in your lap, put your arms around him, love him . . . and take his sticky hands off the steering wheel.

(p. 79)

After this introduction to communication rules, I move on, as appropriate, to more specific recommendations. In what follows, I first outline useful rules and follow these with discussions of the emotional difficulties in adhering to them.

Follow These Rules Before Beginning

1. *Remind yourself of your ultimate goals, and separate them from your immediate, reflex-driven impulses.* This is the premier guideline to keep in mind from beginning to end.
2. *Decide whether you really need to talk. Ask yourself whether changing something in your behavior might improve things substantially.* Unilateral change is an important alternative to difficult conversations. Being aware of this option can give hope to clients whose partners refuse to participate in the process (Weiner-Davis, 2002). Unilateral changes include:

    - *Reward your partner for behavior you like.* Try to "catch" your partner when he or she does what you want and comment on it: "It was a big help to me that you emptied the dishwasher. I really appreciate it." You may feel that you should not have to ask for or reward good behavior, so this may feel forced at first, but rewarding actions that are in the right direction works surprisingly well, not just for the specific, rewarded behavior, but for the overall atmosphere of the relationship.
    - *Do things your partner would like ("unilateral behavioral exchanges").* Start doing things you know your partner would like you to do and resolve not to be discouraged if the initial response is, "It's about time!" or "I told you so!"
    - *Work to increase your personal happiness, independent of the relationship.* If you increase your happiness by taking care of yourself and your life, you will be more pleasant to be with, less likely to draw criticism, less vulnerable to whatever criticism may come, and more accepting of your partner's shortcomings. Ask yourself if your complaint about your spouse is really some displaced problem of your own that you should deal with. Working on your self-esteem, transference allergies, and acceptance of your partner's imperfections can also be accomplished with the help of personal therapy that may then benefit the marriage.

3. *Make a plan.* Not planning is planning to fail. Most people don't prepare; they simply begin talking, either when they are triggered or when they just can't stand it anymore. It is best to clarify beforehand what you hope to accomplish. Anticipate your partner's responses and think about how to

address them. Consider which aspects of the conversation might threaten a positive view of yourself and your partner. Rehearse the conversation, playing both sides.
4. *Remember that there is fair fighting and dirty fighting.* Dirty fighting may feel good in the short run, but will not be good in the long term.
5. *Be aware of your hot buttons.* If one of these is the issue, acknowledge this when you begin, "I know I'm more sensitive about this than most people, but . . ."
6. *Don't put off talking for too long.* Soft start-ups and perfect timing are preferable, but some criticisms can't be sugarcoated and some need to be addressed promptly. Remind yourself that avoiding conflict altogether causes devitalization and unhappiness in marriage (Hawkins & Booth, 2005). If you wait too long, you may become so full of resentment that you explode counterproductively.
7. *Don't expect quick or easy solutions.* Expect and plan for the likelihood that your partner will see things differently and may behave in aggravating ways.

Only One Person Speaks at a Time

Therapists should clarify to clients the distinct roles of speaker and listener and stress that a person should take on only one of these roles at a time. Just as baseball teams alternate playing offense (batting) and defense (pitching/fielding), and never do both simultaneously, so spouses must take turns speaking and listening. When clients are consciously aware of which role they are playing, they are better able to concentrate on the specific demands of that role. One way to help clients take turns is to use a tangible prop to designate who has "the floor"—I use a small pillow—and encourage them to use such a prop at home.

Listening Is Active and Empathic

I discuss skillful listening before skillful speaking because it is more important in facilitating couple communication and preventing negative cycles. Active and empathic listening is not easy. It is a frequent casualty of negative interaction cycles, as indicated by the quip that, "The only people who really listen to an argument are the neighbors!" It means not just letting your partner speak, but refraining from silently constructing rebuttals or counterattacks at the same time. Ideally, the listener has one goal: to understand the partner's position from the partner's perspective; in laboratory experiments, accuracy of empathy correlates with, among other things, reduced physical and psychological aggression between partners (Cohen, Schulz, Liu, Halassa, & Waldinger, 2015). This creative work of empathic immersion is what makes active listening "active." In this book for therapists, these are obvious points, but they must be stated explicitly to clients, along with suggestions concerning how to succeed.

Following Michael White (2009), I encourage clients to describe a time when someone took a strong "embodied interest" in them, demonstrating deep understanding, support, and compassion. Recalling such occasions can help them identify with and behave like that person—as an active, supportive listener.

The Benefits of Empathic Listening

Clients learn the benefits of active listening firsthand after becoming better listeners in our offices. We can motivate them in this effort by mentioning the following benefits, when they are relevant.

- Much of the panic that powers negative cycles derives from feeling alone and unheard. When people are upset, often they just want someone to listen and validate their feelings. When those needs are met, calm and reason return. Further discussion or problem solving may not be needed. Genuine apologies are only possible when you fully understand the details of how your partner experienced an offense.
- Although empathy and assertiveness may seem incompatible, that is a mistaken dichotomy. Even in very contentious bargaining, it is essential that those on each side understand what their opponents consider their vital interests and why. Listening carefully to the other side helps one to make one's own case more coherently, comprehensively, and understandably.
- A person who has been able to speak and feel heard is more willing to allow his or her partner to do the same.
- Active listening helps, regardless of whether subsequent steps by the listener include sympathetic validation ("Oh, now I see why you were so upset"), apology ("I'm so sorry I let you down"), or continued disagreement and negotiation ("OK, now I think I understand your side; let me try to explain mine").
- Detailed, empathic listening is not just for difficult conversations. Applied to one's partner's reporting of the events of the day—from stresses to triumphs—it is the stuff of intimacy and closeness.

Rules for the Listener[6]

1. *Try hard to put yourself in your partner's shoes; tune in to his or her channel.* Try to feel what the speaker is feeling. Remember or imagine being in a similar position. Think about what hidden issues are active and what hot buttons have been pushed. Above all, listen "with an open heart," as you would with a good friend who is upset (Fishbane, 2010).

2. *Don't interrupt.* There are exceptions to this rule (described below), but there should be only minor interruptions of the main event: allowing your partner to speak and be heard.
3. *Hold your problem solving.* Because solutions might provide immediate relief, it is tempting to offer them, but this temptation must be resisted. Instead, problem solving must wait until the speaker has had time to ventilate and feel heard, and because productive problem solving must be informed by a detailed understanding of the issues. Rushing to problem solving (done more frequently by men) is one of the most common ways to short-circuit optimal listening. By contrast, following this recommendation to wait often leads to rapid improvement in couple communication. Asking clients to recall a time when they experienced unsolicited advice as unwelcome can help make this point stick.
4. *If you feel like objecting or rebutting, or are just waiting your turn to do so, don't; think of yourself, instead, as a news reporter.* Good reporters don't have to agree with a violent criminal or a despot; they need to get their stories and expose their thinking. Rather than imagining yourself as a courtroom lawyer jumping up to shout, "I object, Your Honor!" think of yourself as a reporter trying to get the inside story.
5. *If you think your partner has the facts wrong, it is usually preferable to let his or her version of the story stand, and remain curious about why the facts have been misrepresented—for instance, to express the intensity of hurt feelings.* The inclination to rebut is based on the regressive, erroneous belief that if something is not refuted immediately, it is "admitted into evidence" and has been tacitly accepted as fact.
6. *Don't cross-examine.* Again, don't play the courtroom lawyer: "You seem to think this is my fault. But surely you must agree that you made far more mistakes than I did!" Your goal should be to learn from your partner, not to prove him or her wrong.
7. *If your partner's position seems overly harsh, unfair, or irrational, assume that upsetting underlying issues have been activated, and try to discover what they are.* View your partner's painful insults as indicators of intense distress rather than as how he or she really judges your character. Remember that people only yell after their conventional requests have failed.
8. *Don't be fooled or put off by an intense argument over a seemingly trivial matter. Use it to point you toward important concerns that, almost certainly, explain the intensity.*
9. *Keep in mind that there is almost always truth on both sides of a heated argument; try hard to learn the truth on the other side.*
10. *Check your understanding from time to time by paraphrasing what you've heard.* For instance, "If I understand you correctly, you were really angry when I ... because ... ." Don't wait too long to do this, lest you be seen as just waiting to make your rebuttal. Don't assume that your partner will interpret

your lack of protest as assent. When people are upset, they're looking for validation, even if it is simply an acknowledgment that their message has been received.

11. *When paraphrasing, begin by stating the main feeling that is preoccupying your partner.* For instance, "You were really sad when ..." Doing this almost guarantees getting off to a good start.
12. *When paraphrasing, try to state the "moral" of the story your partner is relating.* This will help you avoid becoming bogged down in disputes over "the facts," since errors and exaggerations are actually clues to the main message.
13. *When paraphrasing, be sure to maintain eye contact and watch your partner's body language.* Body language is a good indicator of whether you are on target.
14. *Do not force your partner to go on and on about things you would concede to be true.* This is one of those times to interrupt, by saying, "That's a good point," "Yes, I was late," or "You're absolutely right, I was wrong to do that!" Listeners commonly accept that they must *wait their turn*, but then wait impassively, with poker faces, possibly fearing that conceding anything will weaken their positions. This generates needless anxiety in speakers who will think they need to keep making their case about a particular point. Congregants in some Baptist churches offer an excellent example of active listening, showing their agreement with the preacher with frequent exclamations of "Amen!" There are far too few "amens" when troubled couples talk to each other.[7]
15. *If you are in partial agreement with what your partner has said, try to build on that, rather than emphasizing its flaws; use "and" rather than "but."* "I certainly agree we need to do something about our finances, *and* I think we might extend your suggestion by ..."
16. *When you don't agree with your partner, be sure to show you have received the message about what the problem is.* If you can do so honestly, say that you agree that your partner has a legitimate right to feel differently from you: "Although it doesn't bother me so much to be kept waiting, you are justified in being upset."
17. *Answer your partner's invisible questions:* "Are my feelings OK?" "Do you understand them?" "Do you care about them?" *"Do you care about me?"* (Stone et al., 2010).
18. *Recast intense attacks on you as attacks on the problem, and restate what you have come to see as that problem from your partner's perspective* (Fisher et al., 2011).
19. *If you find yourself struggling to follow the listening rules because of difficult emotions, try to identify, manage, and make use of your feelings.* Listeners should consider which relationship hot buttons might have come online and, most of all, try to meet the emotional challenges of being a good listener, which we will discuss next.

The Emotional Challenges of Empathic Listening

Using the active, empathic listening rules just described usually results in more cooperation and less defensiveness, as they directly counter many of the common pitfalls of maladaptive discussions, such as invalidation, stonewalling, and contempt (Markman, Stanley, & Blumberg, 2001). As productive conversation continues, both participants will find it easier to manage their emotions. Improved communication via empathic listening can unfreeze distancing partners who have become convinced that their partners cannot be reasoned with or influenced. While such partners may have seemed to be listening before, many have only been passively acquiescing, all the while secretly building resentment as they waited for their pursuing spouses to tire of the conversation. Therapists who instruct such contemptuous distancers to take an *active* stance in listening can often show them that their partners' seeming irrationality and intransigence lessens when they are being accurately understood.

While the benefits of active listening can be almost instantaneous, the challenge for most listeners will be to cope constructively with the emotions stirred up as they listen. As we have discussed in previous chapters, profound concerns—often hidden and unconscious—may be aroused in difficult conversations. *Once therapists have spelled out the rules as targets to aim at, their task will be to help clients manage the emotional challenges these rules present.* Just as having a target in sports (a basket, a fairway, a strike zone) assists both coach and player in working toward mastery, so defining the goals for active listening helps us identify constraints and work toward improvement.

The fundamental emotional challenge for the active listener is to maintain an empathic connection with someone who is upset, often, specifically, with you. To do this, the listener must be able to be distressed enough to care—including to care to make the effort to understand—but not so distressed as to need to flee or silence the speaker. Empathy requires us to put ourselves in the other person's situation without becoming overwhelmed. If your wife cries when she tells you her mother has been diagnosed with cancer, or your husband rages about his boss, you must not be too upset to listen because you can't stand to see your wife cry or your husband yell. Listening to strong emotions like hopelessness, anger, and anxiety present specific (countertransference) challenges, which can become our focus when we are helping clients become better active listeners.

To help clients (more often men) to be better listeners, I remind them of the scene from the film, *A League of Their Own,* where Jimmy Dugan (Tom Hanks), the manager of a professional women's baseball team, insults one of his players: "Well I was just wonderin' why you would throw home when we got a two-run lead. You let the tying run get on second base and we lost the lead because of you! Start using your head! That's the lump that's three feet above your ass!" When she bursts into tears, Dugan famously declares, "There's no crying in baseball!" Dugan's patently absurd attempt to banish distressing feelings allows me to point out that some clients have similar troubles managing specific distressing emotions and try, instead, to declare them illegal. I then work with them, as discussed in Chapter 9 on projective identification, to help them contain their own distressing feelings.

That said, therapists should keep in mind that it can be challenging to remain empathic with a person who voices the same complaints ("My boss is so mean!" "My mother always asks me to do too much!" "I hate my job!") day after day. In such situations, we should be empathic with, and lend support to, listeners who are understandably motivated to try to persuade speakers to change behaviors that lead to the chronic stress.

Listening to Criticism

Criticism may be fair or unfair. If the speaker's critique is legitimate, the ideal listener will be able to accept personal responsibility without becoming overwhelmed by guilt or shame. *Difficult conversations are difficult because they force us not just to face another person, but to face ourselves*—"Maybe I *am* too selfish," or "My brother's right: No woman *has* ever loved me." Because such conversations force us to look at ourselves in the mirror, many clients are tempted to either look away or rebuff the spouse who is forcing them to look. They must learn, however, that "Working to keep negative information about ourselves out of awareness during a difficult conversation is like trying to swim without getting wet!" (Stone et al., 2010, p. 112). Whatever it is that is there, we have to face it.

In the case of unfair criticism, the ideal listener will be able to manage the feeling of being unfairly blamed by realizing that the criticism conceals some other issue. The listener can then try to discover what is actually upsetting the speaker.

Besides helping listeners manage their emotions (as discussed in the psychodynamics chapters, for instance, by uncovering a sensitivity to being told what to do), therapists can offer several educational suggestions. One is to propose that clients visualize setting a physical boundary between themselves and their critics—a fence (Fishbane, 2010) or a windshield (Real, 2007). Or we can teach clients to recast strong personal attacks as attacks on the problem. Here, the assumption is that the vociferous attack reflects the erroneous belief that the listener is perversely opposing some sensible solution. The listener can respond, instead, by depersonalizing the attack and clarifying the actual disagreement about how to move ahead.

Most generally, helping listeners meet the challenges of listening shows them that they can "consider the other without the automatic fear of losing themselves" (Ringstrom, 2014, p. 203).

How Long Should Speakers Speak and Listeners Listen?

Speakers should be encouraged not to speak too long. This makes it easier for listeners to paraphrase, to keep up in the conversation, and to wait their turn. Nonetheless, many speakers have a hard time confining themselves to a few sentences or even a few paragraphs. This is especially true when they have pent-up, emotionally intense things to say. If we loosen the requirement that speakers should always speak briefly and that listeners should paraphrase often, couples may find it easier to stick to our conversational rules outside our offices. Discussions in which speaker and listener alternate frequently feel safer, but they can also feel overly controlled and sterile, with the result that partners feel they never really get to vent or present their case.

A related rule modification allows listeners to cut in judiciously to report their distress about having to listen for too long. As Wile (2013b) aptly notes:

> But the more you force yourself to sit there quietly while your partner misrepresents you, lectures you, or makes unfair charges, the angrier and more dispirited you become and the less you'll be able to listen. By the time you get a chance to talk, you may have built up so much resentment that you throw a tantrum. Or you may have become so demoralized that you no longer feel like saying anything at all. So here's the problem: If you interrupt your partner, he or she may become an angry or dispirited person who can't listen; if you don't interrupt your partner, you may become an angry or dispirited person who can't listen.
>
> *(para. 13–14)*

In an ideal world, partners would adjust the frequency of their back-and-forth comments to address these complications; in real life, some imperfection can be expected.

Rules for Opening Difficult Conversations

According to Gottman and Levenson (1999), the outcome of an argument can be predicted 96% of the time from watching only the first three minutes, so the opening is critical.

1. *Be prepared (as previously described).*
2. *Get permission to talk and choose a good time to do so.* Couples should not try to talk when either person is too tired or has been drinking, or when children are within earshot. E-mail and text-messaging are not acceptable workarounds.
3. *If you expect an extended conversation, set an upper limit on how long you will talk.* Knowing that a challenging conversation has a time limit makes it

easier to agree to talk and to participate, as in, "I'd like to find a free hour for us to talk about Matthew's school work."

4. *Tell your spouse that your relationship is important to you.* Say that it's far more important than who washes the dishes or who walks the dog.
5. *Own your requests, rather than cloaking them in appeals to virtue or logic.* I-statements, when used correctly, remind speakers not to hide behind rules, virtue, or absolutes, and encourage them to acknowledge the feelings they are expressing are *theirs*, as in "I was hurt when you forgot my birthday." People who don't get this point will misuse them, as in, "I feel that you're a jerk!"
6. *Criticize your spouse's actions, not his or her character.* "Be hard on the problem, soft on the person" (Fisher et al., 1981). It's easier to change "what you do with your dirty clothes" than "how thoughtless you are."
7. *When requesting a change, state clearly what you want the other to do the next time the situation arises.* Criticism is easier to accept if a solution is offered; "would likes" are easier to listen to than "don't likes."
8. *When giving feedback, stress that you are open to persuasion ("Correct me if I'm wrong . . .") and that you are taking responsibility for your own feelings about what you thought happened ("What it seemed like to me . . .").*
9. *To make a simple request for change, use a "criticism sandwich." Begin with a compliment, say what you would like done differently, and end on a positive note.* My wife is a master at this. Even when I see what's coming, her sugar helps the medicine go down: "Art, you're such a good father to help Cindy with her geometry homework. I do think, though, that she doesn't need to learn the whole course this week. I'm sure you understand she also needs time for her other assignments. Thanks, Honey."
10. *For somewhat more detailed, but still relatively brief, complaints, use Real's "feedback wheel" (2007):*

    a. Describe what you saw or heard, as if a video camera had recorded it.
    b. Describe what you "made up" about this, how you interpreted what you observed.
    c. Describe how you felt, based on your observations and construal.
    d. Describe what you want to happen next, what your partner can do differently in the future.

    For example: "(a) Just now when you were on the phone with Becky for ten minutes when I was waiting to watch a video with you, (b) I 'made up' that I'm not very important to you. (c) This made me angry with you and a bit anxious about our relationship. (d) The next time, I'd appreciate if you would end the call more quickly or, if it's something that can't wait, tell me and then go back to the call." The first step carefully presents objective facts that, hopefully, are not in dispute. The next two steps—"what you made of it" and your feelings—cannot be contested, since it is only the speaker who knows his or her thoughts and feelings. "What should happen in the future" *can* be discussed, and this discussion has begun with the speaker offering a solution. Real's format may seem somewhat stiff, but sticking to it is precisely what makes it safe and, therefore, more likely to be productive.

11. *For most difficult conversations—ones that deal with more extensive, emotionally challenging issues—begin by narrating "the third story" (Stone et al., 2010, pp. 147–162).* The "first story" is your story, the "second" is your partner's, and the "third" is the situation as you imagine a neutral mediator would see it. Talk like a mediator right from the beginning, aiming to outline the gap between the two of you and your divergent stories. For instance, "Jane, you and I seem to have different beliefs about how much money to save." When doing this, you need not soften too much how you feel when telling *your* story, but you must be clear that you know the other person sees things quite differently, and that you are hoping to hear more about those differences. Keep an open mind, reminding yourself that even your version of the third story is *your* version. Although we may *say* that we believe there are two sides to every story, when we are upset, deep down most of us feel sure that we are right and that our partner is selfish, naïve, controlling, or irrational. As noted by Stone et al., this is frequently because we make sense inside the story we are telling ourselves, while we generally haven't yet heard our partner's story.[8]

12. *Emphasize that your first goal is to have a "learning conversation" (Stone et al., 2010). This tells your partner, up front, that you want to hear his or her thoughts.* Since listening is far more disarming than speaking, you will optimize success by working the listening agenda into your opening remarks.

13. *Emphasize that your next goal is to solve the problem, and that you need your partner's help to do that.* This clarifies that neither partner *is* the problem, but both are involved in the shared project of solving the problem. You want to look forward, not back. This means fighting the impulse to take an adversarial approach. In a business setting, each side knows, and is committed to, its own interests. In order to make a deal everyone can accept, each side must learn what is important to the other. We can also apply this model to difficult marital disputes.

14. *If your "story" regarding your partner is very negative, ask your partner to help you understand him or her more favorably.* An example from Stone et al.: "The story I'm telling in my head about what is going on is that you are being inconsiderate. At some level I know that's unfair to you, and I need you to help me put things in better perspective" (2010, p. 156). Once the conversation is underway, the Rules for Continuing Difficult Conversations (below) will prove helpful.

The Emotional Challenge of Opening Difficult Conversations: Assertiveness

When beginning a difficult conversation, many clients avoid voicing their desires directly. They may revert, instead, to citing others who agree with them ("My sister also thinks you should be ashamed of yourself for not visiting my mother!"), especially experts ("Dr. Expert says that husbands ought to . . ."). They may appeal to fairness ("Considering what I've done for you, this isn't asking so much") or love ("If you really loved me, you would . . ."), or they may combine insults with appeals to absolutes ("Any sane person would see it this way!"). Clients sometimes overplay anger or summon crocodile tears—what Greenberg and Goldman (2008) call "instrumental emotions"—or exaggerate psychiatric symptoms or physical disability to manipulate a partner (Haley, 1976). *Most such appeals to friends, relatives, authorities, ethics, and pity serve to conceal the act of asking, the relativism of the request, and the fear of refusal.*

By contrast, when partners believe they have a right to be heard, they are better able to deliver their messages clearly, and their partners are less likely to have to guess what they're saying. Healthy self-regard also allows partners to seek change sooner, before their frustration gives way to rage. Paradoxically, intense anger and fear of its destructiveness may inhibit assertiveness.

Building on this understanding of assertiveness, therapists can assist clients who shy away from asking for change directly. Perhaps they don't feel entitled to ask for what they want. Often, we will uncover internal conflict and negative expectations. Some may be afraid of the power of their anger. Others, anticipating (often correctly) that their partner will not be immediately accommodating, fear the distressing feelings that may ensue. In particular, many fear the pain of narcissistic injury if their partners fail to regard their needs as legitimate and important.

In general, by uncovering specific fears and expectations and teaching ways to succeed without bloodshed, we can help clients ask for what they want, rather than merely encouraging them to stand up for what the therapist or friends and relations see as their rights. In one assertiveness-inhibited couple I treated, both husband and wife feared stating their needs directly, leading to misunderstanding, anger, and disappointment. The husband, we learned, feared traumatizing his wife as he and others in his family had felt traumatized by his domineering, narcissistic father. The wife feared becoming like her mother, who had imposed her idiosyncratic religious preferences on the family. Uncovering these fears, rather than just prescribing directness, helped move the couple away from their fears toward a far happier marriage.

There is considerable variability in just what helps people overcome inhibitions about asserting themselves. For some, simple validation and encouragement will start them moving in the right direction. For others—whose friends constantly exhort them to stop putting up with considerable unfairness in their lives—simple encouragement and skills training are insufficient, and individual psychoanalytically oriented therapy may prove beneficial (see Summers, 1999, pp. 215–250).

Feeling entitled to assert one's desires and feelings helps clients to begin difficult conversations *and* to carry them through. This may sometimes include calling the other out for behaving badly: "Please stop talking to me like that. I'm trying really hard to listen to you and understand why you're upset."

Knowing and following the rules for communicating will further boost partners' confidence in speaking out, because the therapist-given rules give legitimacy to self-assertion and because the rules make successful self-assertion more likely.

Rules for Continuing Difficult Conversations

1. *Rather than merely examining the "facts"—about which you two may well disagree—try to discover where your divergent stories come from.* Be curious. "Help me understand how you see things." "What is most important to you in this discussion?" "Is there something I could do that would make it easier for you to say yes?" (Questions from Fisher & Shapiro, 2005.) Partners must learn to fight their own skepticism, and turn "How can he think that?" into "I wonder what information he has that I don't."
2. *Don't mind-read.* Most people do not like being told what they are feeling, thinking, or trying to do. When arguments erupt over whether a spouse is truly angry, sad, or anxious, it is best to simply share one's observations: "You seem not to want to talk to me tonight; I'm wondering if you're still angry over what happened yesterday." "Your voice is quavering; I'm wondering what you're feeling." As noted by Wile (2012), mind-reading is sometimes really about feelings the speaker is trying to conceal from himself and from others:

    > Mind-reading is often an expression of feelings put in the form of assertions about the other person's feelings. It's a fear or worry stated as a fact. "You're bored to death" might mean "I'm worried I'm boring you." "Why are you so angry at me?" might mean: "I'm worried that you're angry at me. I know I've been withdrawn lately, and I'd be angry if you had disappeared on me that way."
    >
    > *(para. 23)*

3. *Be skeptical and curious about your own story.* Don't assume it's as obvious and unbiased as you initially think.
4. *Take responsibility for your contributions to the problem—sooner, rather than later.*
5. *Don't present your conclusions as truth.* Arguing conclusions is both common and pointless, as in "Couples therapy won't help!" versus "Yes, it will!" Such disputes go nowhere, in part, because neither partner can make a persuasive

argument without addressing the data and thinking that led to the opposite conclusion.

6. *Share the feelings that led to your conclusions by reporting them, rather than venting them.* Much of your story will be unknown to your partner, including your feelings. Trying to avoid mentioning your hurt feelings so as not to damage your relationship risks not letting your partner know what has really been bothering you. But do not assume that your feelings are immutable; they may change as you develop a more complex narrative.

7. *Abandon blame: instead, map the contribution system.* When blame is the goal, understanding is often a casualty. Blaming raises questions about who is responsible, how that person's actions should be judged (e.g., do they reflect a lack of competence or compassion or ethics?), and what punishment he or she deserves (Stone et al., 2010). Blame interferes with understanding by inviting the accused parties to defend themselves, rather than to help solve the problem. Instead of working to assign blame, couples should shift to the softer project of discovering "contributions." Searching for contributions aims couples productively forward to consider what they can do next and how they can prevent the situation from recurring.

8. *Avoid certain language choices*:

    - *Don't use hyperbole: "You always . . ."* or *"You never . . ."* Such statements are rarely true, and can be refuted with a single counterexample. "You often . . ." is less inflammatory.
    - *Don't use one-sided arguments that leave out obvious truths.*
    - *Don't swear or attack the other person's character.*
    - *Don't argue that others agree with you.* Some don't and, in any case, it's irrelevant.
    - *Don't argue that others do it your way.* Again, some don't and it's irrelevant.
    - *Don't argue that you should be forgiven or that the topic should be dropped because your partner is guilty of something similar or equally bad:* Two wrongs don't make a right.
    - *Don't argue from, "Look what I've done for you. You should do this for me."* That may not have been part of the bargain.
    - *Don't argue from, "I do this for you. You should do it for me."* Your circumstances may differ.
    - *Don't argue from, "If you really loved me, you would . . ."* which can easily be countered with, "If you really loved me, you wouldn't ask me to . . ."
    - *Don't argue from absolutes or "shoulds."* There is almost always a countervailing principle.

9. *Convey respect and appreciation; recognize your partner's status, expertise, and positive contributions.*

10. *Stay on topic.* Unrelated and tangential complaints detract from the central issue. This does not exclude mentioning thematically related events, but the

speaker should be clear: "The reason I'm bringing up something that happened ten years ago is that I think it really illustrates what I'm upset about now."

11. *Be concise.* You don't need to say everything all at once. Allow your partner to process and respond to what you have to say, point by point.
12. *Ignore your partner's (distracting) inflammatory comments.* Let these fly metaphorically over your head. Do register the intensity of the feelings behind them.
13. *Ask your partner to paraphrase what you've said so that you both know whether you've been understood.* This asks the other to assume the role of active listener. Even if your partner is way off in understanding you, this request may motivate them to listen more carefully.
14. *Ask your partner for help:* "We seem to have hit a dead end. What do you think we should do?"
15. *Monitor your body language, tone of voice, and couple process, and consider discussing them.* Are you making eye contact, showing interest, registering agreement, giving encouragement or, conversely, tuning out, raising your voice, or conveying impatience or disrespect? This doesn't mean that you should fake your behavior or feelings, but that you should know what they are since your partner will be experiencing them along with whatever content you're trying to convey. Should the process be deteriorating, stop and refocus on the process and underlying hurt feelings. Rather than continuing to debate the facts, say something like, "I'm getting upset about how we're talking to each other. What's that about? What can we do about this?" Then ask yourself, and try to discuss with your partner, what is *really* upsetting you that is making talking so difficult. Here, I am encouraging clients to do what I suggest couple therapists do when the process goes south: to shift from a focus on concrete problem solving to a focus on process and underlying issues.
16. *If you think your partner's core negative image has become activated, work to dispel his or her fear.* "You may be worried that I'm saying that it's my way or the highway like your father did, but I'm really open to hearing what you think." But beware of making angry statements of the form, "I'm NOT your mother!"
17. *Use humor and other repair maneuvers to soften the process, but not as a defense or to express veiled hostility.*
18. *If the conversation isn't going well, return to fundamentals, and try the options below, in the order listed:*

    (a) *Work harder at empathy; unilaterally, take the role of empathic listener and follow the advice for the optimal listener.*
    (b) *Work harder at understanding what is most upsetting you, and share your thoughts with your partner.*

(c) *Recall the tactics for optimal repair conversations and unilaterally shift into repair mode.*
(d) *Work to soothe yourself. If this fails, propose a timeout.*

19. *If the conversation ends without a satisfactory resolution, take a break and try again another time.* Difficult conversations are only rarely one-time events. They are better conceptualized as ongoing dialogs.

Further Emotional Challenges for the Speaker

The overall emotional challenge for the speaker is to convey a need, complaint, or hurt clearly and succinctly, without resorting to simplistic, one-sided, self-righteous, blame-filled narratives. We covered some challenges to doing this above, in the discussion of assertiveness. People who have trouble asking for things in general will have a hard time "asking nicely" and persistently should they meet resistance.

Speakers who have less trouble with assertiveness must contain the inclination to go on and on, adding one complaint on top of another, (seemingly) strengthening their cases with more and more evidence. Many clients will have to refrain from exaggerating or leaving out details that would make the account more balanced. When emotions run high, speakers must resist the urge to attack in anger or to break off the discussion in a huff. Much of couple therapy involves not so much teaching clients sound rules for speaking, but helping them follow the rules we advocate.

Too Many Rules?

Having nearly completed reading this section, you may be thinking, "How in blazes can I possibly teach all those rules to my clients? I can't even remember them myself!" Of course, there are too many rules here for a single lesson—for therapists or for clients. However, given the complexity of human behavior, the number of ways things can go wrong in difficult conversations is staggering, so that the number of ways to tackle these errors effectively is almost equally numerous. So, do not despair! No therapist needs to teach all the rules to all clients. After teaching some fundamentals, you should only teach the rules that apply to your clients' specific missteps.

In order to help clients learn and retain the rules, I give them handouts that state the rules and the reasoning behind them. (Feel free to copy material from this chapter.) While it is impossible and counterproductive to have all the rules in mind while carrying on a difficult conversation, over time and with practice, many clients find the rules come to make sense and become automatic.

The Impact of Teaching Speaking and Listening Rules

When couples adhere to these prescriptive communication rules, what occurs frequently surprises them and convinces them of their value. Simply put, when they stick to these apparently constraining formats, they will almost always reach greater depths of emotional expression, understanding, and felt connection. EFT and psychodynamic couple therapists should note that these deeper, transformative states routinely emerge when couples hold themselves to positive rules for difficult conversations. As common defenses are blocked and empathic listening is encouraged, spouses feel safe to unburden themselves about their deepest worries, injuries, and concerns. Teaching speaking and listening rules to couples is almost universally helpful, as it quickly blocks their natural inclinations to be forming rebuttals rather than listening closely to what their partners are saying. Not infrequently, clients experience greater intimacy than they have in a very long time, sometimes more than they have ever experienced together.

As partners struggle to adhere to these rules, they see just how hard it is to keep one's own agenda out of their attempts at empathic paraphrasing and how attentive they must be in order to summarize what they hear each other say.

Teaching specific rules is especially useful for clients who have given up on their efforts to interact with their angry or tearful partners. Such clients have become convinced that nothing they can do will help. As a result, they remain passive, which induces their partners to intensify what amount to cries for help. Teaching communication rules is one of the quickest ways I have found to challenge such transference helplessness.

Teaching skills also helps convince the partners of such previously passive spouses that their spouses have been passive because they believed nothing would work, rather than because they did not love them or care about the marriage. The experience of seeing the rules help the passive spouse to engage routinely counters the pursuing partner's negative transference expectations.

Most generally, teaching communication rules can facilitate behaviors that disconfirm patient negative transferences. As noted by Wachtel (2014) in his theory of "cyclical psychodynamics," change can begin with either changed behavior or changed beliefs, with change in one leading to change in the other. Here, improved communication behavior is followed by better working models of the partners.

Tasneem and Anil: Teaching Communication Rules

Tasneem, a petite, well-mannered, soft-spoken elementary school teacher, always seemed at a loss when listening to Anil, her domineering cardiac surgeon husband. While Anil's previous psychodynamic psychotherapy had been very helpful, he still had some areas of sensitivity and was highly reactive when

Tasneem touched them. In most couple sessions, Anil would talk circles around Tasneem, storming at her insensitivity and stupidity. His criticisms were almost always that she wasn't doing enough for him and that she wasn't appreciative of what he did for her. At his worst, Anil would suggest that he was going to leave her for a woman who would be able to meet his needs.

Tasneem's approach to these tirades was to wait until Anil gave her an opening. She would then offer a quiet, rather sanctimonious, rebuttal of some selected facts on which he had based his criticisms.

After I coached her in active listening, she became much more capable of managing his critical attacks by meeting them with sincere efforts at understanding, rather than with invalidation and rebuttal. This was a big help to him, as he experienced her as truly listening—unlike his parents, but like what he had appreciated in his individual therapist. Tasneem's newfound competence simultaneously helped her realize she did not need to be a passive target of verbal abuse, as she had been as a child when her revered father had berated her. Teaching Tasneem ways to start difficult conversations, especially the use of the "third story," also gave her the courage to act, rather than waiting passively when she wanted some changes in their marriage.

Final Thoughts About Teaching Communication Skills

With clients like Anil and Tasneem, parental failures not only resulted in pessimism about the possibility of success in interpersonal tight spots, they have simultaneously failed to offer models for how to cope with such challenges. Children whose parents did not know how to manage emotional distress within and between people will not have learned those skills from their parents and may never have learned them elsewhere. Some clients, in identification with their parents, will have learned counterproductive behaviors. Others will have had parents who managed conflict well, but who (appropriately) did so outside the hearing of their children, and these children, too, may not have learned how to manage conflict. Consequently, in situations of deficient or maladaptive learning, I now believe it essential to teach constructive behavior explicitly.

Having learned communication skills in our offices, do couples actually use them? Some of my clients make conscious use of the skills outside my office, and others do not. Even if they don't use the rules formally or precisely, most of them internalize the essential, underlying principles: They are aware that they should slow down, that they must be careful when they come to a fork in the road, and that their behavior can help or hurt their relationship. They know that they must take turns listening empathically and speaking respectfully. And many make an effort to remain calm, curious, and caring. It is not perfection, but it is progress. In the next two chapters we add some additional educational interventions that will help clients manage difficult discussions.

Notes

1 Because the majority of the interventions in Part IV were developed by therapists who identify themselves as "behavioral," I have titled it Behavioral/Educational Upgrades. Absent that history, I would have designated the section Relationship Educational Upgrades. While all couple therapists seek "behavioral change" (e.g., less swearing and more cooperating), what differentiates the interventions in this section is not so much their focus on "behaviors," but the way they seek to influence clients to alter their behaviors, namely by direct instruction.
2 See Stanley, Bradbury, and Markman (2000) for a more extensive rebuttal of Gottman's dismissal of teaching relationship skills because they are not observed in healthy, non-clinical couples. Gottman, himself, implicitly contradicts this critique of skills training, since his books and programs are full of admonitions to couples about how to relate productively (e.g., Gottman & Silver, 1999).
3 A study of 51 happily married couples by Rauer and Volling (2013) supports the critical importance of being "caring" during difficult conversations. The authors found that relatively frequent bad behavior (dominance, denial, or conflict) by one or both partners in a problem-solving discussion could be neutralized or compensated for by high levels of partner support.
4 In their wonderful book on parenting, Siegel and Bryson (2015) make recommendations for approaching a misbehaving child that are strikingly similar to my Three Cs. They emphasize helping (caring for) the child via empathic connection which requires parents to restrain their reflexive negative reactions (remain calm) and, instead, "Chase the why" (become curious).
5 In one study, encouraging couples to be "relationship aware"—by simply having them watch and discuss commercial films depicting other couples—was shown to be as effective in improving marital happiness and longevity as more extensive relationship education interventions (Rogge et al., 2013).
6 The communication rules here owe much to Markman, Stanley, and Blumberg (2001) and their speaker–listener technique (summarized here). **Rules for the speaker:** Speak for yourself. Don't be a mind reader. Don't go on and on. Stop and let the listener paraphrase. **Rules for the listener:** Paraphrase what you hear. Focus on what the speaker is saying. Don't rebut. **Rules for both:** The speaker has the floor. Share the floor. No problem solving.
7 This recommendation fits with the observation by Gottman et al. (1998) that the ratio of positive statements to negative among "masters of relationships" was 5:1 during conflict conversations, compared to distressed couples, whose ratio was 1:1. This finding is often mistakenly quoted as applying to periods between fights, but was actually observed during prescribed conflict conversations. This finding of the benefits of positivity during conflict has been replicated many times (Bradbury & Karney, 2010, pp. 336–339).
8 Elaborating the "third story" is widely recommended. IBCT therapists refer to helping clients take a position of "unified detachment" (Baucom et al., 2008). Psychoanalyst Jessica Benjamin (2004) describes how therapeutic impasses that have collapsed into "doer and done to" interactions can be repaired by working toward a co-constructed "third" that includes the perspectives of both parties. And experimental support comes from a study by Finkel and colleagues (2013) in which 120 non-clinical couples were randomized to receive or not receive instructions to review couple disagreements "from the perspective of a neutral third party who wants the best for all involved," to reflect on what made it hard for them to do this, and to try harder to do it going forward. Two years later, the couples who had carried out the interventions showed clear benefits.

12
TEACHING EMOTION REGULATION

In the last chapter, I cited remaining calm as one of the emotional challenges that arises in difficult conversations. This is hard to do and is a major reason we couple therapists are in business. In this chapter, I discuss educational interventions that can help clients gain control of their emotions *in the moment*, precisely when they are losing control. These techniques work for all negative emotions, including anxiety, hopelessness, and (most important) reactive anger. They help to down-regulate overwhelming emotional reactions, thereby enabling individuals to access more adaptive thoughts and actions.

Focusing on the Dysregulated Partner

The self-control and self-soothing skills I cover here target the spouse who is upset, out of control, or stonewalling, and place more responsibility for marital strife on him or her. Dysregulated clients often describe themselves as being "overtaken" by overwhelming feelings, or say their anger "flared up," blaming their partner as the inciting cause. We need to help them own their feelings and also examine what was going on inside them that they used to justify losing control (Goldner, 2004).

Brent Atkinson (2005), one of the leading proponents of teaching emotion regulation skills, explains the value of this approach:

> Often, therapists make progress with couples by going back and forth, softening one partner a little bit, then softening the other, then back to the first partner, and so on. As each partner experiences the other as a bit more willing to give, they become more willing themselves, and things gradually get better . . . It is possible for marriage therapy to

"succeed" without either partner developing any more ability to respond well when feeling misunderstood or mistreated . . . Those who believe that things improved because the therapist got their partners to change often leave couples therapy with an uneasy feeling about their progress. They feel relieved that their partners finally got a clue but also feel just as unable to influence the state of their relationship as they did before therapy. Each of them is haunted by the unspoken question, "What's to keep my partner from starting to treat me poorly again?"[1]

(pp. 5–6)

Steven Stosny (2005, 2006), who has spent his career working successfully with violent men, believes that success depends on helping abusers accept personal responsibility for regulating their emotions. He faults approaches that emphasize teaching victims to be more firm with their boundaries, calling it "the therapeutic equivalent of a judge dismissing your lawsuit against vandals because you failed to put up a 'Do Not Vandalize' sign" (2006, p. 58). He is similarly unimpressed by attempts to teach victims to be less provocative, noting that many perpetrators will react (paradoxically) negatively, viewing such cautious behavior as inherently shaming. Stosny also points out the pitfalls of using insight-oriented work with abusers who may try to pin the blame for further abuse on their painful or deficient childhood: "I know I was mean to you, but with what I've been through, you have to cut me some slack." At bottom, Stosny does not see partner abuse as a systemic or relationship problem, but as due to an intrapsychic deficiency of the abusers who are unable to contain feelings of shame, guilt, or inadequacy.

Goldner, Atkinson, and Stosny have all had considerable experience and success in this area—Stosny with perhaps the most difficult subjects—and their work suggests that we add emotion regulation as an upgrade to our model for doing couple therapy.

Some History of Emotion Regulation in Psychotherapy

Most psychoanalysts consider the ability to calm oneself under fire—like the ability to manage being alone—to be an important outcome of an extensive therapeutic experience (Gehrie, 2011; Wachtel & Wachtel, 1986). Other psychologists have been interested in teaching *specific techniques* for self-control. These include sports psychologists who work to help athletes steady themselves during competition (Gallwey, 1974; Rotella, 1995). In the field of couple therapy, the appeal of coaching people to manage their emotions in the moment derives, in part, from Gottman, Coan, Carrera, and Swanson's (1998) finding that many people become "flooded" and unable to think during difficult conversations. Although this is a common experience and, thus, not really a discovery, Gottman's scholarly focus brought it out of the background of common sense and into the foreground of scientific study.

Interest in the moment-to-moment ability to contain emotional storms has also been stimulated by advances in neuroimaging that allow us to study the brains of people in the throes of powerful emotions. We now know that emotional conditioning happens not only unconsciously, but separately from—and generally faster than—the cortical processing of events (LeDoux, 1996; studies reviewed in Atkinson, 2005)—via pathways LeDoux aptly calls the "low road," which he contrasts with the slower "high road" to the cortex. Thus, our deep-brain, fight-or-flight, intense emotional responses get a head start on our thinking selves. We also know that cortical centers in our frontal lobes exert control over our lower limbic emotional structures. Dan Siegel (2010), a leading investigator in this field, offers a powerful visual image of this: Think of your hand as your brain, with your thumb being the amygdala, and the rest of the fingers being the frontal cortex. When the fingers cover the thumb, your unruly feelings are controlled; when they are raised, you have "flipped your lid" and the thumb/amygdala is unrestrained.

While knowing specific facts about neurophysiology is not yet essential to couple therapy, such "neuroeducation" (Fishbane, 2013) can help clients be less judgmental and more proactive. They can now think, "My amygdala is overreacting, but I know how to calm it down," rather than, "I am a bad, angry person." As Atkinson (2010) points out, such imagery "has a way of softening blame as clients begin to understand that the brain, in its natural, unruly state, does things that its 'owner' may not really want or approve of" (p. 182).

D. Siegel (2010), Solomon and Tatkin (2011), and others interested in the physiology of emotional control have also focused on attachment theory (since children first learn to regulate their emotions through close connection with their caregivers). Therapists who see disrupted secure attachment as the central issue for couples can focus therapy either on partners who fail to provide adequate attachment support (as emphasized by Susan Johnson, 1996), or, the topic of this chapter, on helping the person who has become distraught and dysregulated.

Others have taken inspiration from Buddhist teaching, which stresses the ability to cope with life's adversities through skillful mental practices. An abundance of writing applies "mindfulness" to helping people manage distress during intense conversations, in particular, and in life, generally (Atkinson, 2013; Davison, 2013; Hanson & Mendius, 2009; D. Siegel, 2010; Tolle, 1999). *Mindfulness* can be defined as self-regulated, present-moment awareness that welcomes all experiences, without preconception or judgment, while accepting what is with curiosity and compassion. The ability to be engaged like this in the moment has been found to reduce anxiety and other distressing reactions to past events, current stresses, and future worries (Crapuchettes & Beauvoir, 2011). Mindfulness strategies help people to become more comfortable in the moment, partly by focusing on immediate bodily sensations and partly by clarifying the distinction between experiences and the experiencing self.

Additional valuable contributions to the subject of emotion regulation come from the research of Marsha Linehan and her co-workers (Linehan, 1993; Fruzzetti, 2006) in the development of the school of psychotherapy now known as Dialectical Behavior Therapy (DBT). DBT originated as a set of strategies to help patients with borderline personality disorder to manage their feelings. Because clients in the heat of difficult conversations often resemble dysregulated borderline patients, it is not surprising that techniques developed for one group can help the other. When treating couples in which one partner either qualifies for a borderline diagnosis or simply has great difficulty containing emotions, teaching self-soothing techniques early in couple therapy is especially helpful (Goldman & Greenberg, 2013).

Linehan (1993) notes a particular transference roadblock that arises when one works to help emotionally volatile clients gain control over their feelings:

> Many borderline individuals come from environments where everyone else exhibits almost perfect cognitive control of their emotions. Moreover, these very same others have exhibited both intolerance and strong disapproval of the individual's inability to exhibit similar control. Often, borderline clients will resist any attempt to control their emotions, because such control would imply that other people are right and they are wrong for feeling the way they do. Thus emotion regulation skills can be taught only in a context of emotional self-validation.
>
> *(p. 84)*

Following Linehan's guidance, if we are to succeed in teaching emotion regulation to emotionally volatile clients, we must first acknowledge the validity of their intense feelings.

When studying this vast field—which is both historically ancient and rapidly emerging—one discovers many methods and tactics. All aim to help people take greater responsibility for their emotional reactions and behavior—for feelings of disappointment, shame, guilt, anxiety, sadness, and loneliness at times when expectations are not being met or when feared scenarios are in the offing. Many methods have been proposed to help people calm and soothe themselves; what follows are the ones I have personally found most effective in my work with couples.

Methods for Emotion Regulation/Self-Soothing

1. *Become aware (mindful) of your feelings, name them, and wonder, without judgment, where they are coming from.* Psychoanalysts, mindfulness teachers, DBT therapists, neuroscience influenced therapists, and sports psychologists all instruct clients to slow down and focus nonjudgmentally on simply

describing what is happening as a way to establish some distance when a person becomes overwhelmed by powerful emotions.

In psychoanalysis, this nonjudgmental state is central to free association, and achieving this ability is an important interim goal of psychoanalysis. Just as Freud did, the DBT-informed couple therapist Alan Fruzzetti (2006) recommends that clients focus on "describing rather than judging." This nonjudgmental attitude is also central to "distress tolerance," defined by Linehan (1993) as being able "to perceive one's environment without putting demands on it to be different, to experience your current emotional state without attempting to change it, and to observe your own thoughts and action patterns without attempting to stop or control them" (p. 96). Dan Siegel (2010) encourages a state of mind that he calls "mindsight," a form of calm introspection that allows people to perceive themselves and their partners more objectively. Whatever one calls it, this ability to maintain a nonjudgmental, observing ego during challenging conversations is beneficial. Most often, achieving this state will take considerable work prior to and outside such conversations, whether it be in psychoanalytic psychotherapy or mindfulness meditation.[2]

The self-soothing mindfulness achieves comes about through consciously shifting attention from reflexive, catastrophic evaluations evoked by powerful feelings to detached, nonjudgmental observations.[3] Having attained some distance from their feelings, clients are better able to examine them. *Clients should next name their feelings, as in Siegel's (2010) aphorism "Name it to tame it."* This enables them to become curious about the source and appropriateness of their feelings. Neuroscience influenced therapists, like Atkinson, encourage clients to treat emotional states as if they had minds of their own. The goal is to teach clients to *register* the emotion and then adopt an observational distance that allows them to visualize its informative value while questioning its all-or-nothing, must-act-right-now significance.

This strategy also counters the tendency of some clients to run from their feelings entirely, or to tell themselves not to feel what they are feeling. Instead, by becoming mindful of their feelings, they can move from a mind teeming with feelings ("emotion mind," in DBT terms) to one in which thought can be brought to bear on those feelings ("wise mind").

Certain forms of reflexive, unsettling judgment—"This isn't fair! Why is this happening to me?"—can generally be suspended temporarily. Some patients, however, will need to be assured that this nonjudgmental attitude does not signify ultimate approval. Attempts to suspend judgment and "just observe" will enable them to imagine other perspectives and conclusions, rather than the same old, uniformly negative ones, for example, "I was assuming that he doesn't care, but now I see that although he looks tired, he is actually trying to help me."

2. *Take some deep breaths and relax your muscles.* Deep breathing has been advocated by Buddhists for centuries and by sports psychologists more recently. The activation of the vagus nerve through deep breathing tends to be calming; this can be enhanced through a conscious effort to relax the muscles, which almost invariably become tense in preparation for fight or flight.
3. *Calm yourself by shifting your attention away from what is upsetting you.* Unlike the strategy of mindful, non-critical observation of what is distressing, this amounts to taking a brief timeout. *Shift your attention to some neutral or positively experienced object in your immediate environment—to colors, sounds, or specific objects.* Golfers, for example, are advised to shift their attention to the natural beauty of the course. *Change the subject briefly.* This tactic, which people often employ spontaneously and unconsciously, can be used consciously to restore one's composure. *Take a short break.* Skilled negotiators recommend taking a bathroom break when emotions get out of control. Sports psychologists recommend retying your shoelaces or removing an imaginary pebble from your shoe. Basketball coaches call a team timeout.
4. *Soothe the other person; shift to empathic listening or, better still, to compassionate concern ("caring").* This is a particularly good way to change your focus of attention. Besides shifting your attention away from your personal hurt, this strategy helps calm you by calming your partner who will usually become less provocative. Equally important, if you succeed in seeing things through your partner's eyes, he or she will appear less malevolent, which will decrease your agitation.[4]
5. *Think about whether some personal hot button (core negative image, transference allergy) is in play.* Identifying one may reduce your distress with your partner.
6. *Refocus on your goal and recall your core values.* The discussion in Chapter 11 concerning the fork in the road is relevant here. Students of difficult conversations uniformly advise shifting to a more planful state of mind, which will help hold threatening emotions at bay.
7. *Don't be excessively distracted by your still-powerful feelings.* Just as you can continue to give a speech despite anxiety or keep running when you feel like quitting, so you can stay in a difficult discussion despite being distraught, knowing that the distress is a normal physiological state. To help athletes function under pressure, sports psychologists both normalize the feelings (the distracting uproar of spectators and the swirling thoughts about success and failure) and advise focusing on the goal at hand (making the free throw or sinking the putt). Therapists can help clients work to improve their "affect tolerance," so that they can function even when they are emotionally activated. It is helpful to point out that "self-soothing"—by whatever means—rarely brings one back to a neutral affective state. Accepting this and remaining steadfast despite residual distress counts as an important component of self-soothing.

8. *Tell yourself, "I've been in this situation before and I can handle it."* This is similar to knowing you can function despite being upset or anxious. Recognizing that you have weathered past storms or recalling past successes promotes confidence in dealing with a current challenge. Sports psychologists advocate practicing under imagined pressure—the free throw to win the league championship—so that when the real situation occurs and the game is on the line, athletes can recall that they can perform competently under pressure. This advice from sports psychology reminds us of the value of rehearsing difficult conversations, since rehearsal will leave a positive memory of holding to one's ideas in the face of expected opposition and distressing emotions.
9. *Imagine a physical boundary between you and your partner, allowing you to accept or reject your partner's hurtful words.* The specific image might be a sheet of plexiglass (Hanson & Mendius, 2009), a windshield (Fisher & Shapiro, 2005; Real, 2007), or a fence (Fishbane, 2010). Alternatively, it might be a tree that bends, but doesn't break, as the wind of your partner's anger passes through its leaves (Hanson & Mendius, 2009). These images concretize the psychological truth that our feelings are not the inevitable result of others' characterizations, but depend, also, on our own assessments.
10. *Remind yourself that it is normal for your partner to want things his or her way.* This is not a crime.

Mutual Regulation of Emotion

When couple dances spiral toward dysregulation, partners can also get help down-regulating from each other, the basis for the following suggestions.

11. *When your tactics for self-soothing are insufficiently calming, ask your partner for help. Knowing that empathy will probably be beneficial, ask your partner to tune in to what's driving your distress.* Once clients have been taught communication rules, dysregulated spouses can appeal to their partners to adhere more closely to those rules.
12. *Monitor your partner's emotional state. When you see him or her overheating, think about what has helped in the past and try it.* As noted above, this can be doubly effective because it helps to soothe both partners. *Much of couple therapy can be seen as providing spouses with owners' manuals for their partners, manuals that describe what might help their partners feel less agitated and more content.* Therapists can point out, explicitly, what decreases a partner's distress: "When your wife starts repeating the same complaint over and over, it can help to cut in and tell her that you understand what she's saying and how it makes her feel."
13. *When nothing is working, suggest a timeout.*

Timeouts

If the couple reaches a stalemate or continues to escalate, it can be beneficial to call a timeout. It took me a while to recognize the value of timeouts. Having grown up in a family of conflict-avoiders, I later found salvation in psychoanalysis, which advocated uncovering the feelings and motives that cause trouble if left hidden. This motivated me to become a therapist and helped in my personal life. While the pursuit of hidden issues worked for me personally, I eventually learned that when couples were outside my office and became flooded with emotion, it was often preferable for them to take a break, rather than press on and make matters worse. Encouraging couples to take timeouts and teaching them how have been important upgrades to my practice. In authorizing and advocating for the use of timeouts, we should tailor the discussion to our audience: Distancers need to hear that they must return to talk in the near future; pursuers need to hear that the conversation will resume and not be forgotten. Here are some practical rules for timeouts.

Rules for Timeouts

1. *When things still aren't working and your emotions are out of control—despite your efforts to have a learning conversation, to manage your emotions, and to fight fair—say so and request a timeout to allow you to recover your ability to think clearly and collaborate productively.*
2. *Consider calling a timeout in the following circumstances: when the conversation has gone on for more than an hour without progress, when it is late at night, when one person has something important to do the next day, or when either of you has been drinking heavily.* Most people know that productive conversation under such circumstances is unlikely, but I find it helpful to give clients permission to act on that knowledge.
3. *Take responsibility for calling the timeout and speak respectfully.* Do not say, "You need a timeout!" Say, instead, "I think a timeout would help us regroup."
4. *Include a specific time for reconvening.* "I think I could resume in about an hour," or "I think we should call it a night and continue this discussion tomorrow after dinner [or next Tuesday in our therapist's office] when we can think more productively." This is crucial in allaying pursuing partners' fears that a timeout is a ruse for dropping the discussion for good.
5. *During the recess, calm yourself and review the situation.* Listen to music, take a bath, read a book, take a walk, meditate, or talk to a trusted friend (one you know will steady you and offer sensible feedback). Once your emotions settle sufficiently, think about what to say when the discussion resumes. Writing a letter to your partner may help you focus your thoughts and is an opportunity to vent your anger and let some of it go, but don't send it!

Remind yourself of your constructive goals, reflect on hidden issues, and resolve not to repeat earlier mistakes.
6. *Consider that a formal repair conversation may be a prerequisite to returning full-on to the conversation that required the timeout.*

The Emotional Challenges of Calling a Timeout

Many people find it hard to let go, to not have the last word, or to go to bed without having convinced their partners of their logic or essential goodness. Some people will think they are weak if they withdraw from the battle or allow their partners' accusations to hang in the air, uncontested. Many believe that if they could just get their spouses to admit to being wrong, then the problem would be solved and emotional equilibrium would be restored. Others become so angry that they cannot stop attacking. These are considerable challenges, especially for adversarial couples when neither partner wants to retreat. For these couples, timeouts can be singularly beneficial—including in preventing physical violence as their cycles escalate. For all couples, timeouts will be employed more often and more successfully after therapists spend some time discussing the couple's specific emotional roadblocks to using them.

Charles and Julie: Teaching Emotion Regulation

Married for 25 years, Charles and Julie—both highly educated, responsible professionals—came to me in the wake of a serious episode of physical violence, Charles having hit Julie during a row in their home. Recently separated, they were on the verge of divorce. The source of conflict was Charles's relationship with Samantha, his business partner, with whom Julie suspected he was having an affair. For various reasons, I came to believe that Charles was not having a sexual affair with Samantha, but that their relationship was functionally similar because it preoccupied Charles and reduced the time he spent with his wife.

Julie came to our first session armed with a detailed written record of the many events over the previous several years that, in her mind, pointed to an affair. Julie was dramatic and emotional, frequently bursting into tears as she attacked her husband's integrity. She was aware that his distancing from her aggravated her insecurity and provoked her into incessant interrogations. But what was she to do? She kept catching him in lies! And after he hit her for the second time, she told him he had to move out and then consulted a divorce attorney.

Charles—thoughtful, quiet, beaten-down, and mildly depressed—was a severe conflict-avoider. He confessed his intense anxiety and shame about his handling of these events, and professed his deep love and appreciation of Julie. Facing Julie's onslaught in my office, Charles alternated between listening respectfully and trying to rebut Julie's claims, one-by-one, as she raised them.

He admitted to having hidden important things from her, not only concerning his relationship with Samantha (which he described as painfully entangled, but not sexual), but also regarding financial matters that had not gone well. He knew his deceits made things worse, giving Julie more reasons not to trust him. He felt hounded by her and her frequent phone calls, which interrupted his work and rubbed his nose in his misbehavior. He didn't really understand why he had hit her, but explained that it seemed the only way to stop her verbal attack, other than leaving the scene—which he had done on many occasions.

I then identified the steps in their pursuer–distancer cycle: Charles's absences and secrecy about shameful events had stoked Julie's insecurities, and those insecurities had led her to hound him. He then distanced still more, and so on. In this worsening emotional situation, Charles had resorted to physical violence to try to stop Julie's verbal assault. Both readily agreed with this formulation. My identifying the enemy as a systems problem and expressing hope for their relationship helped calm them enough so that we could continue.

To illustrate some educational interventions aimed at emotion regulation, I will focus on the first four months of therapy that moved from cycle identification to emotion regulation to exploration of hidden issues (especially his sensitivity to shame and hers to abandonment). The therapy continued for another year past this opening phase, with their deepening of understanding of those issues, a gradual return of trust, and considerable practical planning about what to do about finances and Samantha.

After identifying the steps in their cycle, I focused on Charles's trouble managing his shame and guilt when Julie would attack him or cry. We agreed that his reflexive strategy of countering Julie's attacks on his integrity with factual rebuttals was not effective. In keeping with Charles's own theory about her interpersonal insecurity, I suggested that what might work better was to help Julie to feel close to him in the moment, and that he might accomplish this by trying to remain "calm, curious, and caring" when she began criticizing him.

I was concerned that there might be more violence or an impulsive divorce so—following Stosny's (2005) studies on the benefits to abusive men of imagining their wives as victims needing to be protected—I helped Charles work with his shame at not being able to provide assistance when his wife was upset. My idea was that if I could get Charles to help Julie manage *her* emotions, he would be better able to manage his shame sensitivity and simultaneously calm Julie's attachment insecurity. Knowing that Charles had served as a medic in wartime, I called upon that side of him to do better in the presence of his wife's tears. I told him that when Julie became emotional and sobbed loudly, he should try to remain calm and concerned, as he had with wounded soldiers. Just as Charles had not run from wounded soldiers' blood, so he should not run from his wounded wife's tears. I acknowledged that maintaining his composure while he was upset and under verbal attack would be difficult, but told him I thought he could succeed in this situation as he had under enemy fire.

Since Julie had a low threshold for tears, I had ample opportunity to model remaining calm for Charles as I talked her down myself, trying to understand the nature of her tears and the hopelessness that they communicated. After challenging Charles to persevere and showing him that it could be done, I began to teach him the concrete skills—especially empathic listening—that I thought would help him to calm them both. When Charles stopped defending himself and proposing simplistic solutions to their problems, Julie finally felt heard.

By learning to better manage his emotions, Charles had now created some space that allowed him to make further compassionate comments to Julie. He told her that he could imagine how lonely she felt when he worked late, especially when it was with Samantha and how, even though he had told her not to worry, she had a right to do so under the circumstances. Touched by her husband's reaching out to her with genuine feeling, Julie burst into tears again, but these were tears of happiness and relief. Both Julie and Charles could see that this was what she had longed for from him: reassurance that he loved her and cared about her. I told them that what really worked in situations of undue anxiety about affairs was real connection between the partners—the kind of connection they were now feeling. And what most convinced them was not my pronouncement, but the experienced reality it described.

This was not a one-time event; I repeated this sequence again and again, as I showed Charles how to deal with his struggle to comfort his sobbing wife. Along the way, we saw the extreme cultural—possibly even biological—differences between them when it came to showing emotions: Julie came from a family in which both men and women were frequent criers; in Charles's family, no one—not even his sisters—had cried at their beloved father's funeral.

In addition to helping Charles to manage his feelings when Julie attacked him or began to cry, I worked on his assertiveness. For Charles to really be *for* Julie, he would have to stand up *against* Samantha, someone who was placing inordinate demands on his time and money. It took a long time and a lot of work until Charles felt better about himself, more able to identify his angry feelings when they emerged, and less afraid that voicing his displeasure would damage others. I strove to help him feel that he had a right to be more selective in choosing whom he would attend to. Being more selective, he found the emotional energy he needed to respond to Julie when she needed it and less need to wall himself off by escaping to work or the gym. Eventually, despite some negative business consequences, he ended his interactions with Samantha for good.

As I worked with Charles, I also had my eye on Julie's contributions to their dance. I sought to help her manage her emotional storms better, independent of help from Charles. At the end of our first session, I had directed them to limit contact and conflict when they were outside my office—a form of therapist-prescribed timeout—but Julie was not complying. She called Charles more frequently than we had agreed to and, when he retreated and failed to call her at an appointed time, she gave him an ultimatum: "Go out with me tonight or our marriage is off!" When Charles was slow to respond to her ultimatum, she called me and left a message that she was going ahead with the divorce.

In the session that followed, I repeated my observations about their negative interaction cycle and drew them into discussing how Julie's ultimatum and Charles's response fit that model. I pointed out how hard it had been for Julie to contain her feelings of being unloved when she was separated from Charles and didn't get the contact he had promised. While empathizing with Julie, I also asked her to consider why she gave her husband so much power to determine whether she was lovable. Julie replied that she and her individual therapist were also puzzling over this and mentioned that while she understood the women's lib quip that "A woman needs a man like a fish needs a bicycle," she felt helpless to act accordingly. By encouraging her to keep working on that problem, which would actually give her more "relational power" (Fishbane, 2010), I implicitly affirmed that Charles was not solely responsible for Julie's attachment distress, something both of them knew intellectually, but neither really believed emotionally.

I challenged Julie to talk with Charles and me even when she was anxious or sad (as described above), and to remain curious about what her underlying fears and assumptions really were. As with Charles, I was trying to show her that she could hang in when she was upset and derive self-esteem from being able to do so. Beyond that, I wanted to teach Julie, more specifically, how to regulate her feelings better. I suggested that when she was upset, she should try to "*Become aware (mindful) of your feelings, name them, and wonder, without judgment, where they are coming from.*" I emphasized the importance of taking up a nonjudgmental stance and seeking simply to observe her feelings. I also recommended taking deep breaths and trying to relax her muscles. I reinforced her nonjudgmental inquiry whenever she became distressed. All of this helped, and allowed us to pursue what I call an *individual psychodynamic therapy in a dyad* or a *witnessed individual therapy*. We could now talk about previous times when she had been painfully alone with her feelings and had felt rejected by others, and about how these experiences sensitized her to distress when separated from Charles. This case not only brings to life some of the recommendations and benefits concerning teaching skills to regulate emotions, but also illustrates how teaching relationship skills is always embedded in a comprehensive approach to the couple that includes their interpersonal process and psychodynamics.

Pharmacotherapy to Assist with Emotion Regulation

In many cases, psychotropic medications can assist clients in controlling their emotions better, both generally and when under fire from their spouses.

Though not the focus of this book, many patients with high levels of anxiety, depression, or irritability will benefit from medical/psychiatric interventions, including anxiolytic and antidepressant medications.

We turn now to the topic of teaching couples better ways to work out concrete solutions to their problems. With Charles and Julie, this included developing plans for managing their finances, dealing with Samantha, and deciding how much time they would spend together.

Notes

1 While he makes a good point here, Atkinson unduly minimizes the benefits of gradual softening. Softening allows couples to encounter each other in new, transformative ways and to develop more complex and sympathetic views of each other. One can hardly respond empathically—which Atkinson agrees is crucial to responsible, skillful communicating—without really "getting" what is bothering one's partner.
2 Kornfield's (2008) Meditation for Beginners is an excellent, concise introduction to mindfulness meditation. It comes with a CD to guide listeners through different forms of meditation.
3 This path to self-calming resembles the Cognitive Behavioral Therapy (CBT) mode of helping clients to de-catastrophize and then tame the unrealistic fears that constrain their lives. The difference is that the skill we are discussing now requires only that clients take up a nonjudgmental frame of mind; as such, it is antecedent to whatever conclusions are subsequently reached. Nonetheless, CBT can work synergistically with mindfulness practice (Davison, 2013).
4 Consistent with this recommendation, based on his belief that the fundamental problem of abusive husbands is feeling disrespected, Steven Stosny (2005) challenges them when they are losing it to do something to improve their self-respect, that is, to help their partners feel better, just as they would if their partner had been attacked (by someone else) or had been in an accident.

13
TEACHING PROBLEM-SOLVING AND NEGOTIATION SKILLS

> Like it or not, you are a negotiator.
>
> Fisher, Ury, & Patton, *Getting To Yes (2011)*

Background

Research summarized in Kelly, Fincham, and Beach (2003) confirms clinicians' experience that distressed couples do less constructive problem solving than happy couples. Consequently, I included the PREP problem-solving template (Markman et al., 2001) in the *Marriage 101* course curriculum. I also began to teach it to my clients and to try it out in my own marriage. I was impressed by improved results and began to read more widely about the subject. PREP lays out the following step-by-step sequence:

- Preliminary *problem discussion,* using the speaker–listener technique.
- *Agenda setting:* narrowing the scope of the discussion.
- *Brainstorming:* opening up the discussion to all possible solutions.
- *Plan specification:* working toward agreement and compromise.
- *Follow-up:* assessing results and modifying solutions.

This sequence remains the valuable scaffolding onto which I have added contributions from other experts and from my own experience. Although such structured problem solving was not something I learned during psychiatric residency or psychoanalytic training, it has proved quite valuable in my ability to help couples work out acceptable compromises and practical solutions to complex life problems. Introduced after we have worked on couple process and underlying issues, it addresses the question, "Now that we know how we feel about this issue, what do we *do* about it?"

Hold Your Problem Solving!

The first thing to know and to teach couples about problem solving—codified as a rule in the speaker–listener technique—is not to attempt it too soon. One non-trivial reason for this is that, in many cases, *restraining early problem solving in favor of listening will frequently render additional efforts to come up with compromises or solutions unnecessary.* My own daily observations and formal research by others (Markman et al., 2001) show that many heated arguments end amicably as soon as people feel heard.

In more complicated situations, successful problem solving in couple therapy should still be preceded by empathic listening and by therapeutic work on the topics covered previously in this book: underlying hopes, fears, and defenses, and the ways these contribute to negative interaction cycles.

In all cases, for negotiations to succeed, partners must first understand better what is at stake, including possible conflicts within themselves about the topic being discussed. Indeed, the most important component of the famous recommendations for "getting to yes" in negotiations (Fisher et al., 2011) requires both sides to state their underlying interests in detail, as illustrated by a story of two men quarreling in a library:

> One wants the window open and the other wants it closed. They bicker back and forth about how much to leave it open: a crack, halfway, three-quarters of the way. No solution satisfies both. Enter the librarian. She asks one why he wants the window open: "To get some fresh air." She asks the other why he wants it closed: "To avoid the draft." After thinking a minute, she opens wide a window in the next room, bringing in fresh air without a draft.
>
> *(p. 42)*

A couple I treated illustrates the same point: Discussing whether or not to purchase a summer cottage became more tractable after we learned that the husband feared that his wife wanted to buy it so as to be away from him, and that the wife resented the idea that her husband's larger salary seemed to give him more votes in making this decision. Like this couple, *many couples seem willing to fight to the death over seemingly superficial or easily-decided decisions until they become aware of the deeper issues that lend symbolic weight to the topic.*

This problem of not really understanding what is at issue is also the basis of Wile's (1981) important critique of superficial behavioral "contingency contracting" (trading). He cites an example from the behavioral literature in which a wife agreed to give her husband a glass of beer when he arrived home in return for his spending ten minutes playing with their kids. On the surface, this deal might seem sensible but, as Wile notes, the couple and their therapist failed to wonder why the wife did not initially want to give him the beer and why the husband got no satisfaction from playing with his children. *In general, when someone is not doing something spontaneously, it is important to try to discover—before attempting problem solving—what is making performance aversive.*

Finally, in many cases, the *process* whereby partners propose and respond to possible suggestions will also need work before they can have productive problem-solving discussions. For instance, one husband feared that his wife would contemptuously reject any less-than-perfect suggestion he might propose to any topic under discussion. This was a powerful, negative paternal transference expectation, unfortunately confirmed by many painful interactions with his wife, and readily observed by me during the therapy. After we exposed his transactional fear and his own defensive perfectionism diminished, he became able to offer suggestions in a more collegial tone of voice. His wife could then hear his suggestions as contributions, and we were able to move forward with constructive problem solving.

Couples Who Require Problem Solving

Many conflicts persist after both sides have been heard, and these must be decided one way or another. Numerous couples present to us with disagreements about major life decisions, with the expectation that we will help to resolve them. Common impasses occur over whether to have a child (or have more children), how to parent a difficult child, whether to take elderly parents into their home, whether to relocate, or whether to make a major purchase. In such cases, we become mediators between people with competing values, goals, and ideas about how to settle differences. Sometimes, after hearing each other's deepest concerns, partners will not need formal skills training to work out solutions, as documented by Johnson and Greenberg (1985), in what they call the "consolidation phase" of EFT. Others may need more specific guidance. As with managing other aspects of "difficult conversations," there are strategies—many of them time-tested and formally researched—that facilitate better solutions. These strategies can be learned, by therapists and clients alike.

The Benefits of Concrete Solutions

Therapists sometimes lose sight of the substantial emotional benefits that accrue when people finally decide how to handle a chronic problem. We often celebrate cathartic, emotionally intense sessions in which clients uncover fears deeply rooted in childhood experiences, preferring them to sessions in which they find a workable compromise. Concrete solutions may be less dramatic, but they provide hope, demonstrate that therapy has tangible results, and build the therapeutic alliance (Pinsof, 1995). In addition, they end the obsessing and indecision that wear people down and prevent them from getting on with their lives.

Solving practical problems can also reduce the persistent negative conceptions (transferences) that partners have of each other. I have seen many couples get along far better after they establish a night-time routine—who helps with homework, when the children go to bed—that leaves time for them to be together. The result is not only more pleasant evenings, but spouses who stop viewing each other as uncooperative, selfish, or uninterested in spending time together.

Even though a final decision usually requires both partners to compromise, and even though it can do only so much to rein in problems with children, in-laws, or finances, couples are generally happier because they undertook this work. If we can free them from the acrimony of their negative dancing, we can provide a positive experience of working together that will build feelings of trust, intimacy, and shared identity.

Stalling

As I've noted earlier, interminable battles over who is to blame for a bad situation may serve as defenses against the challenging tasks of working toward, and living with, an attempted solution. Faced with significant, concrete challenges for which there are no obvious, perfect solutions, couples may stall, unconsciously reverting to the familiar, though destructive, habit of assigning blame. When this happens, therapists should interrupt the couple's defensive blame game and direct them toward the more challenging task of coming up with acceptable solutions to difficult problems.

Avoiding Shortcuts

It may be tempting to evade the challenges of negotiation by letting inertia, tradition, gender, power, or disability "decide," but solutions should not routinely be determined this way. It will not do for the person who is more concerned about cleanliness to always do the dishes, or for the person who seldom wants sex to control its frequency. Couples have to put in the energy to work out solutions that address the needs of both partners.

The Emotional Challenges of Negotiation and Problem Solving

In addition to the anxiety of not knowing exactly what to do, which can lead to stalling, *the principal emotional challenge for couples trying to find solutions to their problems is addressing their competing interests while still remaining a team.* As a negotiation proceeds, partners face the internal ethical dilemma of how much to assert their needs and preferred solutions when these may unsettle their partners: "Assertion without empathy risks escalating conflict, while empathy without assertion risks jeopardizing one's legitimate concerns" (Mnookin et al., 2000, p. 4). A balance must be struck between accepting influence and capitulating.

Lessons from Social Science: Fairness

The field of couple therapy can learn from the extensive literature on negotiation in economics, politics, and social science, including "game theory," which spans these fields. Students in these disciplines have examined "social dilemmas" or "mixed-motive interactions" that force individuals to choose between maximizing selfish interests and maximizing collective ones. For our purposes, one of the most important, though not terribly surprising, findings is that groups become deadlocked when they are unable to agree on what is fair (Komorita & Parks, 1995). As we might also expect, groups have more trouble avoiding deadlock when members are more interdependent—as with our couples—and when decisions involve greater novelty or risk (Rusbult & Van Lange, 2003).

Knowing that it is desirable to find solutions that optimize fairness and fair play—while avoiding inequitable shortcuts based on tradition or gender—will not tell us whose desires and ideas should prevail. This awareness can, however, help us to keep these targets in view and remind couples that they can never safely omit issues of fairness from their negotiations. Indeed, this awareness is one reason we should recommend that couples begin most difficult conversations with the "third story," which explicitly acknowledges the presence of two partners with divergent views who must arrive at a solution acceptable to both.

Principled Negotiation: Getting to Yes for Couples

We discussed some of the ins and outs of power-sharing in Chapter 3, including the challenge of breaking ties in a two-person political system ("the co-captains problem"). Fisher, Ury, and Patton, the authors of *Getting To Yes* (2011), probably the best-known book on negotiation, begin their discussion with a critique of "positional bargaining" (e.g., when a buyer and seller haggle over the price of a house with each focused solely on the price) and show this to be decidedly inferior to "principled negotiation" or "negotiation on the merits."

Positional bargaining has many of the same unfortunate consequences as negative interaction cycles. In both situations, "positions" tend to become rigid and polarized. In both, a new "interest"—maintaining self-esteem and saving face—emerges or increases, and this development impedes progress. In both situations, important underlying concerns (hidden issues) remain concealed by the surface conflict. Positional bargaining interferes with discovering how compromises, trades, and other beneficial possibilities might be worked out. Unlike the zero-sum game of positional bargaining, principled negotiation can sometimes arrive at win–win solutions, as in the example of the two men arguing over whether to open a window. When negotiators change the game to principled negotiation, the process generally improves. Released from dependence on their petulant, adversarial positions, partners are better able to remain on task.

In principled negotiation, parties attempt to (a) separate the people from the problem (being hard on the problem and soft on the people); (b) focus on interests, not positions; (c) formulate multiple options; and (d) agree that the result be based on objective standards or principles.

This last point, which gives the method its name, is especially relevant to our question of how to arrive at fair solutions. In principled negotiation, negotiators remain curious, rather than certain, about what principles to employ. They inquire, "Can you tell me the principle behind your planned action, or desired outcome?" and assert, "We would like to settle this [conflict] on the basis of independent standards, not on who can do what to whom" (Fisher et al., 2011, p. 122).

Debating couples may do well to agree on some external method for reaching decisions—say, by consulting experts in the field ("Let's agree to take our financial advisor's advice on how best to save for college"), outside evaluators ("For the next month, we'll try your plan. When the month is over, we'll see if Sally's teacher says her homework is improving"), or by simply agreeing to take turns making the decision ("Tonight, I get to pick the restaurant; next week, you can choose").

Deciding who qualifies as an external arbiter is not so simple. Spouses frequently cite the opinions of others (friends, family, therapists) in order to strengthen their positions. Because these outsiders are routinely biased (or are viewed as such), this tactic may inflame the discussion. Such appeals to outsiders tend to backfire and commonly serve to mask the challenges of "asking for things," so I often counsel against making them. Nonetheless, as long as couples are aware of these complications, they can still work to identify informative external referees and standards.

Patience and Acceptance of Structure

To succeed in negotiations, parties must be patient. Decisions that may appear to be easy often take time, and partners will have to accept this as the cost of being in their relationship. Couples who follow the specific steps I recommend below must also accept that it will not feel natural. As noted by Jacobson and Christensen (1998), "Problem-solving is a specialized activity ... It is not expected to be spontaneous, natural, relaxing or enjoyable, in the way that regular communication is" (p. 181). As with other rules for handling difficult conversations, some suggestions are designed explicitly to keep things under control and, as a result, couples will sometimes feel constrained and notice that their speech becomes uncharacteristically formal. This is to be expected, if not enjoyed. Greater acceptance of these practices will come when partners attain results superior to those they had achieved previously in their unstructured free-for-all.

Having noted the importance of problem definition, fairness, principles, patience, and structure, I now offer step-by-step suggestions to help couples reach equitable, efficacious, and lasting solutions to their concrete problems. These were culled from the literature and have been field-tested in my office. They are written from the clients' perspective so that they can be used as handouts.

Practical Suggestions for Couple Negotiations and Problem Solving

Step 1: Before problem solving

1. *Hold your problem solving until underlying issues have become clear and (hopefully) less intense.*
2. *Pick a time free of distractions, when you both have the emotional energy that will be required. Neither of you should start out upset. Limit the discussion to no more than 60 minutes per session.*
3. *Limit yourself to one problem or, if the problem is large and complex, try to break it into components. Consider carving out one piece of the problem to see if you can make progress on that.*
4. *Commit to following the rules for difficult conversations and try to remain calm, curious, and caring.*

Step 2a: Problem-solving formula for simple problems

5. *If the problem is minor, use the following short formula:*
   a. *Begin with a soft start-up—a compliment or recognition of the other person's perspective.*
   b. *State your problem/request.*
   c. *Ask, "What might we do about this?"*
   d. *If you don't like your partner's proposed solution, don't just criticize it; instead, thank your partner for the proposal, state your reasons for disagreeing, and ask for another suggestion.*
   e. *Repeat until you are satisfied.*

   Example: "I know you love listening to music, but when you play it that loud, I have a hard time reading. What could we do about this?" This formula resembles the "criticism sandwich," in being relatively easy for the listener to hear and easy for the speaker to remember. It begins collaboratively and invites brainstorming while remaining committed to improving the status quo. For more complex problems, a more extensive approach begins with the next step.

Step 2b: Problem definition for more difficult problems

6. *Work hard to define the problem clearly. State your goals before getting bogged down debating the pros and cons of possible solutions. In most*

couple situations, this step will follow and blend into a "difficult conversation" where, ideally, each person's concerns have been fully expressed and acknowledged.

One reason a *formal* problem-definition phase is particularly beneficial for couples is that most partners coming to therapy semi-consciously define the "problem" simply as "My partner should change," or "My partner should stop asking me to change." This amounts to a positional argument that has resulted in a standoff.

Another reason to avoid moving too quickly to discussing solutions is that—without quite knowing it—partners will proceed to discuss somewhat different problems. The resulting discussion will be muddled and frustrating. Similarly, if the problem is not clearly defined, the proposed solution is unlikely to "scratch the real itch." What we then observe are discussions of solutions that become derailed as they drift back to discussions of problem definition. Nonetheless, while defining problems clearly before working on solutions is desirable, sometimes partners will only become fully aware of what is at stake when specific solutions are being discussed.

7. *Be clear about when, where, and under what circumstances the problem occurs, ideally defining your complaint in behavioral terms.* This is an important contribution of behavioral approaches to couple therapy, since they stress that requests for change are more effective when they address behavior, not character.
8. *Be clear about why it is important to you,* going beyond merely stating the behavioral basics.
9. *Be clear about how important or unimportant it is to you; consider using a scale from 1 to 10.* By doing this, you can flag the great importance of an issue without having to raise your voice or use other inflammatory tactics, or you can alert your partner that the issue is *not* a big deal for you.
10. *At the conclusion of this problem-definition phase, write the problem down.*

Step 3: Brainstorming

11. *After defining the problem, brainstorm to come up with possible solutions.* Keep in mind that this is "inventing," not "deciding." Allow yourselves to be creative and playful. Try hard to create an atmosphere where even impossible or ridiculous "solutions" can be heard. There should be no "ownership" of proposed ideas, as in, "John, I'm surprised to

hear you suggest that [stupid] idea!" Try to come up with some solutions targeted to meet your partner's needs as well as your own.

12. *Write down all possible solutions.* This is surprisingly helpful and frequently omitted by participants eager to state their views. It not only makes repetition less likely, but it adds an element of planful formality. It will help structure the subsequent discussion of pros and cons, as each written suggestion gets a hearing. One partner should record the options, whether they are brainstorming at home or in the consulting room.
13. *Wait until you have listed all the solutions you can imagine before discussing the relative merits of any of them.* Shooting down options too early may inhibit the creative process and eliminate their possible partial contributions—say, if they speak humorously to an important need.
14. *Do not limit yourself to what you can think of at the moment. Consider consulting outside experts, self-help books, friends, or family members who have faced a similar problem, or other data sources relevant to brainstorming.* Parents arguing over which school a child should attend, for example, should research their options before solidifying their choice.

Step 4a: Evaluating options and working toward agreement

15. *Review your options and discuss their pros and cons.* Include a review of your prior experiences with the various options, together with the experiences of others who have faced similar problems. It may turn out that each of you has had a previously undisclosed bad experience with some course of action. For instance, having grown up with a controlling father may make you leery of setting firm limits on your children, while having had overly lenient parents may make you fear too little parental control.
16. *Look for opportunities that build on your differences.* This suggestion may seem surprising in a text on couple therapy, where it is almost axiomatic that couple problems derive from couple differences. Nonetheless, it turns out that successful negotiating frequently benefits from differences. As noted by Mnookin et al. (2000), in any trade, it is precisely the differences that make the trade possible: a vegetarian with a chicken and a carnivore with a large vegetable garden will find trading beneficial. Understanding that one person cares little about some aspect of a problem while the other cares greatly will facilitate compromising and trading ("I don't really care

which of the movies you've suggested we go to, but I really want to go to this restaurant afterward").

17. *Invite your partner to convince you of the superiority of his or her solution, and reserve the right not to be persuaded. Explain your reservations, and state what would persuade you.* "I understand that you really think we should ground Sally for the weekend, but I'm still not convinced. Let me show you where I have trouble following your reasoning . . ."
18. *Ask what, if anything, would persuade your partner to accept your solution.*
19. *Ask what standards are relevant to a "principled solution."* Consider agreeing on an outside referee or expert to settle your dispute. Alternatively, you can look for "comparables" in your community. In real estate, you might say, "I know you want me to pay more for this house, but that's not what comparable houses are going for." So, in family situations, you might say, "I know you think that punishing Michael this way is appropriate, but let's see what other parents in his grade consider fair and appropriate."

    The search for standards and principles can also help when partners discover that they have different, unconscious, default standards (e.g., about the "right" way to celebrate a child's birthday). Uncovering these may lead to a better understanding of the impasse.

    In many situations, the problem is that no single standard applies. As with debates in constitutional law, there are often competing standards. For example, in the case of Tom and Jennifer in Chapter 4, their debate over whether to leave Chicago involved the competing standards of family loyalty (stay put) versus economic opportunity (move elsewhere).
20. *If no shared solution appeals to both of you, suggest a compromise.* When you do this, be wary of conceding too much ("soft negotiating") or asking for too much, since the lack of fairness of either course may create resentment and noncompliance.
21. *If you are having trouble reaching a compromise, point out the costs of not doing so.* For instance, "If we fail to agree on *some* plan for dealing with Jim's drug problem, we'll never improve the current situation."
22. *If no compromise is possible, agree to follow one person's solution for a specified time.* Years ago, family therapists noticed that when one parent "complained from the sidelines" about a problem, it could help to put that parent fully in charge of fixing it. If nothing else, the know-it-all parent came to understand just how difficult the

problem was to solve. Should the problem yield to the solution proposed, how nice! If not, the partners can return to the drawing board with more information.

23. *Do not accept a solution that you feel is extremely unlikely to work or last.* Sometimes, a trial period will make your point, but other times, the cost will be too high.
24. *Do not accept a solution that will make you or your partner inordinately angry or resentful.* Most solutions will leave one or both partners somewhat disappointed. When one partner continues to see the negotiated agreement as unfair or offers only grudging acceptance, however, the apparent resolution is unlikely to last and will diminish marital harmony.
25. *Do not accept a solution that you do not intend to carry out.*
26. *Establish criteria for evaluating success and discuss them before finalizing your plan.* While criteria for success will vary with the situation, partners should keep in mind that successful agreements should (a) meet the legitimate interests of the parties; (b) resolve conflicting interests fairly; (c) improve or, at minimum, not damage the relationship; (d) take the interests of others outside the couple into account; and (e) prove durable (criteria modified from Fisher et al., 2011).
27. *Set a time when you will reconvene to assess outcomes.*
28. *Be clear that you both understand the negotiated solution, and write it down.* In some cases, sign a formal agreement.
29. *Review how the problem-solving session went.* Skilled negotiators recommend that after every such meeting, the parties review WW and DD: *w*hat *w*orked and what they would *d*o *d*ifferently (Fisher & Shapiro, 2005).

Step 4b: What to do if there is still no agreement

30. *Consider the alternatives for both of you should you not reach an agreement, your BATNAs (best alternatives to a negotiated agreement).* This may mean simply continuing on with the status quo, with the advantage of knowing that you have thoroughly explored the alternatives and, possibly, that the grass might not be greener elsewhere. If you decide to walk away without agreement, you should state why you are doing so, and should be willing to accept the consequences.

© 2016, *A Roadmap for Couple Therapy: Integrating Systemic, Psychodynamic, and Behavioral Approaches,* Arthur C. Nielsen, Routledge

31. *When you reach your limit, instead of saying, "Enough is enough!" (which is likely to make matters worse), summarize the situation as you see it, including what actions you will take in the absence of an agreement and the likely consequences of no resolution.* Say something like, "Here's what I see. Here's its impact on me. Here's its impact on us. You may disagree with my perceptions or feel that your behavior is justified. Our current way of interacting doesn't work *for me*. I am asking you to change this behavior. If it continues nonetheless, here is what I'm going to do" (modified from Fisher & Shapiro, 2005).

Step 5: Trial period and follow-up evaluation

Even though conducting a follow-up assessment seems like an obvious step, it is often neglected. Careful review not only allows couples to learn from their experience, but it allows them to work more as a team, tackling an external adversary even if it is not defeated on the first attempt.

32. *Reward and encourage each other for carrying out the plan.* Adequate implementation may depend on this.
33. *Assess your results.* Evaluate outcomes using the agreed-upon criteria. If you didn't discuss formal criteria before, work them out based on what you have experienced. Don't be too hard on yourselves. Many plans fail the first few times they are tried. Rather than expecting perfection from the start, give yourselves permission to make mistakes and refine solutions as you go. Remember: If this problem had been easy to solve, you wouldn't have engaged in this formal process in the first place.
34. *Allow several attempts before you declare the plan a failure.* Rather than changing your entire plan, consider how you might improve implementation.
35. *Revise your plan based on what you have learned.* In ongoing therapy, therapists can assist in this assessment phase, helping couples refine their understanding of the problem while working toward solutions, compromises, and acceptance.

Fred and Beth: Problem Solving

As their interpersonal process improved, Beth was able to express her desire for more help with the children in a way that Fred could now hear. When he responded helpfully to her requests, she was delighted. I was able to build on this and teach them some of the formal problem-solving steps just described, including problem definition and brainstorming, in particular. Armed with these, they successfully worked out some aspects of parenting that had bedeviled them for years. Their formal collaboration, both in and outside my office, produced a clear set of expectations for homework, sleepovers, and household chores that they both agreed to monitor and enforce. As with other couples, the brainstorming phase was particularly useful. As they laid out all the options they could think of, Fred was forced to see the limitations of his previous, insufficiently formulated ideas. They also had some fun and grew closer—as they imagined draconian punishments for their unruly teenagers.

This success with problem solving allowed me to continue to challenge Fred's underlying (transference) certainty that nothing he did had an impact on Beth's moods. He had to admit that she was clearly happier. In this lessening of his negative expectancy, we see the important interdependence of intrapsychic change and behavioral change—here, with behavioral change leading the way, following successful, structured problem solving.

14
ENCOURAGING POSITIVE EXPERIENCES

> There has been a hidden assumption in couple therapy: If we adequately deal with couples' conflicts, a sort of vacuum will be created, and all the positive affects will rush in to fill this void. We suggest that this assumption is wrong. Positive affect systems need to be built separately in therapy.
>
> J. M. Gottman & J. S. Gottman (2010, p. 149)

When working to resuscitate marriages, we usually need to do more than help couples to fight fair. That sort of success might lead to amicable roommates, but it will prove insufficient for clients who were once lovers. With this distinction in mind, researchers interested in "positive psychology" have distinguished between "flourishing" marriages and devitalized or otherwise unhappy marriages (Fincham & Rogge, 2010; Fowers & Owenz, 2010; Gottman, 2011; Pines, 1996; Wallerstein & Blakeslee, 1995). Flourishing marriages are characterized by considerable amounts of pleasurable time spent together (including satisfying sex and recreational activities), by shared goals, and by a sense of "we-ness." From these studies and the experiences of a diverse array of therapists (Atkinson, 2005, 2010; Dimidjian, Martell, & Christensen, 2008; Greenberg & Goldman, 2008; Leone, 2008; Pines, 1996), it is clear that therapists should urge troubled couples to bring friendship, fun, and shared pleasure back into their relationships, sooner rather than later. Because couples are usually too wary to move in this direction spontaneously, much of this work will be initiated and guided by therapists, which is why this is a behavioral/educational upgrade.

Further Research-Based Rationale

Couples do not marry to become better at managing conflicts, but because of the pleasures they experience during courtship—pleasures they hope will continue going forward. There are other aims, to be sure—financial stability, procreation, social identity—but, by and large, couples will remain happy only to the extent that they continue to enjoy each other's company. Losing the pleasures of being together is not only unpleasant, but actually dangerous, since Gottman and Levenson (1999) found "drifting apart" to be a more common contributing cause of divorce (60%) than intense fighting (40%).[1] While many "devitalized" or "burned out" couples do *not* divorce, they remain unhappily married, leading lonely parallel lives, at risk for divorce when their children leave home.

John Gottman frequently cites his finding (Gottman & Levenson, 1999) that, *during conflict discussions*, his healthy couples showed a 5:1 ratio of positive to negative interactions, whereas the ratio for his unhappy or divorcing couples was only 1:1. More recently, he and his wife/collaborator have stressed the importance of marital positivity—in conflictual *and* nonconflictual interactions—in assuring that the benefits of couple therapy will last. In addition to companionship and intimacy, they noted the importance of "building and savoring the positive affect systems (e.g., play, fun, humor, exploration, adventure, romance, passion, good sex)" (Gottman & Gottman, 2010, p. 140).

In studies by Barbara Fredrikson, "the most flourishing individuals, the most flourishing marriages, and the most flourishing work groups . . . all show ratios [of positive to negative emotions] greater than three to one" (cited by Lyubomirsky, 2013, p. 56). Such positive ratios, sometimes described as having "money in the love bank," help to buffer the impact of inevitable negative events (Keyes & Haidt, 2003; Pines, 1996). They may be necessarily greater than one-to-one because of our inclination to be more impressed by negative events than by positive ones and to become inured to the ongoing benefits we derive from our partners.

Positive emotions and interactions do more than just cancel out negative ones, however. Atkinson (2005) and Panksepp (1998) highlight differences between pleasurable neural circuits and aversive ones, and students of positive psychology distinguish between rewarding (positive and desired) and punishing (negative and unwelcome) experiences. They sensibly reject the idea that "processes by which relationships are satisfying and beneficial are simply the inverse of, or reflect nothing more than the absence of, the processes by which relationships are distressing and harmful" (Reis & Gable, 2003, p. 131).

Making use of this growing research literature on happiness and flourishing, I will now discuss interventions to facilitate positive couple experiences.

Pleasurable First Steps: Friendship and Intimacy

Summarizing their extensive research on marriage, Markman et al. (2001) note that "people from all walks of life, of all ages, both men and women, say that the most important goal for their marriage is to have a friend and to be a friend" (p. 217), and add, "One of the most significant changes in our work with couples . . . has been to make friendship a high priority" (p. 227). After hearing Howard Markman and Scott Stanley make this point at a SmartMarriages Conference in 2002, I began working with couples to foster "friendship" and other positive aspects of marriage more directly—and earlier—than I had before.

To some extent, I had already been trying to help couples become better friends, by fostering the honesty and vulnerable self-disclosure that brought alienated, distant partners together as they learned about each other's inner lives and responded more positively. What was new was working to help couples have pleasurable, conflict-free, out-of-the-office experiences together, ones like they had had when courting.

Becoming the Ballroom Dance Instructor

Although couples often said they wanted to have fun together, few of them did so spontaneously. Without my direction, encouragement, and structuring, most couples played it safe and maintained their distance, neither of them wanting to risk rejection and disappointment by expressing their positive desires.

This holding back was easiest to see with the many couples who had stopped having sex before coming to therapy. With these couples, sexual encounters simply failed to return spontaneously after overt conflict had lessened and cordial feelings had returned. While clients came to trust their partners to fight fair, they remained reluctant to trust them with their strong, literally naked, desires for love and affection. To return such couples to predominantly positive emotional states, I found that I had to become the ballroom dance instructor of frightened middle schoolers, the instructor who declares that it is now time to choose a partner and master the anxieties of dancing together. I began to direct couples' attention to their lack of shared pleasurable activities. And, even if they were not complaining openly about their absent sex lives, I began asking about that, too. All in all, I now make reviving pleasure an explicit goal, one only slightly less important than improving negative interaction cycles.[2]

Timing

Once you have this goal in mind, timing is critical. Begin such activities too soon and couples will only experience more acrimony and disappointment. Wait too long and therapy will drag on without couples reaping the benefits pleasurable activities can bring. So, fairly soon after therapy has begun, and after I have established a reasonable therapeutic alliance, I begin to assess the couple's likelihood of success in planned, positive experiences. I do this by tracking their overall emotional tone—observed and reported—to see whether it is sufficiently amicable to support positive activities. When I feel they are ready, I encourage them in the project and help them brainstorm. Good activities for fostering *friendship* are pretty simple: dinner out, a movie, an evening walk. The goal is for the couple to spend more time alone, free from the demands of work, household, and children.

Discuss Constraints

Just as discussions aimed at increasing closeness in the consulting room predictably lead to discussions of constraints, so do discussions of plans for friendly contact outside the office. Some constraints are external (finding babysitters), and some are internal (trusting that others can watch the children safely). These days, the most common external constraints are time demands (Doherty, 2003). As noted by Singer and Skerrett (2014):

> What is hard for couples to see is that buried in the seeming inevitability of their routine is a series of choices that express their relative amount of attention and commitment to their own relationship. How they structure their time reflects what needs they are putting first—the needs of the couple or the needs of employers, children, in-laws, and so on.
>
> *(p. 73)*

Because much of the time spent with work, children, and extended family *is* necessary, it is easy to use these responsibilities to rationalize avoiding spending time together. Many spouses allow dutiful service to extended family, work, or community to come between them. Others let their children come between them, literally, letting them sleep in the parental bed, thus inhibiting sex. Still others will need help to cut back on outside activities that have provided the satisfactions they have not been getting from their marriages.

The most important *internal* constraint blocking spending friendly time together is the fear that painful emotions will emerge, especially in public. We have all seen such couples in restaurants, either creating angry scenes or sitting in painful defensive silence. Should a partner mention a fear of such a silence, we can label it as a fear of taking chances, with silence protecting a vulnerable self from the risk of disapproving or indifferent responses. More generally, we should attempt to discover and discuss feared scenarios.

No Fighting or Practical Discussions Allowed

To make success more likely, I tell couples they must not discuss anything controversial while on their dates. Should a dispute arise, the couple should change the subject and save the discussion for our next therapy session. This rule is essential if we are to create opportunities for good times while we are still working on troubling issues in therapy. Most couples at this phase of therapy are already avoiding conflict outside their therapy hours, but they are generally avoiding intimacy, too. When we encourage them to spend unstructured time together, they are bound to fear that conflict will break out as it does in therapy. Banning conflict offers hope that they can put their differences aside and focus, instead, on having some nonconflictual good times.

Equally important, couples are not to use this time to discuss practical issues (when to remodel the kitchen, the best preschool for their daughter). Even when such discussions might not lead to arguing, this is no way for the couple to spend their precious time alone.

Designating Times for Difficult Conversations

The flip side of proscribing problem solving during date nights is to work with couples to designate times when they *will* discuss problems. Many couples have no system for doing this and only discuss serious issues when they can't avoid it any longer, usually at inopportune times. Again, more than I did in my free-form Couple Therapy 1.0 days, I ask couples to describe their routines for discussing serious matters, and we work to improve them. I suggest that they reserve specific times for conflict discussions: no more than 30 minutes a day, and certainly not the last thing before going to bed. For communicating straightforward practical matters ("I set up dinner with the Doyles for this Friday at 7" or "Your doctor called to say . . ."), I recommend written notes, texts, or emails, which save time and increase communication reliability.

The Anticipatory Benefits of Scheduling

Couples with substantial marital problems usually are not scheduling pleasurable time together, including time for sex. Once they resume scheduling good times together ("On Saturday night, we're going to dinner and a movie" or "On Wednesday after the kids are in bed, we will make love"), they will get pleasure not only from the planned events, but also from anticipating them (Lyubomirsky, 2013). This will help buffer difficulties in the days preceding the event and reduce nagging from partners unsure about whether they will have their needs met. Clients who still believe that spontaneity is necessary for romance will need our help to let go of this ideal so they can reap the benefits of scheduling.

Talking Like Friends

Beyond barring fighting and problem solving during planned enjoyable activities, I encourage couples to "talk like friends." To induce a sense of safety, fun, and reflection, I suggest that they imagine themselves as close, childhood friends on a campout or at a slumber party, lying on their backs staring at the stars or the ceiling, sharing their thoughts and talking into the night. I encourage them to share the prosaic stuff of their daily lives: good news, funny stories, observations about their day. As their therapy progresses, I also encourage them to share their dreams for the future, as well as their actual dreams from the previous night. Clients who are particularly intimacy-challenged can be taught to ask questions and to provide emotional support. The goal is to clear some space for them to rediscover each other's positive characteristics and renew their marital bond.

Daily Reviews and "Turning Toward" Each Other

I work to help couples not only schedule pleasurable, special times away from home, but also to plan routine, daily conversations so that they can stay in touch when their busy lives threaten to pull them apart. Ideally, they will set a more-or-less regular time for doing this. A helpful formula is for partners to report the high and low experiences of their day. This guarantees that the conversation will not just dwell on day-to-day logistics, such as who will call the electrician or respond to the Smiths' dinner invitation. Couples who "turn toward" each other (Gottman, 2011) and express interest in each other's "life projects" (Kernberg, 2011) have better outcomes (Driver, 2007), as their conversations are what you would expect from good friends.[3]

Couples often make the same mistakes in such daily reviews as they do in more difficult conversations: Listeners are too passive or offer premature or unwelcome advice; speakers fail to consider the needs of their listeners. Both speakers and listeners fear showing themselves fully. In such cases, therapists can work—in the ways already described—to help couples do better, so they can reap the many benefits of an improved long-term friendship.

Fun, Novelty, and Play

As emphasized by Weingarten (1991), "intimacy" should not be defined narrowly as self-disclosure during deep conversations, but can arise from a wide variety of shared activities that "co-create meaning." Markman et al. (2001), in a national telephone survey of married couples, found—unsurprisingly—that "the amount of fun partners had together emerged as a key factor in predicting their overall marital happiness" (p. 256).

What counts as "fun" often involves novelty, as shown in both naturalistic and experimental studies, which have found that novelty consistently jumpstarts positive emotions (Aron, Norman, Aron, McKenna, & Heyman, 2000; Bradbury & Karney, 2010; Lyubomirsky, 2013; Pines, 1996). This is the flipside of the observation that couples' efforts to guarantee emotional safety in their relationships often lead to deadening boredom and loneliness, with extramarital affairs a frequent untoward result (Mitchell, 2002; Perel, 2006). Consequently, when I ask couples to come up with fun activities to do together, I try to get them out of their routines and ruts, so as to provide them the pleasure of novelty.

Closely related to the concept of novelty is that of "play." When the brain's "PLAY circuit" is active, internal opioids are released throughout the brain, and these correlate with pleasure and with the desire to continue contact with the partner (Panksepp, 1998). When I brainstorm with couples, I specifically ask them to think about what they did playfully for fun in the past: when they were children, before they met each other, during their courtship, and before they had children. I also have them consider what appeals to them when they scan the newspaper for upcoming events.

The activities they come up with will require varying amounts of money, effort, courage, and time, but whatever they choose should help them to re-experience the pleasure of doing things together. Just as I do when we brainstorm about practical problems, I encourage a creative atmosphere, open to *all* suggestions *before* discussing their pros and cons. Ideally, the discussions themselves will be fun. Since some couples benefit from hearing what others do for fun, I have listed some suggestions in Table 14.1.

Table 14.1 Enjoyable Activities to Share

- Go for a walk or a jog.
- Cook together.
- Garden together.
- Play cards or a board game.
- Read a short story or book out loud and discuss it. Alternate who reads.
- Go biking, bowling, canoeing, ice skating, or cross-country skiing.
- Go dancing.
- Attend a public lecture.
- Attend a concert, play, or movie.
- Explore your city as if you were tourists, and see the sights and museums you've never taken time to explore.
- Go camping and/or hiking.
- Learn or play a sport.
- Take a class: cooking, dance, "continuing education," whatever.
- Join or organize a book or movie discussion group.
- Join a community theater group.
- Participate in a community service project, like Habitat for Humanity.
- Participate in a project or group organized by your religious community.
- Participate in a political campaign or event.
- Learn a language.
- Travel—ideally, somewhere new; if possible, to a country where your new language is spoken.

After couples come up with some promising ideas, it is frequently necessary to help them discuss impediments to engaging in them. As discussed above, some obstacles will be realistic and some will be rationalizations for maintaining a safe distance. While it would be nice if couples rapidly got onboard and stayed there, my experience is that it takes considerable persistence and encouragement from me before partners are willing to take the risks that will allow them to bring playfulness and fun back into their relationships.

Fun, Play, and Affection in the Consulting Room

While encouraging pleasurable activities outside the office, I also look for chances to foster moments of fun, play, and affection during sessions. Sometimes, such good feelings emerge when we laugh together or briefly discuss positive developments in the news or in their lives—a welcome respite from the difficult emotional work of the therapy. When appropriate, I tell illustrative jokes or use humorous examples from my own life—revealing myself as a fellow human who struggles with life's challenges and as someone who can find humor in his own missteps. Partners who fear that therapy will be relentlessly serious and painful appreciate this more relaxed atmosphere, which helps them expose their own faults and foibles and allows them to be more open to fun and affection.

Many couples I see have grown wary of touching each other. Others have always avoided it, because their families rarely hugged or touched. When I feel the time is propitious, I may suggest that clients hold hands or hug each other during a session and then ask them to reflect on the experience. It is almost always instructive. Most often, it is beneficial and may be quite moving. When a spouse shows apprehension or awkwardness, however, this is useful to discuss.

Handholding, Hugging, and Sex

For many couples, physical contact is slow to return, but extremely beneficial when it does. Encouraging handholding or hugging in the office can get the ball rolling, and sometimes it continues at home. More frequently, I need to sell handholding a little more, so I cite MRI studies showing positive benefits (Coan, Schaefer, & Davidson, 2006). These studies measured functional MRIs of married women as they received a warning of an oncoming electric shock. When they held their husbands' hands, both their subjective and brain responses of fear and distress were significantly reduced, compared to holding the hand of a male stranger.

Obviously, and in keeping with the ineffectiveness of holding hands with strangers, handholding is not merely physical, but also symbolic, conveying emotional support and connection. So it is even more intriguing to learn that the benefits of handholding varied as a function of marital quality, with better marital quality correlating with greater attenuation of the fear response. Further, this beneficial effect could be induced by successful couple therapy (Greenman & Johnson, 2013). To this finding, I would add my experience that once couple relationships become "positive enough," *additional* handholding will further improve attachment and positivity in the relationship.

I have found similar benefits after I have successfully encouraged other forms of physical contact, specifically hugging and sex. I prescribe hugs using Stosny's (2006) formula of "6 x 6": six hugs a day for a minimum of six seconds each. I suggest that couples do this whenever they meet or separate and, following David Schnarch's (1997) recommendation, I advise them to "hug until calm." Or they can follow Peter Fraenkel's (2011) advice to touch base—for 60-seconds, six times a day—via hugging, kissing, back massages, phone calls, or texts—whatever works to establish frequent episodes of positive connection throughout the day.

As with other homework assignments, it is surprising how often couples do not follow through on this advice and how valuable it is to discuss why not. When discussing impediments, therapists can point out that 36 seconds a day is an insignificant *time* demand and then explore the *emotional* demands that are interfering. When couples succeed in "6 x 6" or in simply hugging when greeting, when parting, and when it feels necessary ("I need a hug!"), they almost universally feel greater connection, warmth, and support.

Having experienced the pleasures and safety of holding hands and hugging, couples can move on (as most of us do as adolescents), to more erotic forms of physical contact. Unlike handholding or hugging, sex can bring up fears of physical inadequacy related to attractiveness or performance.

Even with couples who have not complained initially of sexual dissatisfaction, sexual contact is often slow to return, so therapists need to be proactive in assisting with the revival of sexual pleasure. When we succeed, much good feeling will be generated, and hope for the future of the relationship will increase dramatically. Beyond the mutual pleasure, satisfying sex will reassure the partners that they are acceptable and that they are capable of giving and receiving pleasure. It will lessen their fear of rivals (real or imagined), and enhance their identities as men and women. Thanks to our knowledge of brain biochemistry, we can tell them that the increase in oxytocin that attends sexual contact will strengthen their bond and decrease aggression (Panksepp, 1998). Even after we have convinced them of the value of restoring sexual contact, however, continuing sexual inhibition may require our focused attention.[4]

Compliments and Other Loving Actions

"If you want to love big, you have to think small, every day" (Stosny, 2006, p. 287). Unlike the planned, big-ticket events we discussed earlier in this chapter (date nights, vacations, sexual encounters), spouses need to give to each other in small ways, on a daily basis. What Stosny has in mind are small acts of love that behavior therapists have identified when they ask partners to pay more attention to each other's needs in "behavior exchanges" or on "love days"—actions like fixing broken things around the house or cooking a partner's favorite dish for dinner (see Jacobson & Christensen, 1998, pp. 151–169).

Behavioral couple therapists have long emphasized learning, and then performing, the *specific actions* each partner finds pleasing. To facilitate this, I ask partners to describe on my intake questionnaire what makes them "feel loved" and what they believe makes their partner "feel loved." Most clients answer the former with relatively concrete actions—"Talk to me more" "Have more sex" "Tell me I'm attractive" "Help out more with our kids"—but they do not always know what concrete actions make their partners feel specially loved. Identifying these behaviors as goals and exploring how to achieve them can help create more positive feeling between the partners. Knowing that more is at stake symbolically when doing certain routine actions may also help partners perform these acts more conscientiously and reliably.

In marriage, many routine actions that benefit both partners (making the bed, picking up the dry cleaning, paying the bills) recede into the background where they hardly register and become taken for granted. As Lyubomirsky (2013), our expert on human happiness, noted, "We are prone to take for granted pretty much everything positive that happens to us" (p. 18). And when we are mad at our spouses, we are even less likely to compliment them or express gratitude for such services. Consequently, I work not just to reduce negativity and to identify positive desirable behaviors, but to help couples voice their appreciation more frequently for commonplace undertakings. I encourage direct expressions of love and specialness ("It makes me feel so good when you tell me I look great!") and explicit compliments for daily actions performed on the couple's behalf ("Thanks so much for that delicious dinner"). I model this behavior ("That was an insightful connection"), complimenting partners myself and pointing out how much they enjoy such affirmation. I challenge partners (more often men) who say that no one should be complimented for things they are "supposed" to do, who act according to the unconscious principle that, "I've told you that I love you. If I change my mind, I'll let you know!" Such people need to be more vocal with their appreciation and less abstemious with their verbal hugs.

When I feel confident that it's true, I sometimes encourage clients to tell their partners they are "the most important person in the world" to them. I stage this forcefully, asking each person to look directly into the other's eyes. As when instructing couples to hold hands, this directive almost universally gets people over their fearful relationship hump and moves them toward a deeper appreciation of their indispensable value to each other.

Facilitating Positive Couple Identity (We-ness)

As noted by Singer and Skerrett (2014), "Current research in social and clinical psychology suggests that one of the strongest predictors of marital stability and happiness is the couple's ability to build and maintain a sense of We-ness" (p. 2). This goes beyond shared positive experiences; a shared couple identity contributes to a willingness to sacrifice for, and remain committed to, each other—in sickness and in health, for richer, for poorer—which, in turn, correlate with relationship stability (Stanley & Markman, 1992; Stanley, Rhodes, & Whitton, 2010). Additionally, Gottman's early research (Buehlman, Gottman, & Katz, 1992) showed not only that we-ness strongly predicted marital success, but that couples who "glorified the struggle" of their lives together also did better. In developing a shared couple identity, partners are involved in the "co-creation of meaning" (Weingarten, 1991), building a positive social identity through their marriage—a valuable asset in an era when that can be hard to achieve.[5]

Many shared activities can count toward this goal, ranging from the mundane to the more existentially significant. Some, like raising children and creating a household, are prosaic, but provide a vital background structure. Others include sharing significant holidays (religious, secular, and couple-specific), rituals (birthdays, Christenings and confirmations, bar and bat mitzvahs, graduations, weddings, funerals, family reunions), and traditions (holiday parties, games, shared cooking, watching a favorite video at the same time each year). All of these bind couples and families together in the fabric of their shared lives. They can also be the source of dispute and strife and may lead couples to therapy when these important shared events are threatened.

When disputes over life plans (whether to have another child, whether to move to the suburbs) or traditions (what religion to raise a child in, whose parents to visit at Thanksgiving) bring couples to treatment, we must understand that their importance extends beyond the particular issues at hand to the partners' lifelong dreams and expectations (recall Dick and Tina's struggle over celebrating Christmas in Chapter 6).

Encouraging Friendships With Others

Over the years, I have learned the significance of couples' friends for good and for ill. The majority of couples who come with severe and long-standing marital problems have been avoiding their friends. Most clients do not want to air their dirty laundry in public and do not feel that they can pull off a charade. Sometimes, work or family responsibilities have reduced healthy social connection. Social isolation then robs the couple not only of the *pleasures* of being with friends (pleasure being the topic of this chapter), but interferes with the kind of buffering and community support we all need as we face life's challenges. When one partner complains of needing more verbal intimacy, as is common in many marriages, the situation is often being exacerbated by isolation from friends. (On the other hand, some friends can have a destabilizing impact on marriages that they think should end, and therapists should be alert to this possibility.) Helping couples to re-establish and re-invigorate their social networks will, therefore, be beneficial.

Therapist Follow-up and Review

Therapists should be sure to follow up and inquire about how planned positive events (conversations, date nights, hugs, compliments, dinners with friends) actually went. Not only are couples slow to initiate positive activities, they frequently do not report their successes or failures. Successes are often considered unworthy of "therapeutic" discussion, while failures are avoided due to shame. We should be sure to ask how things went and to help the couple learn from their experiences.

Fred and Beth: Fostering Shared Pleasurable Activities and Friendships

In my fifth couple session with Fred and Beth, I brought up the topic of shared pleasurable activities. I learned that they had enjoyed dinners out with each other and that these had fallen off due to marital tensions. Socializing with friends had also become infrequent. Fred said that Beth had become especially sad when her closest friend had recently moved to a distant city, and I now realized that this had contributed to their marital deterioration. As we brainstormed, it emerged that each of them secretly longed for the more adventurous and varied social and recreational life they had previously enjoyed, especially before their children were born.

We then discussed how to re-establish their social life and how to carve out time for date nights and weekend camping. We encountered some impediments to doing so (Fred's fear that he had "nothing in common" with some of Beth's friends, Beth's fear that Fred found her boring). We talked about bringing back other forms of previously shared pleasure, such as playing jointly with their kids, fixing up their home, and going dancing together. As the couple engaged in these activities in the months that followed, the fun and pleasure they experienced was palpable and countered their prior dread that their marriage had irrevocably soured and that they could never be happy together again.

As with other couples, Fred and Beth had sex infrequently. Before their sex life could come back, however, they had to develop more confidence that they could please each other, in general, and that being vulnerable was safe. When most of the external disagreements that had brought them to therapy had been settled, and after learning that sex was still a rare event, I encouraged handholding and then hugging in the office, followed later by sensate focus exercises (Masters & Johnson, 1970; McCarthy & McCarthy, 2003), so as to gradually build confidence in reconnecting physically. In the second year of therapy, when satisfying sex returned, the couple's happiness improved still more. We ended the therapy shortly thereafter. As in other cases, I had the sense that satisfying sex was the final frontier, that achieving it served as a guarantor that the overall tone of the relationship would remain positive.

Circularity, Synergy, and Sequencing

As noted by Gurman (2013) in his discussion of integration in couple therapy, while Emotionally Focused Couple Therapy posits that improved attachment will lead to improved marital satisfaction, increased satisfaction can also lead to improved attachment. More fun, hugs, compliments, sex, and intimate involvement of all kinds can be expected to lead to beneficial changes, not only in couples' attachment, but also in their abilities to fight fair, to understand themselves more deeply, and to accept and forgive each other—the targets of interventions discussed in earlier sections of this book. Indeed, improvement in any area of couple life often leads to improvement in others. The practical questions then become how to sequence possible interventions and how to customize them to specific couples. While all roads may lead to Rome, some will get us there faster! In the final section of this book, I discuss some general guidelines for conducting therapy and for sequencing the interventions discussed previously.

Notes

1 In keeping with this bivariate view of marital unhappiness, a cluster analysis by Paul Amato (2010) found two pathways to divorce: (1) a high level of conflict and unhappiness, and (2) a low level of commitment. Presumably, the low-commitment group included couples who had lost the satisfactions of being together.
2 Wachtel (2014, p. 47) has called attention to the tendency of therapists to become "session-centric," prioritizing patterns observed in the consulting room, while other patterns of daily life get insufficient attention. One area of life that can remain relatively silent is what goes on, if anything, that might be more positive in the couple's relationship than the usually conflicted discussions occurring in therapy.
3 Driver (2007) analyzed 600 hours' worth of couples' 10-minute dinnertime conversations and recorded responses to "bids for emotional connection," that is, "verbal and nonverbal attempts to get one's partner's attention, conversation, interest, enthusiasm, humor, affection, playfulness, emotional support, etc." She found that "couples who stayed together after 6 years had initially (in the first year of marriage) turned toward one another's bids for emotional connection about 86% of the time, whereas couples who later divorced had turned toward their partner's bids only 33% of the time."
4 These issues are discussed in more detail in Leiblum (2007); Levine (1999); Levine, Risen, and Althof (2010); Margolies (2001); B. McCarthy and E. McCarthy (2003); B.W. McCarthy and Thestrup (2008); Perel (2006); and Risen (2010).
5 An important reason that many same-sex couples reacted emotionally on learning they would be allowed to wed relates not so much to gaining certain legal rights (like visitation in hospitals), but to being granted entry into the affirmative social identity of marriage.

PART V
Sequencing Interventions and Concluding Remarks

15
GENERAL GUIDELINES AND THE SEQUENCING OF INTERVENTIONS

> It remains much easier to create a generic model of what to do than to state the order in which to proceed with those activities.
>
> *Jay Lebow (1997, p. 10)*

Couple therapy engages us in a complex, recursive process of interlocking activities: data gathering, hypothesizing, planning, sharing our ideas with clients, and processing their feedback. These activities proceed almost simultaneously, allowing us to continuously refine our working models of what the problem is and what we can do to help. This complexity can be both stimulating and overwhelming. While much of what I do now in couple therapy has become automatic, some attitudes and behaviors require constant vigilance, even after many years. In this chapter, I offer some overarching recommendations for conducting therapy, and then discuss the sequencing of interventions in detail.

Collaboration and the Therapist's Mindset

Many research studies demonstrate the vital importance of a positive therapeutic alliance in couple therapy (Lebow, 2014; Sparks, 2015; Sprenkle, Davis, & Lebow, 2009), and process studies show that therapists do better when they individualize their treatments so as to optimize the alliance (Norcross & Beutler, 2015).[1] Consequently, an overarching concern when doing couple therapy is to maintain and strengthen collaboration between ourselves and our clients. This will frequently influence our choice of interventions.

Thinking of our alliance as a bridge between my clients and me, I continuously assess its strength to see how much weight it can bear. When

I meet client intransigence (resistance), I know I must slow down and examine the trouble. In most cases, clients are protecting themselves from some anticipated danger. In others, *I* am off track. Working with such impasses requires tact and humility, and often bears unexpected fruit, including when clients learn that I can accept their critiques. Like a good personal trainer or athletic coach, I often push a bit more than clients might like, but not so much as to do damage, and always with an eye toward our alliance. When facing resistance, I remind myself of how hard it has been for me to make significant life changes, and I may share some of my own struggles with clients—sometimes with humor, sometimes with sorrow. To create an atmosphere of teamwork, when we hit an impasse, I often solicit clients' help in finding our way out, balancing my role as expert with the necessity of having them make the therapy their own. Finding that balance is sometimes quite challenging.

Since the alliance also hinges on my state of mind, I monitor my own collaborative inclinations. I note times when I want to fight with a client or flee the scene (Wile, 2002), and I give myself the same advice that I give my clients: Try to remain calm, curious, and caring. Curiosity, which helps me remain calm and caring, begins with an empathic attempt to put myself in my clients' shoes, including by paying attention to the frequently distressing feelings they evoke in me. Curiosity can suffer if I feel too sure that I know what is going on; so I try to keep my mind open and capable of generating new hypotheses and testing them against ensuing evidence. This helps especially in situations where what has worked in the past, even many times with many couples, is not working with the couple I am seeing today.

As concerns "caring," I endeavor to maintain a warm, benevolent feeling toward clients and to convey an explicit desire to help them comprehend and reduce their suffering—again, attitudes unsurprisingly associated with client satisfaction and improvement (e.g., Bowman & Fine, 2000). Warmth can fall victim to clients who give their spouses or me a hard time, however, or simply when I become confused or distressed. When I repeatedly feel annoyed with a client, I work hard to understand where my feelings are coming from, so as to contain them and then use them productively.

Over the years, I have tempered my ideas about how much change is possible. Consequently, I focus on what I think can be improved and, as I teach clients, try to accept what can't. Such professional humility frees me to be less defensive when clients complain about results.

Finally, when a therapy stalls, I go back to basics. I try to discover what I may have missed, how I may be making things worse, and what other options I have. I review my notes, especially those from early and high-intensity sessions. I look systematically at biopsychosocial variables I may have overlooked or underestimated. I assess the couple's process, psychodynamics, and skills. And I talk to colleagues and read about other approaches that might help.

Categories of Interventions

Table 15.1 lists the main categories of couple therapy interventions I have described in previous chapters. These interventions are like pieces on a chessboard or tools in a toolbox, each with its own strengths, functions, and limitations. Our challenge is to know how to make them work together and in what order.

Table 15.1 Categories of Couple Therapy Interventions

- Allow the partners to talk to each other, with minimal assistance from the therapist, about problems that concern them (Couple Therapy 1.0).
- Focus on their interpersonal process, especially their negative interaction cycles.
- Focus on their psychodynamics: underlying issues (hopes and fears), personal meanings, transferences and defenses, and attempts to cope via projective identification.
- Focus on acceptance and forgiveness.
- Teach communication skills.
- Teach emotion regulation skills.
- Teach problem-solving and negotiation skills.
- Teach and work out adaptive, domain-specific solutions to particular problems.
- Discuss and encourage positive activities.

Overview of Sequencing

The sequencing of interventions depends on the details of the problem at hand and on the stage of therapy. Some moves will get us off to a good start and others will have to wait. While couple therapy will always be an unpredictable, nonlinear activity—unlike building a bridge, for which steps can be outlined in advance—experience and research show that therapy goes better if therapists pay attention to sequence, notwithstanding the varying sequences recommended by different schools of therapy.

As noted by Scheinkman (2008), a sequencing map can be useful for beginners and experienced therapists alike. For beginners, often flooded with too many options, it offers direction. For experienced therapists, with their ingrained personal preferences, it offers an alternative array of options.

The ideal sequencing map should be relatively comprehensive—allowing improvisational use of diverse interventions as required by specific circumstances—but not so complex or encyclopedic as to give practitioners brain freeze. The ideal map should also prioritize interventions that are most likely to work and to work quickly (Pinsof, 1995). Unlike some therapists, I do not assume that the most expeditious therapy will necessarily begin with attention to behavior, to surface concerns, or to medications, since sometimes these just delay getting to the heart of the matter. In what follows, I describe my sequencing preferences and their rationale, including (a) what to try first, (b) what to try next should that prove insufficient, and (c) what to do when success has created the foundation for further work. Figure 15.1 provides a visual summary of sequencing options, beginning at the top and moving as indicated by the arrows.

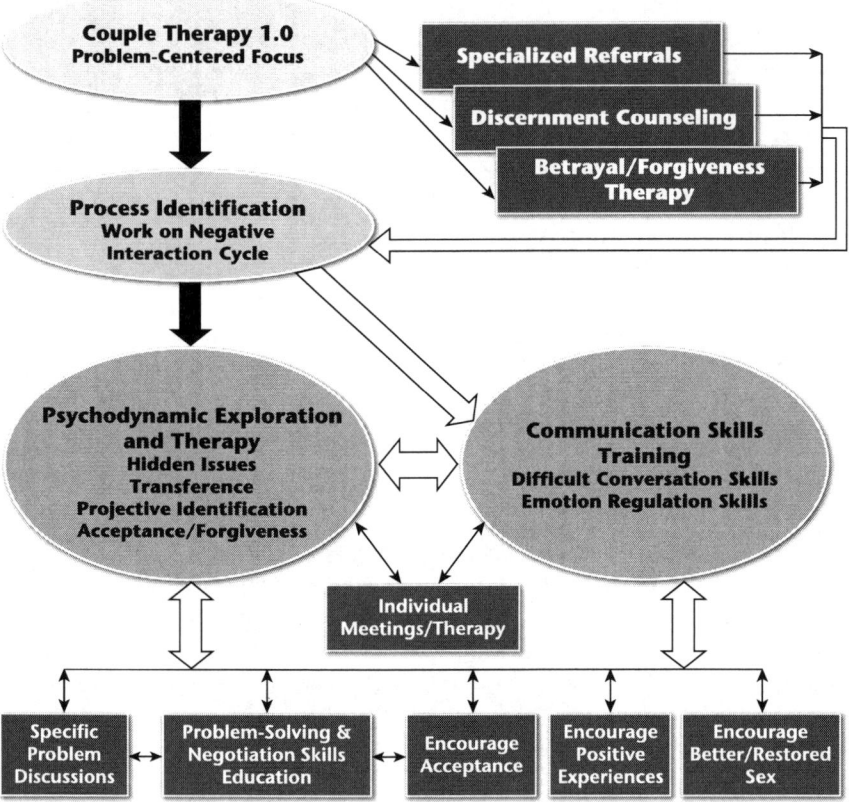

FIGURE 15.1 Sequencing Couple Therapy Interventions. In general, interventions flow from top to bottom and then horizontally, as indicated, with the ovals representing the earlier and more important options. Rectangles at the top represent a rapid alteration of the conjoint format. Those at the bottom represent therapeutic foci made possible by earlier interventions. The exception is the rectangle of individual therapy or individual meetings with the couple therapist, which may be a necessary or concurrent step supporting the entire enterprise.

Couple Therapy 1.0 Interventions

I begin with the conjoint format of therapist and couple meeting to discuss the couple's presenting problems. This will be foundational to all that follows and offers a measure of structure, safety, and hope in the context of a professional, helping relationship.

1. *Begin with the couple's choice of a problem to discuss.* It is almost always best to start the therapy itself, and most subsequent sessions, with the client's choice of a pressing problem. I reserve the option of bringing up topics that have been avoided or that seem promising, and I will sometimes steer partners to more workable topics early on, leaving more difficult issues until later, when their relationship to each other and to therapy is stronger.
2. *Allow the couple to begin to talk unassisted.* After the topic has been opened, encourage the partners to talk to each other about it.[2] If they are doing well, utilizing only the symbolic holding provided by the therapeutic setting and the minimal structuring offered by your presence, allow the dialog to progress and enjoy watching the couple move forward to the next step of minimally assisted problem solving. If things are not going well, proceed to options further down the list. This illustrates an important general principle: *If they are doing well on their own, stay out of it.* As noted by Pinsof (1995), "Excessive therapist competence leads to an underadequate and underachieving patient system," one that is too dependent on the therapist (p. 104).
3. *Attempt assisted problem solving.* Some couples begin talking reasonably well about a delimited topic (parenting a difficult teenager, coping with an aging relative), but then bog down because they have too little information or insufficient problem-solving skills. In such circumstances, I offer the practical assistance the couple appears to need, while helping them to hear each other's feelings and positions more completely. It may be that extensive therapy will not be required if they can succeed with the help of minimal practical mediation and guidance. The test of this is whether the couple actually works out a compromise or solution themselves.

Ancillary or Modified Treatment Formats Based on Presenting Problems

In some situations, the typical conjoint format must be modified immediately.

4. *If divorce seems imminent because one partner is only tenuously committed to the marriage, propose "discernment counseling."* Doherty (2011) has developed an important treatment modification for "mixed-agenda couples" on the brink of divorce, when one (the "leaning out" partner) strongly inclines toward divorce and the other (the "leaning in" partner) wants the marriage

to continue. If after several conjoint couple sessions, the mixed agenda becomes clear, the therapist should begin to work simultaneously with each client separately. The goals are for the partners (a) to develop narratives of their contributions to the marital problems and (b) to *discern* whether or not to stay in the marriage and continue conjoint therapy aimed at improving it. If the partners decide not to go forward, we turn our attention to mourning the marriage and managing the divorce.

Doherty notes that such cases are common and offers his approach to overcoming the structural weaknesses of the usual model of conjoint couple therapy that interfere with success. Fearing that honesty will only increase their partner's hurt or anger, leaning out partners are unwilling to discuss the details of their ambivalence. They may go through the motions and then use the failed therapy to further justify leaving. Leaning in spouses, fearing that honesty will make their partners more determined to leave, will also hold back. Therapists who press ahead make three common errors: pursuing the leaning out spouse too much, agreeing that the marriage cannot be revived, or trying to do couple therapy without a clear contract. Having made all of these mistakes, I now achieve superior results by employing Doherty's format.

The downside of the discernment counseling format is that complications can arise regarding confidential information and uncertainty about whose interests the therapist sees as uppermost. Nonetheless, by having far more direct and transactional information, the couple therapist working separately with both partners has a considerable advantage over the less challenging alternative of each partner working with his or her individual therapist. I have found several months of discernment counseling to be superior to other options. For more information, see the *Minnesota Couples on the Brink Project*'s website: www.cehd.umn.edu/fsos/projects/mcb/couples.asp.

5. *If serious psychopathology, depression, substance abuse, or extensive intimate partner violence are present, make appropriate referrals for specialized treatment; sometimes, this may run concurrently with the couple therapy.*
6. *If betrayal of trust is central at the outset, begin with a conjoint therapy tailored toward forgiveness.*

Negative Process Identification

In most cases, Steps 1 through 3 (Couple Therapy 1.0) will prove inadequate and more assistance will be needed, as follows:

7. *Focus on the couple's interpersonal process.* When minimally structured discussion and practical guidance have failed, I focus on the pathological

group process and identify the steps in the couple's negative interaction cycle. Most of the time, I begin to do this in the first diagnostic session. Almost all contemporary couple therapists begin here. This focus allows us to label the systemic process as the enemy and to suspend work on other presenting problems until the partners improve their manner of relating.

A Fork in the Road

After they have identified the behavioral steps in the couple's negative interaction cycle (e.g., a pursuer–distancer cycle), therapists of different persuasions take different paths. Behaviorally inspired therapists will choose to label specific problems in communication and teach better tactics. Psychoanalytically informed therapists, EFT couple therapists, and others who favor a more experiential approach will focus on the psychodynamic issues that lie below the surface of most "communication problems."

Whichever path we take, if either partner is experiencing too much distress, no new learning or useful dialog will take place. Our job is to help partners to calm down sufficiently to talk to each other safely—sometimes by uncovering and validating deeper emotional concerns, sometimes by teaching rules that direct conversations into less volatile channels. Partners must be relatively calm and receptive for them to engage in problem solving or in planning positive activities.

Sprenkle, Davis, and Lebow (2009), after reviewing many studies of this choice point, concluded that "therapists do better offering insight-oriented procedures to clients who are more self-reflective, introspective, and introverted. Conversely, therapists should offer skill-building and symptom-focused methods to clients who are more impulsive and aggressive" (p. 52).

Consistent with their advice, I take a pragmatic approach tailored to each client's personality style and receptivity. For reasons to be mentioned shortly, I usually begin with a psychodynamic, uncovering approach. Should that prove ineffective, I shift quickly to teaching rules for safe dialog and techniques for emotion regulation. In particular, with high-intensity couples who lack psychological-mindedness, uncovering deeper anxieties—say, about commitment or respect—may be inflammatory. Teaching such couples how to talk more safely will often enable them to access deeper concerns later in the therapy. That said, some volatile couples will not hold still for such practical instruction, so you may need to do some empathic interpreting as a prelude to relationship education.

Psychodynamic Interventions

8. *Focus on underlying issues, personal meanings, transferences, and resistances.* The principal reason to focus here first, before teaching fair-fighting skills,

is because asking people to behave themselves when they don't want to, and don't understand why they should, can feel inauthentic and forced, and may result in a failure to facilitate genuine emotional healing. With this problem of authenticity in mind, my usual preference—after labeling the components of the negative interaction cycle and noting its circularity—is to try to access the deeper, hidden issues that tend to maintain such cycles.

While virtually all couples can use instruction in the optimal ways to handle "difficult conversations," many couples will converse collaboratively soon after the therapist helps them address their underlying concerns. One couple I treated had been fighting endlessly over whether the husband should or should not work harder on his career. This surface disagreement became accessible to discussion soon after I helped them see that the road to compromise was blocked by the emotional issues connected with both the content and the process of their disagreement: the husband feeling shamed and controlled, the wife feeling powerless to avoid reliving the economic hardship she had experienced as a child. In situations like this, uncovering therapy can move things along rapidly, whereas teaching skills like empathic listening can feel like stalling and can actually increase anxiety if partners feel that their complaints remain painfully unaddressed. Indeed, there is suggestive evidence—albeit from research conducted by proponents of this strategy—that choosing this experiential fork in the road yields superior results to choosing behavioral or problem-solving interventions (Johnson & Greenberg, 1985).

The initial goal of the psychodynamic approach is to reduce defensiveness and blame via "reframing" and "making a short story long" as we explore personal meanings and allergic reactions stirred by surface conflicts. Transference hopes and fears and idiographic sensitivities are explored with the goal of elucidating the intense counterproductive behaviors of the negative interaction cycle. Once such an issue is uncovered and reframed in one partner, the other will often become more understanding. When this does not happen, the therapist can work to help him or her react sympathetically, so as to make real dialog and deep intimacy possible. In all cases, therapists can point out that people facing their core negative images or believing that their central needs are not being met will frequently behave badly. Explaining the nearly universal regressive behavior we see in such situations restores hope and facilitates further exploration.

Where to go after the initial exploration of hidden issues depends on the psychodynamics and the content uncovered: Work on projective identification, acceptance, forgiveness, and families of origin usually evolves organically, as specific hidden issues are explored in an increasingly safe setting.

Usually, when I am uncovering psychodynamic issues (meanings, hopes, fears, defenses), my preference is to work in the here-and-now to improve the couple process, prior to exploring historical origins. For instance, I encourage spouses who seem unduly afraid to express themselves to their partners to test out the reality of their fears before I ask them to consider how those fears developed. I do this because it makes corrective experiences more likely, while also making it less likely that the spouse will pile on with, "I've always known you react to me as though I were your mother!"

9. *Work with projective identification.* Viewing couple problems through the lens of projective identification flows naturally out of explorations of unacceptable feelings. Such work holds exceptional promise for effecting long-lasting change. Since projective identification involves motivations to keep the spouse at a distance, successful work here will also improve communication and intimacy. Many couple polarizations spring from the couple *process* itself: Specifically, when each partner voices a part of the truth, but fails to acknowledge the merit of the opposing side, both partners will become more extreme and insistent in maintaining their positions. This type of inductive process can often be interrupted relatively easily by using the "You're Both Right" intervention. When projective identification stems from more characterologically entrenched defensive patterns, however, therapeutic attention must be directed at deeper concerns, since clients aiming to disavow painful states will not so easily concede that "both are right."

10. *Explore each client's family of origin and past history.* Clients will often recall relevant historical material spontaneously as they try to understand specific underlying issues, hopes, and fears. When reviewing historical events, my focus is on how past events are *currently* active and how they shape the present (Breunlin, Pinsof, Russell, & Lebow, 2011; Cooper, 1987). Reviewing formative traumatic life events in detail almost always makes current sensitivities more comprehensible, and that makes everyone more sympathetic. When I feel fairly certain that a current pattern is long-lived, I ask directly about its historical origins: "Has this always been a sensitive area for you? When did it start?" Or, after we have uncovered a particular historical event, I might ask, "How do you think that has affected you and your relationships?"

11. *Work on forgiveness and acceptance.* With some couples, such as those who begin therapy reeling from a recently exposed affair, forgiveness work is necessary from the start, and therapy begins as crisis intervention. This is why I have diagrammed "Betrayal/Forgiveness Therapy" in Figure 15.1 as a separate form of therapy, evolving rapidly out of the limitations of Couple Therapy 1.0. When the chief complaint concerns betrayal, we need to move more quickly past discussion of couple process and follow the treatment guidelines described in Chapter 10. Once things have settled

down, work can proceed in the usual manner, focusing on negative cycles, psychodynamics, and skill deficits, and progressing to discussions of the specific issues that led to the violation of trust. For other couples, specialized forgiveness work will occur later in treatment, when it becomes safe or relevant to bring up a long-past betrayal.

For most couples, work on *acceptance* will almost always come later, after attempts at problem solving and compromise have shown their limitations. To some extent, acceptance is a background theme for all therapeutic interventions, as we work to help clients learn to live with their less-than-perfect partners and their less-than-perfect selves. Working on self-acceptance is also central to reducing projective identification, since partners who can accept negative aspects of themselves no longer need to locate them in their partners.

Behavioral/Educational Interventions

12. *Teach communication and emotion regulation skills.* Early in treatment, I give clients handouts and readings that discuss skillful communication. The readings help us develop a shared vocabulary of do's and don'ts for difficult conversations, presenting the material more systematically and in greater depth than would make sense to do in therapy sessions. They also lend scientific standing to the therapy and locate me in a profession of trustworthy, scientific practitioners.

    Most of my teaching of communication skills then unfolds organically in the context of the couple's discussions, not unlike most lessons in sports, dance, or music, in which individual lessons focus on particular strengths and weaknesses. I offer individualized relationship training when it seems appropriate: communication skills when we encounter recurring maladaptive ways of speaking and listening, emotion regulation skills when emotion tolerance is repeatedly exceeded, and problem-solving and negotiation skills when we discuss specific concrete topics (sex, money, parenting). As indicated by the horizontal arrows in Figure 15.1, there is usually a back and forth focus between psychodynamics and skills education, including moving to explore psychodynamic obstacles to following recommended communication rules.

    As mentioned before, the timing of teaching skills is critical. Too soon, and the therapist may fail to connect with the couple's pain. Too late, and couples may be deprived of powerful tools that can arrest their repetitive negative cycles.

    I teach communication skills more extensively and more systematically in two (sometimes overlapping) situations: with concrete thinkers who are deficient in psychological-mindedness and with emotionally volatile couples. With clients who are non-abstract thinkers less comfortable with—or capable of—introspection, I teach communication skills in a formal manner, early in the treatment. Most of these couples seem grateful for this early shift to relationship education, which offers them explicit rules that help them do better. This is similar to teaching helpful rules of etiquette to people who would be hard-pressed to explain their psychological basis. This also gives these couples a sense of getting something tangible from me, in keeping with their relatively concrete, non-psychological manner of relating.

I also move more quickly to systematic didactic teaching with highly volatile couples, including teaching emotion regulation skills and the nuts and bolts of timeouts. In order to break up the intensity of the conjoint sessions, I sometimes also supplement my work with such emotionally turbulent couples by adding individual sessions.

Specific Problem-Solving Interventions

13. *Work toward resolution of specific tangible problems.* Once we have a more workable interpersonal process, we can begin to target concrete areas of couple conflict. Of course, all along, couples will have been discussing *some* specific topics that have elicited conflict and hard feelings, even as I tried to focus their attention on their maladaptive process, their underlying psychodynamics, and their communication skill deficits. But it is only now, after we have cleared away some of the structural constraints to productive problem solving, that couples will make headway on their more thorny and chronic disagreements. Discussing presenting problems in new and satisfactory ways has been shown to be a frequent characteristic of "pivotal moments" in couple therapy (Helmeke & Sprenkle, 2000).

    At this point, we should recall the research that has found that, in the majority of naturally occurring couple arguments, no practical problem solving is required at all. This is because most such dustups arise from partners' inadvertently touching each other's hot buttons. When this has been the core of a couple's deteriorating marriage, therapy is a matter of teaching the partners to better understand each other's sensitivities (via psychodynamic exploration) and to reconnect (via the empathic apologies that are the heart of the recovery conversations described in Chapter 10).

    Nonetheless, in many cases, substantive issues and conflicts will still require attention. But now, having improved their interpersonal process and ability to work together, partners will have a far better chance of making workable decisions than they had when they entered therapy. Remaining mindful of the couple process, the therapist's attention can now shift to the details of the couple's ongoing disputes. This means returning to Steps 1 to 3 and allowing the couple to have another go at problem solving, with the therapist sometimes offering domain-specific suggestions. Couples

in this phase of treatment will also benefit from self-help readings pertaining to the topics they are discussing (step-parenting, financial planning, caring for an aging parent).
14. *Teach problem-solving and negotiation techniques.* Once we have a more workable interpersonal process and have begun to discuss concrete areas of couple conflict, we can again observe how the couple does on their own. Sometimes, it will help to teach problem-solving and negotiation skills over and above rules for talking to each other safely, but I do this only after determining that it will add value. One advantage of doing this at least once during a course of therapy is that clients will then have these skills available to them after therapy has concluded.

Concurrent Interventions

15. *Along the way, encourage positive interactions.* Concurrently, beginning as soon as I believe there is a reasonable chance of success, I encourage date nights and other pleasurable times spent together, time explicitly prescribed to be free from conflict and stress. As discussed in Chapter 14, I help couples brainstorm and work with them to uncover possible impediments. In the process, it is frequently necessary to *challenge other social obligations that stress the couple and interfere with their good times together.*
16. *Along the way, work to restore sexual intimacy.* For many couples, physical and sexual contact may be the final frontier requiring our help. Even when couples do not explicitly complain about sexual problems, therapists should assess sexual satisfaction, both as a measure of how they are doing and as an important target for assistance.
17. *Along the way, consider recommending individual psychotherapy.* For many clients, couple therapy is a minimally stigmatizing way to begin to rework lifelong sensitivities and personality deficits. After a course of couple therapy, many clients will stop blaming their partners, assume more responsibility for their marital problems, and acknowledge that these problems stem from their own ongoing emotional issues. In such cases, referral for individual treatment or psychoanalysis is often welcome, if not a cause for celebration. Requests for individual therapy referrals are fairly common at the termination of a successful couple treatment.

Whether to recommend individual treatment *during* an ongoing treatment is more debatable. My preference is to try not to complicate matters this way and to wait, instead, until couple issues are considerably improved. The main exception is when serious psychiatric or personality pathology either does not seem to be improving or is grossly interfering with the couple work. In such cases, separate individual therapy may be essential to enabling the couple treatment to succeed (Graller, Nielsen, Garber, et al., 2001).

Repetition and Nonlinearity

Although the decision tree that I have presented appears fairly linear, actual therapy is far more circular, chaotic, and repetitive. Important changes take time and practice before they sink in. Clients rarely understand this: They expect their partners will simply change after being told to do so, and they are surprised when therapy takes so much time and patience. We must therefore help clients replace the discouragement of "Here we go again." with the more hopeful attitude of "OK, things are heating up. What have I learned that can make this work out better for both of us?" Therapists also need not become overly discouraged when, week after week, couples make the same mistakes and follow the same patterns. Change is most often slow and difficult.

Mixing Psychodynamic and Relationship/Educational Interventions

While interventions will often follow one after the other in the sequence I described, skillful therapy will sometimes interdigitate intervention types, for instance, moving back and forth between psychodynamic exploration and educational didactic modes (Wachtel, 2014). Leone (2008) provides a good example of this, in her account of how she directed and challenged a husband to be more verbally present, and then elicited his reactions:

> We talked about my direction and encouragement to Mike. Ann said it was one of the first helpful things I'd done in the 18-month treatment ("Finally!"). Mike acknowledged that if I directed him like that too frequently he might start to feel controlled and dominated by me as he did with Ann. However, he said that in this case he had appreciated the direction, especially because it was a suggestion, not an order. He also described a mixed experience of feeling embarrassed that I'd have to tell him something he "should have known," but also pleased or flattered that I'd seen him as capable of doing it. He had imagined I'd be thinking, "This is important stuff. I'd better handle this, Mike will screw it up!" We explored extensively Mike's sense of himself as "not good at these things," and related it to the fact that no one had comforted him or helped him learn how to comfort someone else.
>
> *(p. 95)*

This example also illustrates the benefits of obtaining client feedback. Some clients will eagerly seek and absorb skills training, while others will resist it as superficial or controlling. Some clients will flourish once we begin to explore and integrate past traumatic events; others will resist and never quite see the relevance. Asking clients how they experienced an intervention, as Leone did, can help us tailor our interventions to client receptivity.

Relationship education and psychodynamics are also intertwined when, after teaching a skill, like the speaker–listener technique, we find clients unable to perform it. Here, we must become curious about the underlying dynamics that interfere. *More than most relationship education or behavioral couple therapies, this roadmap emphasizes working with the psychological issues (the psychodynamics) that make it hard for clients to follow adaptive rules for communicating or problem solving.* In doing so, this becomes an integrative therapy practiced with a "psychoanalytic accent" (Wachtel, 2014, p. 110).

In other cases, the psychodynamics become clearer *after* a client successfully follows our directives about better ways to communicate. For example, one sheepish husband who perennially feared displeasing his wife was overjoyed to see how sticking to the role of active listener almost guaranteed him success with her. More powerfully than my prior interpretations, his actual success demonstrated to him the unreality of his inhibiting fears of failure. Both spouses also had corrective experiences after his wife followed the rule that the speaker keep remarks to a manageable minimum. This allowed her fearful husband to experience her as less overwhelming and allowed her to experience him as more responsive (in contrast to her negative expectations, which had powered her off-putting pursuit). *More than most purely psychodynamic approaches, this roadmap employs teaching and encouraging rules for safe communicating to achieve the "softening," lessened defensiveness, and corrective experiences that are the desired outcomes in emotionally focused therapies and in other therapies based on attachment theory or psychodynamics.*

Finally, as noted by Fraenkel (2009), many of our best interventions are *simultaneously* relationship/educational and psychodynamic, and some will advance the goals of almost all schools of couple therapy:

> [T]eaching (or at least encouraging) a couple to use more equitable, non-aggressive communication is simultaneously supported by a cognitive-behavioral theory promoting acquisition of skill; by a feminist couple approach that seeks to promote greater equality and less intimidation between partners; by a structural couple therapy that promotes increased closeness between partners; by emotionally focused couple therapy that values the opportunities for couples to express deeply held, vulnerable emotions; by a psychodynamically-informed couple therapy focused on increasing each partner's capacity to reflect on the mind of the other; by an attachment-based therapy seeking to improve neuro-physiologically determined emotional regulation (Atkinson, 2005); by a family-of-origin approach seeking to interrupt inherited distance-promoting interactions; and by a narrative couple therapy that values opportunities for each

partner to share their respective perspectives in order to attain a more "preferred story."

(p. 238)

Direction Versus Non-Direction

Separate from client feedback and the decision tree I have outlined, we should base our sequencing choices on the immediate structural pros and cons of possible interventions, including the tradeoffs between being directive and providing a safe, non-directive space for client initiative. As has been emphasized for years by psychodynamically informed therapists, if we give direct advice, we may fail to uncover and discuss the ambivalence and anxiety that block authentic action. Whether clients follow our too-soon advice or rebel against it matters little, since important life decisions based on the preferences of others are unlikely to last or suffice. By contrast, our failing to give helpful, timely advice risks depriving clients of the information they need to make educated choices.

Not only do greater or lesser amounts of directiveness impact clients, but pursuing one or the other shapes our own mindsets. When I am in teaching mode, I am trying to be systematic and convincing. When I am allowing space, I experience more of the free-floating curiosity and openness that are the hallmarks of the listening psychoanalyst. Both are useful, but they are somewhat antithetical states of mind. To achieve balance, I try not to allow myself to get too caught up in one to the exclusion of the other.

Still more generally, the relevant dichotomy here is between having a plan for what should happen next and going with the flow. Therapists who lack a plan will become lost and may fail to recognize landmarks they have visited before, whereas therapists with too much of an agenda will miss improvisational opportunities that emerge out of the give-and-take of the moment. As in so many areas of life, the key to optimal functioning is balance.

Notes

1 Separate from individualizing therapy based on client intervention preferences, Norcross and Beutler's review found better outcomes when therapists paid attention to cultural issues, to coping styles, and to clients' motivation for change.
2 A study by Butler, Harper, and Mitchell (2011) supports giving priority to assisting couples with *talking to each other* (what they call "enactments") and offering input as needed, rather than using a more controlled therapist-directed format from the start. The researchers randomly assigned couples to enactments followed by therapist-directed work, or the reverse sequence. Results strongly favored the former.

16
CONCLUDING REMARKS

I began this book by describing a simple model that I called Couple Therapy 1.0. In this model, the therapist helps partners to "talk to each other" in the here-and-now about difficult, unresolved issues. This is the method I began with 40 years ago, and it still serves as the foundation of the more complex model that evolved from it.

My inability to help a significant number of couples using this bare-bones model led me to add modifications and upgrades drawn from my work and from the work of others in the field. The most important upgrade has been to focus early and explicitly on the couple's interpersonal process, their negative interaction cycle. In most cases, this maladaptive dance, in which couples do all the wrong things and gradually escalate to increasing levels of distress and incapacity, must be addressed before specific problems (with finances, children, or sex) can be tackled. Other important upgrades include unpacking the pathological dance by focusing on psychodynamics; working toward acceptance and forgiveness; teaching communication, emotion regulation, and problem-solving skills; and increasing positive couple experiences.

The advantage of the metaphor of upgrades is that these treatment options can be defined, used, and researched independently of their creators and of the often insular schools of thought that promote them. While it might be true that Therapy X is superior to Therapy Y—although this situation is rarely found in the psychotherapy outcome literature—it is more likely that both X and Y have therapeutic value, and we should be asking when to use each and how to integrate them.

In the introduction to this book, I discussed the theoretical advantages of integrating approaches. In subsequent chapters, I presented what I see as the best practices of each approach and my thoughts on how to sequence and integrate them. My hope and belief is that the field of couple therapy will move gradually beyond narrow "one size fits all" models that developed out of the creative work of diverse, creative individuals, and find ways to agree on a more comprehensive model that benefits from that diversity. Ideally, couple therapy will come to look more like modern medicine, whose texts—on surgery, internal medicine, and pediatrics—have no acronyms, branding, or names of proponents in their titles. (Sticklers might mention here that *Harrison's Textbook of Medicine*, *Nelson's Textbook of Pediatrics*, and *Brain's [sic] Diseases of the Nervous System* live on in ever later editions, but will also know that those gentlemen are now all dead and the volumes that bear their names are multi-authored.) This does not mean that practitioners will ever totally agree on methodologies or that we should stop doing research. Honing our craft will be an ongoing process, but we would do well to learn which interventions from our therapeutic toolboxes work best in which situations and to stop offering treatments based more on therapists' insular training than on couples' individual needs.

Therapist Maturity and Well-Being

Success in couple therapy depends on more than the therapist's knowledge of how to use and sequence various techniques. Research on the outcomes of couple therapy consistently finds that therapist factors are crucial—often apparently more important than the interventions applied (Sprenkle, Davis, & Lebow, 2009). A bedrock principle in psychoanalytic training is that personal mental health is indispensable to therapist performance, and that personal therapy is an important—possibly essential—path to that end. As the therapeutic process unfolds, the therapist's maturity and well-being can be decisive, especially when the therapist is challenged to be a container of difficult emotions and when he or she is under fire from critical, demoralized clients. Sensitivity to divergent cultural values and differences is also essential. My final recommendation to my readers, then, is to work on yourself: Read great literature, pay attention to your own areas of distress, make an effort to understand your family of origin, learn about cultures and values other than your own, work on your relationships and other sources of fulfillment, pay attention to what helps *you*, and gain humility as you see how hard it is to change yourself and those you love.

Relationship Education and Client Feedback: Additional Tools

Before closing, I want to mention two promising, additional upgrades to our ability to help couples. The first is the still underutilized opportunity to reach out and work with people before they come to us with relationship problems.

Relationship education programs have been shown to improve communication and conflict management skills, increase commitment and positive feelings about marriage, and reduce chances of divorce (Carroll & Doherty, 2003; Stanley, 2001; Stanley, Amato, Johnson, & Markman, 2006). In my ideal world, we would provide destigmatized, universal relationship education at predictable stages of life, from elementary school through college, prior to weddings and childbirth, and as needed for married couples—just as we offer sex education and childbirth preparation classes. Current exemplars are *The First Dance* program (www.thefirstdance.com) and the *Bringing Baby Home* program (Shapiro & Gottman, 2005; Gottman & Gottman, 2007) designed for couples who are, respectively, about to get married or about to have a baby; and PREP (Markman, Stanley, & Blumberg, 2001; www.prepinc.com), PAIRS (Gordon, 1993; www.pairs.com), Prepare-Enrich (www.prepare-enrich.com), and Relationship Enhancement (Guerney, 1977; www.nire.org), which offer marriage education to those who seek it, before or after they marry. While marriage education has been shown to be beneficial during marriage, reaching people even sooner has advantages, especially in heading off the unions of mismatched couples. Currently, many high schools and some elementary schools offer programs in relationship education, some utilizing components of the previously mentioned programs for adults. Our own *Marriage 101* course offers such education to college students (Nielsen, Pinsof, Rampage, et al., 2004), and contributes to the growing, but still underutilized, field of marriage education for young adults (Lowe, 2003; Lowe, Scott-Lowe, & Markman, 2003; Stanley, 2001).

Finally, I want to flag the promising development of using ongoing (computerized) client feedback to improve the results of couple therapy. Sparks (2015) has reviewed this topic and the extremely positive results of a large-scale, randomized clinical trial in Norway. My colleagues at The Family Institute at Northwestern University are engaged in similar promising research (Pinsof, Breunlin, Russell, & Lebow, 2011). Routine client feedback may be especially helpful in situations where clients are silent about their dissatisfaction with the therapy or therapist and, more generally, may facilitate active participation by all clients in the work.

Book Two

This volume has covered the basic categories of interventions currently available to couple therapists, including recommendations on how to sequence and choose among them. But there is much more to say, especially about the nitty-gritty details of doing therapy. In a second volume—shamelessly plugged here and tentatively titled *Comprehensive Couple Therapy in Practice*—I will discuss (a) how to work with common problems that couples face (including money, children, sex, and extramarital affairs), (b) psycho-pathological complications (including clients with depression or serious personality disorders), and (c) additional practical aspects of doing couple therapy (conducting diagnostic interviews, collaborating with other therapists, and other nuts-and-bolts issues).

Closing Thoughts

Treating couples is an adventure. People share their deepest hurts and fears with us so that we can help them cope with the painful and perplexing issues of their lives. In doing so, they offer us a gift that can enrich our lives, as well. Couple therapy is almost always fascinating and challenging. It is also sometimes terribly sad or utterly frustrating, but even then we have a front-row seat for many of life's otherwise hidden dramas. As we engage with couples, we gain invaluable wisdom and perspective on life. When we make a difference in our clients' lives, we feel the profound satisfaction that comes from serving others and the gratifying feeling that we are on this planet for a reason.

Couple therapy will always be a clinical art form that relies on our ability to synthesize our storehouse of knowledge with our experience, intuition, and wisdom. I hope that the model I have presented here has added substantially to your own personal storehouse and will be of value as you engage in this fascinating, challenging, and most worthwhile enterprise.

REFERENCES

Akhtar, S. (2002). Forgiveness: Origins, dynamics, psychopathology and technical relevance. *Psychoanalytic Quarterly, 71,* 178–212.

Alarcón, R. D., & Frank, J. B. (2011). *The psychotherapy of hope: The legacy of persuasion and healing.* Baltimore, MD: Johns Hopkins University Press.

Amato, P. R. (2010). Research on divorce: Continuing trends and developments. *Journal of Marriage and Family, 72,* 650–666.

Aron, A., Norman, C. C., Aron, E. N., McKenna, C., & Heyman, R. (2000). Couples' shared participation in novel and arousing activities and experienced relationship quality. *Journal of Personality and Social Psychology, 78,* 273–283.

Atkinson, B. (2005). *Emotional intelligence in couples therapy: Advances from neurobiology and the science of intimate relationships.* New York: W. W. Norton.

Atkinson, B. (2010). Rewiring emotional habits: The pragmatic/experiential approach. In A. S. Gurman (Ed.), *Clinical casebook for couple therapy* (4th ed., pp. 181–207). New York: Guilford Press.

Atkinson, B. (2013). Mindfulness training and the cultivation of secure, satisfying couple relationships. *Couple and Family Psychology: Research and Practice, 2,* 73–94.

Basch, M. (1988). *Understanding psychotherapy: The science behind the art.* New York: Basic Books.

Bateson, G. (1972). *Steps to an ecology of mind.* New York: Ballantine Books.

Baucom, D. H., Epstein, N. B., Taillade, J. J., & Kirby, J. S. (2008). Cognitive-behavioral couple therapy. In A. S. Gurman (Ed.), *Clinical handbook of couple therapy* (4th ed., pp. 31–72). New York: Guilford Press.

Baucom, D. H., Hahlweg, K., & Kuschel, A. (2003). Are waiting-list control groups needed in future marital therapy outcome research? *Behavior Therapy, 34,* 179–188.

Baucom, D. H., Snyder, D. K., & Gordon, K. C. (2009). *Helping couples get past the affair: A clinician's guide.* New York: Guilford Press.

Baumeister, R. F., Exline, J. J., & Sommer, K. L. (1998). The victim role, grudge theory, and two dimensions of forgiveness. In E. L. Worthington, Jr. (Ed.),

Dimensions of forgiveness: Psychological research and theological perspectives (pp. 79–104). Philadelphia: John Templeton Press.

Baumeister, R. F., Bratslavsky, E., Finkenauer, C., & Vohs, K. D. (2001). Bad is stronger than good. *Review of General Psychology, 5,* 323–370.

Benjamin, J. (1995). *Like subjects, love objects.* New Haven: Yale University Press.

Benjamin, J. (2004). Beyond doer and done to: An intersubjective view of thirdness. *Psychoanalytic Quarterly, 73,* 5–46.

Bergler, E. (1949). *Conflict in marriage: The unhappy undivorced.* Madison, CT: International Universities Press.

Berkowitz, D. A. (1999). Reversing the negative cycle: Interpreting the mutual influence of adaptive, self-protective measures in the couple. *Psychoanalytic Quarterly, 68,* 559–583.

Betchen, S. J. (2005). *Intrusive partners/elusive mates: The pursuer–distancer dynamic in couples.* New York: Routledge.

Bion, W. (1961). *Experiences in groups.* New York: Basic Books.

Bion, W. (1962). *Learning from experience.* London: Tavistock Publications.

Bowman, L., & Fine, M. (2000). Client perceptions of couples therapy: Helpful and unhelpful aspects. *American Journal of Family Therapy, 28,* 295–310.

Bradbury, T. N., Fincham, F. D., & Beach, S. R. H. (2000). Research on the nature and determinants of marital satisfaction: A decade in review. *Journal of Marriage and the Family, 62,* 964–980.

Bradbury, T. N., & Karney, B. R. (2010). *Intimate relationships.* New York: W. W. Norton.

Breunlin, D. C., Pinsof, W., Russell, W. P., & Lebow, J. (2011). Integrative problem-centered metaframeworks therapy I: Core concepts and hypothesizing. *Family Process, 50,* 293–313.

Booth, A., & Amato, R. (2001). Parental predivorce relations and offspring post-divorce well-being. *Journal of Marriage and Family, 63,* 197–212.

Buehlman, K. T., Gottman, J. M., & Katz, L. F. (1992). How a couple views their past predicts their future: Predicting divorce from an oral history interview. *Journal of Family Psychology, 5,* 295–318.

Butler, M. H., Harper, J. M., & Mitchell, C. B. (2011). A comparison of attachment outcomes in enactment-based versus therapist-centered therapy process modalities in couple therapy. *Family Process, 50,* 203–220.

Carlson, R. G., Guttierrez, D., Daire, A. P., & Hall, K. (2014). Does the frequency of speaker–listener technique use influence relationship satisfaction? *Journal of Psychotherapy Integration, 24,* 25–29.

Carroll, J., & Doherty, W. (2003). Evaluating the effectiveness of premarital prevention programs: A meta-analytic review of outcome research. *Family Relations, 52,* 105–118.

Catherall, D. (1992). Working with projective identification in couples. *Family Process, 31,* 355–367.

Cherlin, A. J. (2004). The deinstitutionalization of American marriage. *Journal of Marriage and Family, 66,* 848–861.

Christensen, A. (2010). A unified protocol for couple therapy. In K. Hahlweg, M. Grawe-Gerber, & D. H. Baucom (Eds.), *Enhancing couples: The shape of couple therapy to come* (pp. 33–46). Gottingen, Germany: Hogrefe.

Christensen, A., & Jacobson, N. (2000). *Reconcilable differences.* New York: Guilford Press.

Coan, J. A., Schaefer, H. S., & Davidson, R. J. (2006). Lending a hand: Social regulation of the neural response to threat. *Psychological Science, 12,* 1032–1039.

Cohen, S., Schulz, M., Liu, S., Halassa, M., & Waldinger, R. J. (2015). Empathic accuracy and aggression in couples: Individual and dyadic links. *Journal of Marriage and Family, 77,* 697–711.

Cohn, D. A., Silver, D. H., Cowan, C. P., Cowan, P. A., & Pearson, J. (1992). Working models of childhood attachment and couple relationships. *Journal of Family Issues, 13,* 432–449.

Colman, A. D., & Bexton, W. H. (Eds.). (1975). *Group relations reader.* Sausalito, CA: GREX.

Coontz, S. (2005). *Marriage, a history: How love conquered marriage.* New York: Penguin Books.

Cooper, A. (1987). Changes in psychoanalytic ideas: Transference interpretation. *Journal of the American Psychoanalytic Association, 35,* 77–98.

Copen, C. E., Daniels, K., Vespa, J., & Mosher, W. D. (2012). First marriages in the United States: Data from the 2006–2010 National Survey of Family Growth. *National Health Statistics Reports, No. 49,* March 22, 2012.

Cordova, J. V., Jacobson, N. S., & Christensen, A. (1998). Acceptance vs. change in behavioral couples therapy: Impact on client communication processes in the therapy session. *Journal of Marital and Family Therapy, 24,* 437–455.

Cornelius, T. I., & Alessi, G. (2007). Behavioral and physiological components of communication training: Does the topic affect outcome? *Journal of Marriage and Family, 69,* 608–620.

Crapuchettes, B., & Beauvoir, F. C. (2011). Relational meditation. *Psychotherapy Networker,* September–October issue, www.psychotherapynetworker.org/magazine/recentissues/2011-septoct/item/1367-relational-meditation, retrieved 11/15/2011.

Cummings, E., & Davies, P. (1994). *Children and marital conflict: The impact of family dispute and resolution.* New York: Guilford Press.

Curran, M., Ogolsky, B., Hazen, N., & Bosch, L. (2011). Understanding marital conflict 7 years later from prenatal representations of marriage. *Family Process,* 50, 221–234.

Davison, T. (2013). *Mindfulness based cognitive-behavioral psychotherapy.* Unpublished booklet available from the author.

Dicks, H. (1967). *Marital tensions.* New York: Basic Books.

Dimen, M. (2003). *Sexuality, intimacy, power.* New York: The Analytic Press.

Dimidjian, S., Martell, C. R., & Christensen, A. (2008). Integrative behavioral couple therapy. In A. S. Gurman (Ed.), *Clinical handbook of couple therapy* (4th ed., pp. 73–103). New York: Guilford Press.

Doherty, W. J. (2003). *Take back your marriage: Sticking together in a world that pulls us apart.* New York: Guilford Press.

Doherty, W. J. (2011). In or out: Treating the mixed-agenda couple. *Psychotherapy Networker, 35,* 45–50, 58–60.

Doherty, W. J., Galston, W. A., Glenn, N. D., Gottman, J., Markey, B., Markman, H. J. . . . & Wallerstein, J. (2002). *Why marriage matters: Twenty-one conclusions from the social sciences. A report from family scholars.* New York: Institute for American Values.

Donovan, J. M. (2003). *Short-term object relations couples therapy.* New York: Brunner-Routledge.

Driver, J. L. (2007). Observations of newlywed interaction in conflict and in everyday life. *Dissertation Abstracts International: Section B: The Sciences and Engineering, 67 (9-B),* 5441.

Durtschi, J. A., Fincham, F. D., Cui, M., Lorenz, F. O., & Conger, R. D. (2011). Dyadic processes in early marriage: Attributions, behavior, and marital quality. *Family Relations, 60,* 421–434.

Edelson, M. (1983). Is testing psychoanalytic hypotheses in the psychoanalytic situation really impossible? *Psychoanalytic Study of the Child, 38,* 61–109.

Eggerichs, E. (2004). *Love and respect: The love she most desires; the respect he desperately needs.* Nashville, TN: Thomas Nelson.

Engel, G. L. (1980). The clinical application of the biopsychosocial model. *American Journal of Psychiatry, 137,* 535–544.

Enright, R. D., & Fitzgibbons, R. P. (2000). *Helping clients to forgive: An empirical guide for resolving anger and restoring hope.* Washington, DC: American Psychological Association.

Fehr, R., Gelfand, M. J., & Nag, M. (2010). The road to forgiveness: A meta-analytic synthesis of its situational and dispositional correlates. *Psychological Bulletin, 136,* 894–914.

Feldman, L. B. (1979). Marital conflict and marital intimacy: An integrative psychodynamic-behavioral-systemic model. *Family Process, 18,* 69–78.

Felmlee, D. H. (1998). "Be careful what you wish for . . .": A quantitative and qualitative investigation of "fatal attractions." *Personal Relationships, 5,* 235–253.

Fincham, F. D., & Beach, S. R. H. (1999). Conflict in marriage: Implications for working with couples. *Annual Review of Psychology, 50,* 47–77.

Fincham, F. D., & Rogge, R. (2010). Understanding relationship quality: Theoretical challenges and new tools for assessment. *Journal of Family Theory and Review, 2,* 227–242.

Finkel, E. J., Slotter, E. B., Luchies, L. B., Walton, G. M., & Gross, J. J. (2013). A brief intervention to promote conflict reappraisal preserves marital quality over time. *Psychological Science, 24,* 1595–1601.

Fishbane, M. D. (2010). Relational empowerment in couple therapy: An integrative approach. In A. S. Gurman (Ed.), *Clinical casebook of couple therapy* (4th ed., pp. 208–231). New York: Guilford Press.

Fishbane, M. D. (2013). *Loving with the brain in mind: Neurobiology and couple therapy.* New York: W.W. Norton.

Fisher, H. (2004). *Why we love: The nature and chemistry of romantic love.* New York: Henry Holt.

Fisher, R., & Shapiro, D. (2005). *Beyond reason: Using emotions as you negotiate.* New York: Penguin Books.

Fisher, R., Ury, W., & Patton, B. (2011). *Getting to yes: Negotiating agreement without giving in* (3rd ed.). New York: Penguin Books.

Fonagy, P. (2000). Attachment and borderline personality disorder. *Journal of the American Psychoanalytic Association, 48,* 1129–1146.

Fosco, G. M., Lippold, M., & Feinberg, M. E. (2014). Interparental boundary problems, parent–adolescent hostility, and adolescent–parent hostility: A family process model of adolescent aggression problems. *Couple and Family Psychology: Research and Practice, 3,* 141–155.

Fowers, B. J., & Owenz, M. B. (2010). A eudaimonic theory of marital quality. *Journal of Family Theory & Review, 2,* 334–352.

Framo, J. L. (1976). Family of origin as a therapeutic resource for adults in marital and family therapy: You can and should go home again. *Family Process, 15,* 193–210.

Frank, J. (1961). *Persuasion and healing*. Baltimore: Johns Hopkins University Press.

Fraenkel, P. (2009). The therapeutic palette: A guide to choice points in integrative couple therapy. *Clinical Social Work Journal, 37*, 234–247.

Fraenkel, P. (2011). *Synch your relationships, save your marriage*. New York: Palgrave MacMillan.

Freud, S. (1920). *Beyond the pleasure principle. Standard Edition (SE), Vol. 18*, 7–64.

Freud, S. (1926). *Inhibitions, symptoms and anxiety. SE, Vol. 20*, 87–174.

Frommer, M. S. (2005). Thinking relationally about forgiveness: Commentary on paper by Stephen Wangh. *Psychoanalytic Dialogues, 15*, 33–45.

Fruzzetti, A. E. (2006). *The high-conflict couple: A dialectical behavior therapy guide to finding peace, intimacy and validation*. Oakland, CA: New Harbinger Publications.

Gallwey, W. T. (1974). *The inner game of tennis: The classic guide to the mental side of peak performance*. New York: Random House.

Gehrie, M. J. (2011). From archaic narcissism to empathy for the self: The evolution of new capacities in psychoanalysis. *Journal of the American Psychoanalytic Association, 59*, 313–333.

Gerson, M-J. (2010). *The embedded self: An integrative psychodynamic and systemic perspective on couples and family therapy* (2nd ed.). New York: Routledge.

Gill, M. M. (1982). *Analysis of transference*. New York: International Universities Press.

Gladwell, M. (2008). *Outliers: The story of success*. New York: Little, Brown.

Gobodo-Madikizela, P. (2008). Trauma, forgiveness and the witnessing dance: Making public spaces intimate. *Journal of Analytical Psychology, 53*, 169–188.

Goldbart, S., & Wallin, D. (1994). *Mapping the terrain of the heart: Passion, tenderness and the capacity to love*. Northvale, NJ: Jason Aronson.

Goldberg, A. (1999). *Being of two minds: The vertical split in psychoanalysis and psychotherapy*. Hillsdale, N.J.: The Analytic Press.

Goldklank, S. (2009). "The Shoop Shoop Song": A guide to psychoanalytic-systemic couple therapy. *Contemporary Psychoanalysis, 45*, 3–25.

Goldman, R. N., & Greenberg, L. S. (2013). Working with identity and self-soothing in Emotion-Focused Therapy for Couples. *Family Process, 52*, 62–82.

Goldner, V. (2004). When love hurts: Treating abusive relationships. *Psychoanalytic Inquiry, 24*, 346–372.

Goldner, V. (2013). Plenary Discussant of "Advances in Couples Therapy and Research," American Family Therapy Academy annual meeting, Chicago, IL, June 2013.

Gordon, L. (1993). *Passage to intimacy*. New York: Fireside/Simon & Schuster.

Gottman, J. M. (2011). *The science of trust: Emotional attunement for couples*. New York: W. W. Norton.

Gottman, J., Coan, J., Carrera, S., & Swanson, C. (1998). Predicting marital happiness and stability from newlywed interactions. *Journal of Marriage and the Family, 60*, 5–22.

Gottman, J. M., & Gottman, J. S. (2007). *And baby makes three*. New York: Three Rivers Press.

Gottman, J. M., & Gottman, J. S. (2010). Gottman method couple therapy. In A. S. Gurman (Ed.), *Clinical handbook of couple therapy* (4th ed., pp. 138–164). New York: Guilford Press.

Gottman, J. M., Katz, L., & Hooven, C. (1996). *Meta-emotion: How families communicate emotionally*. Hillsdale, NJ: Lawrence Erlbaum Associates.

Gottman, J. M., & Levenson, R. W. (1999). What predicts change in marital interaction over time: A study of alternative models. *Family Process, 38,* 143–158.

Gottman, J. M., & Silver, N. (1999). *The seven principles for making marriage work.* New York: Crown.

Graller, J., Nielsen, A. C., Garber, B., Davison, L. G., Gable, L., & Seidenberg, H. (2001). Concurrent therapies: A model for collaboration between psychoanalysts and other therapists. *Journal of the American Psychoanalytic Association, 49,* 587–606.

Gray, J. (1992). *Men are from Mars, women are from Venus: The classic guide to understanding the opposite sex.* New York: HarperCollins.

Gray, P. (1994). *The ego and analysis of defense.* Northvale, NJ: Jason Aronson.

Greenberg, L. S., & Goldman, R. N. (2008). *Emotion-focused couples therapy: The dynamics of emotion, love, and power.* Washington, DC: American Psychological Association.

Greenberg, L. S. & Johnson, S. M. (1988). *Emotionally focused therapy for couples.* New York: Guilford Press.

Greenberg, L. S., Warwar, S. H., & Malcolm, W. M. (2008). Differential effects of Emotion-Focused Therapy and psychoeducation in facilitating forgiveness and letting go of emotional injuries. *Journal of Counseling Psychology, 55,* 185–196.

Greenberg, L. S., Warwar, S. H., & Malcolm, W. M. (2010). Emotion-Focused Couples Therapy and the facilitation of forgiveness. *Journal of Marital and Family Therapy, 36,* 28–42.

Greenman, P. S., & Johnson, S. M. (2013). Process research on emotionally focused therapy (EFT) for couples: Linking theory to practice. *Family Process, 52,* 46–61.

Greenson, R. R. (1967). *The technique and practice of psychoanalysis.* New York: International Universities Press.

Guerney, B. G. (1977). *Relationship enhancement: Skill training programs for therapy, problem prevention, and enrichment.* San Francisco, CA: Jossey-Bass, Inc.

Gurman, A. S. (Ed.). (2008a). *Clinical handbook of couple therapy* (4th ed.). New York: Guilford Press.

Gurman, A. S. (2008b). Integrative couple therapy: A depth psychological approach. In A. S. Gurman (Ed.), *Clinical handbook of couple therapy* (4th ed., pp. 383–423). New York: Guilford Press.

Gurman, A. S. (Ed.). (2010). *Clinical casebook of couple therapy* (4th ed.). New York: Guilford Press.

Gurman, A. S. (2011). Couple therapy research and the practice of couple therapy: Can we talk? *Family Process, 50,* 280–292.

Gurman, A. S. (2013). Behavioral couple therapy: Building a secure base for therapeutic integration. *Family Process, 52,* 115–138.

Gurman, A. S., & Burton, M. (2014). Individual therapy for couple problems: Perspectives and pitfalls. *Journal of Marital and Family Therapy, 40,* 470–483.

Haley, J. (1976). *Problem-solving therapy.* San Francisco: Jossey-Bass.

Hamburg, S. M. (2000). *Will our love last?: A couple's road map.* New York: Scribner.

Hanson, R., & Mendius, R. (2009). *Buddha's brain: Happiness, love, & wisdom.* Oakland, CA: New Harbinger Publications.

Hawkins, D. N., & Booth, A. (2005). Unhappily ever after: Effects of long-term, low-quality marriages on well-being. *Social Forces, 84,* 445–465.

Hazlett, P. S. (2010). Attunement, disruption, and repair: The dance of self and other in emotionally focused couple therapy. In A. S. Gurman (Ed.), *Clinical casebook for couple therapy* (4th ed., pp. 21–43). New York: Guilford Press.

Helmeke, K. B., & Sprenkle, D. H. (2000). Clients' perception of pivotal moments in couples therapy: A qualitative study of change in therapy. *Journal of Marital and Family Therapy, 26,* 469–483.

Hendrix, H. (1988). *Getting the love you want: A guide for couples.* New York: Henry Holt.

Hetherington, E. (2003). Intimate pathways: Changing patterns in close personal relationships across time. *Family Relations, 52,* 318–331.

Horowitz, M. J. (1979). *States of mind: Analysis of change in psychotherapy.* New York: Plenum Medical Book Company.

Jacobson, N. S., & Addis, M. (1993). Research on couples and couples therapy: What do we know? Where are we going? *Journal of Consulting and Clinical Psychology,* 61, 85–93.

Jacobson, N. S., & Christensen, A. (1998). *Acceptance and change in couple therapy: A therapist's guide to transforming relationships.* New York: W.W. Norton.

Johnson, A. M. (1949). Sanctions for superego lacunae of adolescents. In K. R. Eissler (Ed.), *Searchlights on delinquency: New psychoanalytic studies.* Oxford, England: International Universities Press.

Johnson, M. D., & Bradbury, T. N. (2015). Contributions of social learning theory to the promotion of healthy relationships: Asset or liability? *Journal of Family Theory & Review, 7,* 13–27.

Johnson, S. M. (1996). *The practice of emotionally focused marital therapy.* Florence, KY: Brunner/Mazel.

Johnson, S. M. (2008). Emotionally focused couple therapy, Chapter 4 in A. S. Gurman (Ed.), *Clinical handbook of couple therapy* (4th ed., pp. 107–137). New York: Guilford Press.

Johnson, S. M., & Greenberg, L. S. (1985). The differential effects of experiential and problem solving interventions in resolving marital conflict. *The Journal of Consulting & Clinical Psychology, 53,* 175–184.

Johnson, S. M., Makinen, J. A., & Millikin, J. W. (2001). Attachment injuries in couple relationships: A new perspective on impasses in couples therapy. *Journal of Marital and Family Therapy, 27,* 145–155.

Jones, D. (2014). *Love illuminated: Exploring life's most mystifying subject (with the help of 50,000 strangers).* New York: HarperCollins.

Karney, B. R., & Bradbury, T. N. (1995). The longitudinal course of marital quality and stability: A review of theory, method, and research. *Psychological Bulletin, 118,* 3–34.

Kelly, A. B., Fincham, F. D., & Beach, S. R. H. (2003). Communication skills in couples: A review and discussion of emerging perspectives. In J. O. Greene & B. R. Burleson (Eds.), *Handbook of communication and social interaction skills* (pp. 723–751). Mahwah, NJ: Lawrence Erlbaum Associates.

Kernberg, O. (2011). Limitations to the capacity to love. *International Journal of Psychoanalysis, 92,* 1501–1515.

Keyes, C. L. M., & Haidt, J. (Eds.). (2003). *Flourishing: Positive psychology and the life well-lived.* Washington, DC: American Psychological Association.

Kim, H. K., Capaldi, D. M., & Crosby, L. (2007). Generalizability of Gottman and colleagues' affective process models of couples' relationship outcomes. *Journal of Marriage and Family, 69,* 55–72.

Kimmes, J. G., Durtschi, J. A., Clifford, C. E., Knapp, D. J., & Fincham, F. D. (2015). The role of pessimistic attributions in the association between anxious attachment and relationship satisfaction. *Family Relations, 64,* 547–562.

Knudson-Martin, C. (2013). Why power matters: Creating a foundation of mutual support in couple relationships. *Family Process, 52,* 5–18.
Kohut, H. (1971). *The analysis of the self.* New York: International Universities Press.
Kohut, H. (1977). *The restoration of the self.* New York: International Universities Press.
Kohut, H. (1984). *How does analysis cure?* Chicago: University of Chicago Press.
Komorita, S. S., & Parks, C. D. (1995). Interpersonal relations: Mixed-motive interaction. *Annual Review of Psychology, 46,* 183–207.
Kornfield, J. (2008). *Meditation for beginners.* Boulder, CO: Sounds True, Inc.
Kurdek, L.A. (2004). Do gay and lesbian couples really differ from heterosexual married couples? *Journal of Marriage and the Family, 66,* 880–900.
Lansky, M. R. (2007). Unbearable shame, splitting, and forgiveness in the resolution of vengefulness. *Journal of the American Psychoanalytic Association, 55,* 571–593.
Lavner, J. A., & Bradbury, T. N. (2010). Patterns of change in marital satisfaction over the newlywed years. *Journal of Marriage and Family, 72,* 1171–1187.
Lawrence, E., & Brock, R. L. (2010). The North-Going Zax and the South-Going Zax: From impasse to empathic acceptance, in Integrative Behavioral Couple Therapy. In A. S. Gurman (Ed.), *Clinical casebook for couple therapy* (4th ed., pp. 67–89). New York: Guilford Press.
Lebow, J. L. (1997). The integrative revolution in couple and family therapy. *Family Process, 36,* 1–17.
Lebow, J. L. (2014). *Couple and family therapy: An integrative map of the territory.* Washington, DC: American Psychological Association.
Lebow, J. L., Chambers, A. L., Christensen, A., & Johnson, S. M. (2012). Research on the treatment of couple distress. *Journal of Marital and Family Therapy, 38,* 145–168.
LeDoux, J. (1996). *The emotional brain.* New York: Simon & Schuster.
Lee, G. R., Seccombe, K., & Sheehan, C. L. (1991). Marital status and personal happiness: An analysis of trend data. *Journal of Marriage and the Family, 53,* 839–844.
Leiblum, S. R. (Ed.). (2007). *Principles and practice of sex therapy* (4th ed.). New York: Guilford Press.
Leone, C. (2008). Couple therapy from the perspective of self psychology and intersubjectivity theory. *Psychoanalytic Psychology, 25,* 79–98.
Levine, S. B. (1999). *Sexuality in mid-life.* New York: Plenum Press.
Levine, S. B., Risen, C. B., & Althof, S. E. (Eds.). (2010). *Handbook of Clinical Sexuality for Mental Health Professionals* (2nd ed.). New York: Routledge.
Lewis, J. M. (1997). *Marriage as a search for healing: Theory, assessment, and therapy.* New York: Bruner/Mazel.
Lewis, J. T., Parra, G. R., & Cohen, R. (2015). Apologies in close relationships: A review of theory and research. *Journal of Family Theory & Review, 7,* 47–61.
Lichtenberg, J. D., Lachmann, F. M., & Fosshage, J. L. (2011). *Psychoanalysis and motivational systems: A new look.* New York: Routledge.
Linehan, M. M. (1993). *Skills training manual for treating borderline personality disorders.* New York: Guilford Press.
Livingston, M. S. (1995). A self psychologist in Couplesland: Multisubjective approach to transference and countertransference-like phenomena in marital relationships. *Family Process, 34,* 427–439.
Lowe, D. (2003). *Junior college, college, and university based marriage education programs.* Unpublished research, June, 2003, available from the author.
Lowe, D., Scott-Lowe, E., & Markman, H. (2003). *Teaching PREP in a university setting: Using Fighting For Your Marriage in a college course.* Denver, CO: PREP Educational Products.

Luborsky, L. (1990). *Understanding transference*. New York: Basic Books.
Luskin, F. (2002). *Forgive for good*. New York: HarperCollins.
Lyons-Ruth, K. (1999). The two-person unconscious: Intersubjective dialogue, enactive relational representation, and the emergence of new forms of relational organization. *Psychoanalytic Inquiry*, 19, 576–617.
Lyubomirsky, S. (2013). *The myths of happiness: What should make you happy, but doesn't; what shouldn't make you happy, but does*. London: Penguin Books.
Malan, D. H. (1979). *Individual psychotherapy and the science of psychodynamics*. London: Butterworths.
Margolies, E. (2001). *Men with sexual problems and what women can do to help them*. Northvale, NJ: Jason Aronson.
Markman, H., Stanley, S., & Blumberg, S. (2001). *Fighting for your marriage* (2nd ed.). San Francisco: Jossey-Bass.
Masters, W. H., & Johnson, V. E. (1970). *Human sexual inadequacy*. Boston: Little, Brown.
McCarthy, B., & McCarthy, E. (2003). *Rekindling desire: A step-by-step program to help low-sex and no-sex marriages*. New York: Brunner-Routledge.
McCarthy, B. W., & Thestrup, M. (2008). Couple therapy and the treatment of sexual dysfunction. In A. S. Gurman (Ed.), *Clinical handbook of couple therapy* (4th ed., pp. 591–617). New York: Guilford Press.
McCullough, M. E., Pargament, K. I., & Thorsen, C. E. (Eds.). (2000). *Forgiveness: Theory, research, and practice*. New York: Guilford Press.
McGoldrick, M., & Gerson, R. (1985). *Genograms in family assessment*. New York: W.W. Norton.
Middleberg, C. V. (2001). Projective identification in common couple dances. *Journal of Marital and Family Therapy*, 27, 341–352.
Mikulincer, M., Florian, V., Cowan, P. A., & Cowan, C. P. (2002). Attachment security in couple relationships: A systemic model and its implications for family dynamics. *Family Process*, 41, 405–434.
Minuchin, S. (1974). *Families and family therapy*. Cambridge, MA: Harvard University Press.
Minuchin, S., & Fishman, H. C. (1981). *Family therapy techniques*. Cambridge, MA: Harvard University Press.
Mitchell, S. A. (2002). *Can love last? The fate of romance over time*. New York: W.W. Norton.
Mnookin, R. H., Pettet, S. R., & Tulumello, A. S. (2000). *Beyond winning: Negotiating to create value in deals and disputes*. Cambridge, MA: Harvard University Press.
Neff, L. A., & Karney, B. R. (2004). How does context affect intimate relationships? Linking external stress and cognitive processes within marriage. *Personality and Social Psychology Bulletin*, 30, 134–148.
Newman, K. (1996). Winnicott goes to the movies: The false self in *Ordinary People*. *Psychoanalytic Quarterly*, 65, 787–807.
Niehuis, S., Lee, K-H, Reifman, A., Swenson, A., & Hunsaker, S. (2011). Idealization and disillusionment in intimate relationships: A review of theory, method, and research. *Journal of Family Theory & Review*, 3, 273–302.
Nielsen, A.C. (1980). Gestalt and psychoanalytic therapies: Structural analysis and rapprochement. *American Journal of Psychotherapy*, 19, 534–544.
Nielsen, A. C. (2003). Family systems and the psychoanalyst. *The American Psychoanalyst* 37, 10, 12.

Nielsen, A. C. (2005). Couples therapy and the psychoanalyst. *The Analytic Observer. Spring, 2005*, 3–5.
Nielsen, A. C., Pinsof, W., Rampage, C., Solomon, A., & Goldstein, S. (2004). Marriage 101: An integrated academic and experiential undergraduate marriage education course. *Family Relations, 53*, 485–494.
Norcross, J. C., & Beutler, L. E. (2015). A new psychotherapy for each patient: Where practice and research converge. Address at the annual meeting of The Society for the Exploration of Psychotherapy Integration, Baltimore, MD, 6/21/15.
Ogden, T. (1982). *Projective identification and therapeutic technique.* New York: Jason Aronson.
Olson, D. H., & Olson, A. K. (2000). *Empowering couples: Building on your strengths* (2nd ed.). Minneapolis, MN: Life Innovations, Inc.
Orlinsky, D. E., & Ronnestad, M. H. (2005). *How psychotherapists develop: A study of therapeutic work and professional growth.* Washington, DC: American Psychological Association.
Paley, B., Cox, M., Burchinal, M., & Payne, C. (1999). Attachment and marital functioning: Comparison of spouses with continuous-secure, earned-secure, dismissing, and preoccupied stances. *Journal of Family Psychology, 13*, 580–597.
Panksepp, J. (1998). *Affective neuroscience.* New York: Oxford University Press.
Park, S. W., & Auchincloss, E. L. (2006). Psychoanalysis in textbooks of introductory psychology: A review. *Journal of the American Psychoanalytic Association, 54,* 1361–1380.
Perel, E. (2006). *Mating in captivity: Reconciling the erotic with the domestic.* New York: HarperCollins Books.
Perry, J. C., & Bond, M. (2012). Change in defense mechanisms during long-term dynamic psychotherapy and five-year outcomes. *American Journal of Psychiatry, 169*, 916–925.
Pines, A. (1996). *Couple burnout: Causes and cures.* New York: Routledge.
Pines, A. (2005). *Falling in love: Why we choose the lovers we choose* (2nd ed.). New York: Routledge.
Pinsof, W. (1995). *Integrative problem-centered therapy: A synthesis of family, individual, and biological therapies.* New York: Basic Books.
Pinsof, W., Breunlin, D. C., Russell, W. P., & Lebow, J. (2011). Integrative problem-centered metaframeworks therapy II: Planning, conversing and reading feedback. *Family Process, 50*, 314–336.
Pizer, B., & Pizer, S.A. (2006). "The gift of an apple or the twist of an arm": Negotiation in couples and couple therapy. *Psychoanalytic Dialogues, 16*, 71–92.
Proulx, C. M., Helms, H. M., & Buehler, C. (2007). Marital quality and personal well-being: A meta-analysis. *Journal of Marriage and Family, 69*, 576–593.
Racker, H. (1968). *Transference and countertransference.* New York: International Universities Press.
Rampage, C. (2002). Working with gender in couple therapy. In A. S. Gurman & N. Jacobson (Eds.), *Clinical handbook of couple therapy* (3rd ed., pp. 533–545). New York: Guilford Press.
Rauer, A., & Volling, B. (2013). More than one way to be happy: A typology of marital happiness. *Family Process, 52*, 519–534.
Real, T. (2007). *The new rules of marriage.* New York: Ballantine Books.
Reis, H. T., & Gable, S. L. (2003). Toward a positive psychology of relationships. In C. L. M. Keyes & J. Haidt (Eds.), *Flourishing: Positive psychology and the life well-lived* (pp. 129–159). Washington, DC: American Psychological Association.

Ringstrom, P. A. (1994). An intersubjective approach to conjoint therapy. In A. Goldberg (Ed.), *Progress in self psychology* (Vol. 10, pp. 159–182). Hillsdale, NJ: The Analytic Press.

Ringstrom, P. A. (2014). *A relational psychoanalytic approach to couples psychotherapy.* New York: Routledge.

Risen, C. B. (2010). Listening to sexual stories. In S. B. Levine, C. B. Risen, & S. E. Althof (Eds.), *Handbook of clinical sexuality for mental health professionals* (2nd ed., pp. 3–20). New York: Routledge.

Rogge, R. D., Cobb, R. J., Lawrence, E., Johnson, M. D., & Bradbury, T. N. (2013). Is skills training necessary for the primary prevention of marital distress and dissolution? A 3-year experimental study of three interventions. *Journal of Consulting and Clinical Psychology, 81,* 949–961.

Rohrbaugh, M. J. (2014). Old wine in new bottles: Decanting systemic family process research in the era of evidence-based practice. *Family Process, 53,* 434–444.

Rosen, I. C. (2007). Revenge—the hate that dare not speak its name: A psychoanalytic perspective. *Journal of the American Psychoanalytic Association, 55,* 595–620.

Ross, L. (1977). The intuitive psychologist and his shortcomings: Distortions in the attribution process, in L. Berkowitz (Ed.), *Advances in experimental social psychology* (Vol. 10, pp. 174–317). New York: Academic Press.

Rotella, B. (1995). *Golf is not a game of perfect.* New York: Simon & Schuster.

Rusbult, C. E., & Van Lange, P. A. M. (2003). Interdependence, interaction, and relationships. *Annual Review of Psychology, 54,* 351–375.

Sager, C. J. (1994). *Marriage contracts and couple therapy: Hidden forces in intimate relationships.* Northvale, NJ: Jason Aronson.

Sandler, J. (1987). *Projection, identification, projective identification.* Madison, CT: International Universities Press.

Satir, V. (1967). *Conjoint family therapy: A guide to theory and technique.* Palo Alto, CA: Science and Behavior Books.

Scarf, M. (1987). *Intimate partners: Patterns in love and marriage.* New York: Random House.

Scharff, J. S., & Scharff, D. E. (2008). Object relations couple therapy. In A. S. Gurman (Ed.), *Clinical handbook of couple therapy* (4th ed., pp. 167–195). New York: Guilford Press.

Scheinkman, M. (2008). The multi-level approach: A road map for couples therapy. *Family Process, 47,* 197–213.

Scheinkman, M., & Fishbane, M. (2004). The vulnerability cycle: Working with impasses in couple therapy. *Family Process, 43,* 279–299.

Schlessinger, H. J. (1995). The process of interpretation and the moment of change. *Journal of the American Psychoanalytic Association, 43,* 663–688.

Schlessinger, N., & Robbins, F. P. (1983). *A developmental view of the analytic process.* New York: The Analytic Press.

Schnarch, D. (1997). *Passionate marriage: Keeping love and intimacy alive in committed relationships.* New York: Henry Holt.

Schnarch, D. (2011). Removing the masks. *Psychotherapy Networker, 35,* 30–35, 54–55.

Schrodt, P., Witt, P. L., & Shimkowski, J. R. (2013). A meta-analytical review of the demand/withdraw pattern of interaction and its associations with individual, relational, and communicative outcomes. *Communication Monographs, 81,* 28–58.

Seedall R. B., & Wampler, K. S. (2013). An attachment primer for couple therapists: Research and clinical implications. *Journal of Marital and Family Therapy, 39,* 427–440.

Shaddock, D. (1998). *From impasse to intimacy: How understanding unconscious needs can transform relationships*. Northvale, NJ: Jason Aronson.
Shaddock, D. (2000). *Contexts and connections: An intersubjective systems approach to couples therapy*. New York: Basic Books.
Shapiro, A. F., & Gottman, J. (2005). Effects on marriage of a psycho-communicative-education intervention with couples undergoing the transition to parenthood, evaluation at 1-year post intervention. *Journal of Family Communication, 5,* 1–24.
Shapiro, D. (1965). *Neurotic styles*. New York: Basic Books.
Siegel, D. J. (2010). *Mindsight: The new science of personal transformation*. New York: Bantam Books.
Siegel, D. J., & Bryson, T. P. (2015). *No-drama discipline: The whole-brain way to calm the chaos and nurture your child's developing mind*. London: Scribe Publications.
Siegel, J. P. (1992). *Repairing intimacy: An object relations approach to couples therapy*. New York: Jason Aronson.
Siegel, J. P. (2010). A good-enough therapy: An object relations approach. In A. S. Gurman (Ed.), *Clinical casebook for couple therapy* (4th ed., pp. 134–152). New York: Guilford Press.
Singer, J. A., & Skerrett, K. (2014). *Positive couple therapy: Using we-stories to enhance resilience*. New York: Routledge.
Slipp, S. (1988). *The technique and practice of object relations family therapy*. Northvale, NJ: Jason Aronson.
Solomon, M., & Tatkin, S. (2011). *Love and war in intimate relationships: Connection, disconnection, and mutual regulation in couple therapy*. New York: W.W. Norton.
Sparks, J. (2015). The Norway Couple Project: Lessons learned. *Journal of Marital and Family Therapy, 41,* 481–494.
Sprenkle, D. H., Davis, S. D., & Lebow, J. L. (2009). *Common factors in couple & family therapy: The overlooked foundation for effective practice*. New York: Guilford Press.
Spring, J. A. (2004). *How can I forgive you?* New York: HarperCollins.
Stanley, S. (2001). Making a case for premarital education. *Family Relations, 50,* 272–280.
Stanley, S. M., Amato, P. R., Johnson, C. A., & Markman, H. J. (2006). Premarital education, marital quality, and marital stability: Findings from a large, random household survey. *Journal of Family Psychology, 20,* 117–126.
Stanley, S. M., Bradbury, T. N., & Markman, H. J. (2000). Structural flaws in the bridge from basic research on marriage to interventions for couples. *Journal of Marriage and the Family, 62,* 256–264.
Stanley, S. M., & Markman, H. H. J. (1992). Assessing commitment in personal relationships. *Journal of Marriage and the Family, 54,* 595–608.
Stanley, S. M., Markman, H. J., & Whitton, S. (2003). Communication, conflict, and commitment: Insights on the foundations of relationship success from a national survey. *Family Process, 41,* 659–675.
Stanley, S. M., Rhodes, G. K., & Whitton, S. W. (2010). Commitment: Functions, formation, and the securing of romantic attachment. *Journal of Family Theory & Review, 2,* 243–257.
Stern, D. (1985). *The interpersonal world of the infant*. New York: Basic Books.
Stern, D. B. (2006). Opening what has been closed, relaxing what has been clenched: Dissociation and enactment over time in committed relationships. *Psychoanalytic Dialogues, 16,* 747–761.

Stern, S. (1994). Needed relationships and repeated relationships: An integrated relational perspective. *Psychoanalytic Dialogues, 4*, 317–346.
Stolorow, R., Brandshaft, B., & Atwood, G. (1987). *Psychoanalytic treatment: An intersubjective approach.* Hillsdale, NJ: The Analytic Press.
Stone, D., Patton, B., & Heen, S. (2010). *Difficult conversations: How to discuss what matters most* (2nd ed.). New York: Penguin Books.
Stosny, S. (2005). *Treating attachment abuse: A compassionate approach.* New York: Springer Publishing.
Stosny, S. (2006). *You don't have to take it anymore: Turn your resentful, angry, or emotionally abusive relationship into a compassionate, loving one.* New York: Free Press.
Strachey, J. (1934). The nature of the therapeutic action of psycho-analysis. *International Journal of Psycho-Analysis, 15*, 127–159.
Summers, F. L. (1999). *Transcending the self: An object relations model of psychoanalytic therapy.* Hillsdale, NJ: The Analytic Press.
Swindel, R., Heller, K., Pescosolido, B., & Kikuzawa, S. (2000). Responses to nervous breakdowns in America over a 40-year period: Mental health policy implications. *American Psychologist, 55*, 740–749.
Tansey, M. J., & Burke, W. F. (1989). *Understanding countertransference: From projective identification to empathy.* Hillsdale, NJ: The Analytic Press.
Tolle, E. (1999). *The power of now: A guide to spiritual enlightenment.* Novato, CA: New World Library.
Vaillant, G. E. (1993). *The wisdom of the ego.* Cambridge, MA: Harvard University Press.
Wachtel, E. F., & Wachtel, P. L. (1986). *Family dynamics in individual psychotherapy: A guide to clinical strategies.* New York: Guilford Press.
Wachtel, P. L. (2014). *Cyclical psychodynamics and the contextual self: The inner world, the intimate world, and the world of culture and society.* New York: Routledge.
Waite, L., & Gallagher, M. (2000). *The case for marriage: Why married people are happier, healthier, and better off financially.* New York: Doubleday.
Waldinger, R. J., Schulz, M. S., Hauser, S. T., Allen, J. P., & Crowell, J. A. (2004). Reading others' emotions: The role of intuitive judgments in predicting marital satisfaction, quality, and stability. *Journal of Family Psychology, 18*, 58–71.
Wallerstein, J., Lewis, J., & Blakeslee, S. (2000). *The unexpected legacy of divorce: A 25 year landmark study.* New York: Hyperion.
Wallerstein, J., & Blakeslee, S. (1995). *The good marriage.* New York: Warner Books.
Watzlawick, P., Beavin, J. H., & Jackson, D. (1967). *The pragmatics of human communication: A study of interactional patterns, pathologies, and paradoxes.* New York: W.W. Norton.
Weeks, G. R., Odell, M., & Methven, S. (2005). *If only I had known . . . Avoiding common mistakes in couples therapy.* New York: W. W. Norton.
Weiner-Davis, M. (2002). *The divorce remedy.* New York: Simon & Schuster.
Weingarten, K. (1991). The discourses of intimacy: Adding a social constructionist and feminist view. *Family Process, 30*, 285–305.
Weiss, J., & Sampson, H. (1986). *The psychoanalytic process: Theory, clinical observation, and empirical research.* New York: Guilford Press.
Westen, D. (1999). The scientific status of unconscious processes: Is Freud really dead? *Journal of the American Psychoanalytic Association, 47*, 1061–1106.
Whisman, M. A., & Uebelacker, L. A. (2006). Impairment and distress associated with relationship discord in a national sample of married or cohabiting adults. *Journal of Family Psychology, 20*, 369–377.

White, M. (2007). *Maps of narrative practice*. New York: W. W. Norton.

White, M. (2009). Narrative practice and conflict dissolution in couples therapy. *Clinical Social Work Journal, 37,* 200–213.

White, R. (1959). Motivation reconsidered: The concept of competence. *Psychological Review, 6,* 297–333.

Whitehead, B., & Popenoe, D. (2002). *The state of our unions: The social health of marriage in America.* Piscataway, NJ: The National Marriage Project, Rutgers University.

Wile, D. B. (1981). *Couples therapy: A nontraditional approach.* New York: John Wiley & Sons.

Wile, D. B. (1993). *After the fight: Using your disagreements to build a stronger relationship.* New York: Guilford Press.

Wile, D. B. (2002). Collaborative couple therapy. In A. S. Gurman & N.S. Jacobson (Eds.), *Clinical handbook of couple therapy* (3rd ed., pp. 281–307). New York: Guilford Press.

Wile, D.B. (2012). Creating an intimate exchange. Retrieved from *Collaborative Couple Therapy Newsletter,* http://danwile.com/2012/07/creating-an-intimate-exchange/. Retrieved 11/20/12.

Wile, D. B. (2013a). Opening the circle of pursuit and distance. *Family Process, 52,* 19–32.

Wile, D. (2013b). Why the rules of good communication are so difficult to follow. Retrieved from *Collaborative Couple Therapy Newsletter,* http://danwile.com/2013/03/why-the-rules-of-good-communication-are-so-difficult-to-follow/. Retrieved 4/20/13.

Willi, J. (1984). The concept of collusion: A theoretical framework for martial therapy. *Family Process, 23,* 177–186.

Winnicott, D. W. (1960). Ego distortion in terms of true and false self. In *The maturational processes and the facilitating environment: Studies in the theory of emotional development* (pp. 140–152). New York: International Universities Press.

Worthington, E. L., Jr., Sandage, S. J., & Berry, J. W. (2000). Group interventions to promote forgiveness: What researchers and clinicians ought to know. In M. E. McCullough, K. I. Pargament, & C. E. Thoresen (Eds.), *Forgiveness: Theory, research, and practice* (pp. 228–253). New York: Guilford Press.

Worthington, E. L., Jr., & Wade, N. G. (1999). The psychology of unforgiveness and forgiveness and implications for clinical practice. *Journal of Social and Clinical Psychology, 18,* 385–418.

Zeitner, R. M. (2012). *Self within marriage: The foundation for lasting relationships.* New York: Routledge.

Zinner, J. (1989). The implications of projective identification for marital interaction. In J. Scharff (Ed.), *Foundations of Object Relations Family Therapy* (pp. 155–174). Northvale, NJ: Jason Aronson.

Zuccarini, D., Johnson, S. M., Dalgleish, T. L., & Makinen, J. A. (2013). Forgiveness and reconciliation in Emotionally Focused Therapy for Couples: The client change process and therapist interventions. *Journal of Marital and Family Therapy, 39,* 148–162.

INDEX

abandonment 62, 82, 88, 138; jealousy 89; negative interaction cycles 42, 45; parental 120, 144
abuse 90, 164, 171, 207
acceptance 9, 30, 73–4, 154–60, 177, 244, 262; acceptance experiments 158; origins of acceptance theory 152–3; self-acceptance 156, 256; sequencing of interventions 250, 254, 256; unsolvable problems 153
acting out 17, 59, 177
active empathic listening 9, 189–94, 203, 204, 254; benefits of 190–2; emotion regulation 211, 216; emotional challenges of 193–4; listening to criticism 194; problem solving 220
actor-observer bias 25–6
adhesiveness 77–8
"admitting-admitting" couple state 160
adversarial couples 61, 62–3, 135, 137, 214
affairs *see* extramarital affairs
agenda setting 219
aggression 81, 151, 240, 253;
  see also passive-aggression
agreeableness 27
Akhtar, Salman 166, 167
alcohol 7, 17, 28, 33, 76, 172;
  see also substance use
alienation 45, 97

alternate realities 109, 110
Amato, Paul 244n1
ambivalence 94, 98, 100–1, 117, 156, 252, 261; conflict-avoiding couples 72–3; identified-patient couples 76; passive-aggression 58; pursuer–distancer couples 67
anger 33, 56–9, 102, 155; active empathic listening 193; assertiveness inhibited by 198; case examples 11, 53, 54; emotion regulation 206, 209; family of origin work 73; identified-patient couples 76; long-term deterioration of marriage 46; perpetrators of transgressions 163; projective identification 136, 147; punctuation of negative cycles 48; raw wounds after betrayal 177; reframing 95–6; unforgiveness 162
anger management 76, 115
anxiety 15, 33, 155, 261; active empathic listening 193; anxiety disorders 5; dominating–submitting couples 78n2; emotion regulation 206; hidden issues 86, 87; pharmacotherapy 218; polarities of worry 146–7; projective identification 135–6, 139, 141, 146; trauma-related 91
apologies 24, 28, 52, 63, 171–2, 257; active empathic listening 190; childhood experiences of 174–5; extramarital affairs 60; incomplete

159; major betrayals 161; physical violence 167; repair conversations 160; self-acceptance 156
appreciation, voicing 241
arranged marriages 34n2
asking for things 67, 71, 202, 224
assertiveness 28, 190, 198–9, 202, 216
Atkinson, Brent 111, 206–7, 208, 210, 218n1, 233
atonement 172
attachment 34n3, 78n2, 92, 123; abandonment fears 88; attachment theory 35n4, 88, 93, 122, 208, 260; Emotion-Focused Couple Therapy 244; pursuer–distancer couples 66; security 118, 119
attunement 31–2, 184
authenticity 160, 254
autonomy 92, 148, 149
avoidance 12, 32, 61–2, 63, 71–4, 183, 189

Bateson, Gregory 40–1
Baumeister, R. F. 175
behavioral exchanges 188, 241
behavioral therapy 6, 21n2, 152, 205n1, 241; Integrative Behavioral Couple Therapy 119–20, 153, 205n8; sequencing of interventions 253, 256–7; skills training 181; "themes" 107n3
beliefs 165, 166
Benjamin, Jessica 109, 205n8
Bergler, Edmund 23, 107n2
Berkowitz, D. A. 133n4
best alternatives to a negotiated agreement (BATNAs) 229
Betchen, S. J. 78n1
"bids for emotional connection" 244n3
Bion, Wilfred 62, 86, 137
blame 27–8, 43; "blamer softening" 67; blaming the pitcher 59–60, 68; blaming the victim 166–7; contributions as alternative to 200; defensive blame game 222; externalization of 25; mutual blaming 47, 62–3, 86; psychodynamic approach 254
body language 13, 143, 192, 201
borderline personality disorder 209
boredom 72, 76, 186, 237
boundaries, imagining 194, 212

Bradbury, T. N. 23, 34n1, 44, 175, 205n2
brain processes 208, 238
brainstorming 219, 225, 226–7, 231
breathing exercises 211, 217
Breunlin, Douglas 39
Bringing Baby Home program 264
Buddhism 208
burnout, couple 33, 78, 233
Butler, M. H. 261n2

calm, curious, and caring (Three Cs) directive 51, 187, 204, 205n4, 215, 248
calming things down 14
Catherall, Don 137
change 63, 107, 152; acceptance experiments 158; cyclical psychodynamics 203; interdependence of intrapsychic and behavioral 231; requests for 196, 198; resistance to 77–8; unilateral 188
Cherlin, A. J. 4
children 3, 9, 12, 221; abused 90; mother's alliance with 114, 115; parental discipline 30; triangulating couples 61, 74–5; unconsciously enacted scenarios 135
Chinese finger traps 57
Christensen, Andrew 5–6, 44, 152, 153, 157, 224
circular causation 39, 43, 169, 175
client feedback 259–60, 264
co-captains problem 31
co-creation of meaning 92, 237, 242
coaching 17, 19, 207
Cognitive Behavioral Therapy (CBT) 165, 218n3, 260
Cohn, D. A. 34n3
collusion 145
commitment 157, 244n1, 263
common factors 5–6
communication 253, 262; behavioral therapy 6; conflict management 30; negative attitudes 40–1; relationship education 263; skills training 9, 181–6, 203, 204, 250, 256–7, 260; *see also* listening
complementary couples 145
compliments 240–1, 244
compromise 46, 73–4, 152, 155, 158, 219, 222, 227–8
"compulsion to repeat" 24

concern 28
conflict 4, 85; avoidance of 12, 32, 61–2, 63, 71–4, 189; banning 235–6; discussions 233; emotional immaturity 22; "experiments" 21n2; family of origin work 73; managing 30–2; opening up 15; problem-solving interventions 257–8
conflict-avoiding couples 61–2, 71–4
conflictual couples 61, 62–3
conservation of anxiety 139
constraints: on partner empathy 103–4; on positive experiences 235
containment: recipient of projective identification 137–8; TTEO Model 17, 18
contemporaneous interpretations 150
contempt 40, 68, 142, 193
"contingency contracting" 220
contribution system 200
control mastery theory 137
controlling behavior 89–90
Coontz, Stephanie 22–3
core conflictual relationship theme 133n2
core negative image (CNI) 45, 121–3, 125–8, 201, 254
corrective experiences 127, 150–1, 255, 260
countertransference 17, 81, 83, 131–2, 142, 193
couple identity 34, 46, 242
Couple Therapy 1.0 8, 20, 42, 185, 262; basics of 12–17; case example 21; depth psychology 82; negative process 95; sequencing of interventions 250, 251; *see also* Talk To Each Other Model
criticism 21, 40, 44, 152–3; criticism sandwich 196, 225; listening to 194; mutual blaming 63; projective identification 147; Three Cs 51
cross-complaining 43, 62, 187
"cure by marriage" 24–5, 144, 145
Curran, M. 34n4
cycle replacement 51–2

daily reviews 237
dating/marrying the cure 24–5, 144, 145
dating/marrying the problem 144, 145
deception 161, 168, 214–15
deep breathing exercises 211, 217
default settings 121

defenses 87, 95, 203, 220; maturity 35n5; projective identification 134–5, 136; psychodynamic perspective 81; transferences 117
defensive contempt 68
defensiveness 26, 40, 43, 47, 85, 96, 260; case example 115; interpretations 99; psychodynamic approach 254; raw wounds after betrayal 177; siding with the least likeable partner 17
demand–withdraw couples 61; *see also* pursuer–distancer couples
dependency 28, 29, 81, 148
depression 33, 58–9, 71, 155; case examples 53, 104, 105; identified-patient couples 76; pharmacotherapy 218; polarization 147; siding with the least likeable partner 17; specialized treatment 252; trauma-related 91
depth psychology 82, 107n1, 135, 167
desires 9, 82, 91–4, 99, 106, 116–17; *see also* needs
detouring 74
devitalization 61–2, 71, 72, 107n4, 155, 189, 233
diagnosis 12, 46–7
Dialectical Behavior Therapy (DBT) 209, 210
differences, building on 227
"difficult conversations" 10, 181, 190, 195–202, 203, 204, 254; designating time for 236; emotion regulation 209; problem solving 221, 223, 226; sequencing of interventions 250
Dimen, Muriel 152
Dimidjian, S. 119–20, 155
discernment counseling 250, 251–2
disclosure, intimate 67
discussions 233
disputing the facts 51, 187
distress tolerance 210
divorce 4, 27; antecedents of 78; case examples 11, 104; discernment counseling 251–2; drifting apart 233; fear of 88, 91; Gottman's work 40; hopelessness 18; impact of relationship education on 263; parental 83; pathways to 244n1; threats of 44, 62, 217; transferences 118
Doherty, William 32, 251–2
dominating–submitting couples 61, 62, 69–71, 78n2, 83, 89

double transference allergies 122, 126
doubling technique 14, 53, 98
Driver, J. L. 244n3
dysphoric moods 155

Edelson, Marshal 7
ego psychology 137
Emotion-Focused Therapy (EFT) 7, 78n2, 82, 102, 167, 260; attachment 244; communication problems 253; "consolidation phase" 221; loss of love 88; rules for difficult conversations 203; schemas 133n2
emotion regulation 9–10, 102, 206–18, 260, 262; history of 207–9; methods for 209–12; mutual 212; pharmacotherapy 217–18; sequencing of interventions 250, 253, 256, 257; *see also* emotions
emotional immaturity 22, 27
emotions 3, 82; active empathic listening 192, 193–4; attitudes about 113; avoidance of 183; calming things down 14; constructive ways to deal with 6; emotional room temperature 13–14, 102, 185; expressing 15, 20; fear of losing control over 90; instrumental 198; mind-reading 199; polarization 147; positive 233, 237; reframing 95–6; transferences 127, 128–9; trauma-related 91; validation of 86; *see also* emotion regulation
empathic listening 9, 189–94, 203, 204, 254; benefits of 190–2; emotion regulation 211, 216; emotional challenges of 193–4; listening to criticism 194; problem solving 220
empathy 14, 16, 21, 28, 94–5, 122, 156–7; assertion and 222; case example 53; chemical reaction metaphor 47; constraints on 103–4; difficult conversations 201; doubling technique 98; failure of 92–3, 136; forgiveness 162, 168, 178n2; interpretations 99; mutual regulation of emotion 212
enactments 261n2
escalation 14, 42–6, 48, 49, 67, 78, 85
existential polarities 148
expectations: marriage 22–4; psychodynamic perspective 81; transferences 118–19, 123, 127, 128, 203, 221; uncovering 198

experiments, Gestalt 21n2
exploring the past 94, 101
extramarital affairs 25, 28, 33, 154, 161, 165, 237; accepting responsibility for 60; anxiety about 216; complex causation 175; conflict-avoiding couples 72; grievance stories 164; loss of trust 168; sex life after 177; shame and guilt 173–4

facts 112–13, 191, 199; disputing the 51, 187
failed assistance transference 122
failure to soften 103–4, 127, 128–9, 136
fairness 223
family of origin work 51, 57, 73, 124–5, 150, 254, 255, 260
family therapy 41, 74
fatal attraction couples 145–6, 150
fears 9, 45, 82, 87–91, 94, 220; corrective experiences 151, 255; identified-patient couples 77; projective identification 136; psychodynamic perspective 81; of therapist bias 16; transference 116–17, 121, 123, 128–9, 133n4; uncovering 198
feedback formula (Real) 196–7
feedback from clients 259–60, 264
Felmlee, Diane 145
femininity 29
feminist approach 260
Finkel, Eli 205n8
The First Dance program 264
Fishbane, Mona 29
Fisher, Roger 41, 219, 223
flooding 43, 96, 207, 213
flourishing marriages 232, 233
Fonagy, Peter 110
forgiveness 9, 152, 154, 156, 160–77, 244, 252, 262; complexity 167–8; empathy related to 156–7; helping the offender 172–6; homework letters 176; psychology of 161–2; repair conversations 160; sequencing of interventions 250, 254, 255–6; as transaction 169–71; unsolvable problems 153
"Four Horsemen of the Apocalypse" (Gottman) 40
Fraenkel, Peter 6, 111, 112, 240, 260–1
Fredrikson, Barbara 233

Freud, Sigmund 7, 24, 42, 82, 83, 131, 210
friendship 233–5, 237, 242–3
Frommer, M. S. 170–1, 176
frustration 11, 52, 54, 96
Fruzzetti, Alan 96, 158, 210
fun 233, 234, 237–9, 243, 244
functional deafness 43, 51, 63, 96
fundamental attribution error 25–6

game theory 223
gender polarizations 28–9
genetic interpretations 150
genograms 125, 133n5
Gestalt Therapy 21n2
"getting more votes" 51, 187
"getting to yes" 20, 220, 223
Gill, Merton 126
goals 165, 188, 211, 214, 225, 241
Gobodo-Madikizela, P. 170
Goldner, Virginia 28–9, 113, 171, 172, 207
Gottman, John 46, 85, 96, 108–9, 195, 205n7; adhesiveness 78; attunement 31, 184; emotions 113, 207; negative process 40; negative sentiment override 133n3; positive affect 232, 233; skills training 183, 205n2; unsolvable problems 153; "we-ness" 242
Graller, Jack 133n4
gratification, current versus future 148
Gray, John 30
Gray, Paul 100
Greenberg, Leslie 48, 78n2, 82, 86, 99, 101, 127; forgiveness 161, 178n2; homework letters 176; instrumental emotions 198; shame 178n3; skills training 183
grief 91, 141–2
grievance stories 164, 169
grudges 26
guilt 16, 88, 89, 93; abusers 207; apologies 171; blaming others 59; case examples 11, 54, 84, 215; constraints on empathy 103, 104; defenses against 25; emotion regulation 209; grievance stories 164; helping the offender 173–4; perpetrators of transgressions 163; personal responsibility 28; psychodynamic perspective 81; pursuer–distancer couples 68, 69; reframing 96; self-images 45;

sex-related 106; sexual pathology 26; systemic awareness 48
guilt-tripping 31, 65, 98, 114, 155
Gurman, Alan 7, 20–1, 23, 153, 244

Haley, Jay 13
handholding 239–40, 243
happiness 4, 5, 188; expectations about marriage 23; life stresses 32; long-term deterioration 45–6
Harvard Program on Negotiation 183
hate 81
Hazlett, P. S. 120–1
healing 101–2, 171
Heine, Heinrich 166
Hendrix, Harville 120
hidden issues 9, 82, 84–7, 91, 94–104, 215; sequencing of interventions 250, 254
holding 20, 66, 137, 251
holding hands 239–40, 243
homework letters 176
honesty 81, 160, 163, 234, 252
hope 20, 48, 123, 215, 220; post-trauma recovery 163; TTEO Model 17, 18
hopelessness 18, 45, 65; active empathic listening 193; case examples 11, 83–4, 216; emotion regulation 206; pursuer–distancer couples 67; reframing 96; transference allergies 122; unforgiveness 163
hostility 93, 155, 177
hugging 102, 106, 239, 240, 243, 244
human nature 25–7
humility 132, 248, 263
humor 106, 201, 233, 239, 248

I-statements 43, 86, 196
idealization 93–4, 118, 131, 156
identification 128
identified-patient couples 61, 65, 76–7, 78, 137
identity: couple 34, 46, 242; dominating–submitting couples 78n2; injuries to 57; psychodynamic perspective 81; shared 222
immaturity 22, 27
imperfect interactions 156
impulsiveness 27, 253
inaction 139, 142
incompatibilities 29–30, 155

inductions: motivated/unmotivated 138–9; as step in projective indentification 35; via inaction 139
influence 31
injuries, attitudes about past 113–14
insecure attachment 34n3, 119
insults 43, 96, 191
integration (therapy) 5–6
Integrative Behavioral Couple Therapy (IBCT) 119–20, 153, 205n8
interlocking transferences 122–3, 127, 128, 136
interpersonal space 44
interpretations: contemporaneous 150; explanatory 99; genetic 150; reframing 94, 95, 99; transference 126–7
interventions: acceptance experiments 158; blocking the "I'm not your mother!" response 129; blocking the "you know I'm that way!" response 129; categories of 249; contemporaneous interpretations 150; corrective experiences 150–1; criticism sandwich 196, 225; daily reviews 237; disclosing humility 132; educational approach 51; family of origin work 51, 57, 73, 124–5, 150, 254, 255, 260; focusing on the dance 46–7; fraction-of-a-second 100; Fraenkel's Three R's 112; genetic interpretations 150; hold your problem solving 191, 220–1, 225; homework letters 176; "how much, how much" 100; hugging 102, 106, 239, 240, 243, 244; imagining a physical boundary 194, 212; improv game 50; "Life Doesn't Come with Labels" 110–11; "making a better case" 98–9; "making a short story long" 50, 254; "name it to tame it" 210; naming the enemy 46–7; "no wonder" 99; pointing out benefits 150, 157–8; projective identification 149–51; punctuation of negative cycles 48; pursuer–distancer couples 66; reframing 18, 94, 95–7, 99, 128, 254; repair conversations 158–60, 202, 214; sequencing 249–61; siding with the least likeable partner 17, 132; talking like friends 236–7; Three Cs 51, 187, 204, 205n4, 215, 248; "To the Extent That" 48; "You're Both Right" 110, 255; *see also* interpretations; metaphors
intimacy 20, 55, 86, 102; as co-creation of meaning 92, 237; "experiments" 21n2; fear of 87, 91; need for 92; positive experiences 222; projective identification 136; psychodynamic perspective 81; pursuer–distancer couples 66, 67, 68; versus separation 64; unsolvable problems 153
invalidation 43, 45, 82, 193
ironic processes 62, 138
irreconcilable differences 153

Jacobson, Neil 44, 152, 153, 157, 224
jealousy 89
Johnson, Adelaide 74
Johnson, Susan 14, 39, 78n2, 82, 96, 121, 171, 208, 221
Jones, Daniel 34n2

Karney, Benjamin 34n1
Kelly, A. B. 118, 219
Kohut, Heinz 31, 57, 89, 90, 107n4, 123, 126
Kornfield, Jack 218n2

labels, common arguments over 111–12
language, choices to avoid 200
Lansky, Melvin 165–6, 167
Lavner, J. A. 34n1
lead-follow cycles 70
A League of Their Own (film) 193–4
"learning conversations" 197
Lebow, Jay 5, 7, 247, 253
LeDoux, Joseph 208
Leone, Carla 260
Lewis, Jerry M. 34n3, 108
Lichtenberg, J. D. 93
"Life Doesn't Come with Labels" problem/intervention 110–11
Linehan, Marsha 209, 210
listening 9, 99, 189–94, 203, 204, 254; daily reviews 237; duration of 195; emotion regulation 211, 216; problem solving 220; pursuer–distancer couples 157; repair conversations 159
loneliness 91, 114, 139, 209, 237
love 3, 24, 26–7, 82, 86, 92; direct expressions of 241; erosion of 45–6; idealization of 156; loss of 88; need for 115; psychodynamic perspective 81; unconditional 93–4, 117

love match 22–3
Luborsky, Lester 119
Luskin, Fred 163–5, 166, 167, 178n2
Lyubomirsky, Sonja 233, 236, 241

Markman, Howard 45, 84, 133n3, 185, 205n2, 205n6, 233–4, 237
marriage: arranged marriages 34n2; benefits 4; conflict management 30–2; divorce rates 4; emotional maturity 27; flourishing 232; Gottman's work 40; high societal expectations 22–3; incompatibilities 29–30, 155; maintaining positivity 33–4; marriage education 264; prevalence of 4; seeking a cure through 24–5, 144, 145; transferences evoked by 117; unrealistic expectations 22, 23–4
Marriage 101 8, 219, 264
marrying the cure 24–5, 144, 145
marrying the problem 144, 145
masculinity 29
maturity 27–9, 35n5, 93, 156; therapist 263
mediation 17, 18–19
medication 217–18
mentalization 110
meta-emotions 113
metaphors: ballroom dance instructor 234; blaming the pitcher 59–60, 68; caged bird 71; calling for a waiter 49, 65; canoe 50; chemical reaction 47; Chinese finger traps 57; cogwheel 49–50; drowning swimmer 49, 65, 97; firemen 49; hungry person 49; lifeguard 49, 65; "no crying in baseball" 194; nuclear reactor 185; passenger in car for "conservation of anxiety" 139; use of metaphorical language 100; *see also* interventions
Middleberg, C. V. 148, 150
Mikulincer, M. 119
mind-reading 199
mindfulness 208, 210, 218n2, 218n3
Minuchin, Salvador 74, 114
mixed-agenda couples 251–2
Mnookin, R. H. 222, 227
model scenes 120
modeling 14–15, 185
money 3, 9, 12, 30, 140–1, 148
mood disorders 5
moralistic thinking 104
motives 138

mourning 106–7, 130, 141, 157, 163, 165
Moynihan, Daniel Patrick 112
multiple choice questions 100–1
mutual blaming 47, 62–3, 86
mutually-avoiding couples 61, 71–4

nagging 11, 65, 66, 82, 147, 155
narcissistic rage 57, 89, 93, 107n4, 139
narrative couple therapy 102, 260–1
naturalistic studies 184
needs: assertive expression of 198; dependency 148; for empathy 103; frustrated 82, 115, 158; hiding 98; positive transference 124; unconsciously enacted scenarios 135; unmet 66–7, 78, 86, 91–2, 101, 117, 254; *see also* desires
Neff, L. A. 133n3
negative interaction cycles 9, 40–6, 220, 262; adhesiveness of 77–8; case examples 52–5, 83, 217; cycle replacement 51–2; failure of empathy 93; fear of shame 88; frequency of 52; inertia 63; interventions 46–51; labeling 254; maladaptive steps 95; negative process identification 40–2, 250, 252–3; preventing/interrupting 104; psychodynamic perspective 85; unmet desires 91
negative reciprocity 43, 63
negative sentiment override 26, 45, 133n3
negotiation 41, 69, 220; active empathic listening 190; emotional challenges of 222; Harvard Program on Negotiation 183; principled 223–4; sequencing of interventions 250, 256, 258
neuroeducation 208
neuroticism 27
neutrality 16, 17, 21, 70
"nice-guy backlash" 159–60
Niebuhr, Reinhold 154
Niehuis, S. 133n3
"no good time to talk" syndrome 18
noncompliance 58–9, 66, 69, 155
nonjudgmental attitude 209–10, 217, 218n3
Norcross, John C. 261n1
novelty 237–8

object relations theory 137
Olson, A. K. 28, 30, 33, 40
one-up position 168–9

PAIRS 264
Panksepp, Jaak 233
paraphrasing 191–2, 201, 203
parents 54, 66, 83, 84, 106; abandonment by 120, 144; distortion of facts by 112–13; exploring the past 101; identification with 204; projective identification 140, 141; transferences 118, 125–6
passive-aggression 30–1, 45, 58, 152–3, 155; dominating–submitting couples 69, 89; pursuer–distancer couples 65, 105
"pathological dance" 39, 40, 42–51, 56–78, 82, 262; *see also* negative interaction cycles
patience 224
perfectionism 67, 88, 221
perpetual problems *see* unsolvable problems
personality 41, 81
personality disorders 110, 134
pharmacotherapy 217–18
physical boundaries, imagining 194, 212
physical contact 239–40
Pines, Ayala 146
Pinsof, William 51, 251
Pizer, B. 44, 155
planning 188–9, 219
play 135, 233, 238
pleasure principle 24
polarities: amplification of 146–7; centered on other emotions and roles 147–8; existential 148; idiographic 148–9
polarization 43, 45, 109; failure of containment 137; gender 28–9; projective identification 145–9, 255
positional bargaining 223
positive couple experiences 42, 158, 177, 222, 232–44, 250, 258, 262
positive psychology 232
positivity 33–4, 205n7, 233
power 3, 31; dominating–submitting couples 61, 62, 69–71; relational 63, 217
PREP problem-solving template 219; relationship education 264
Prepare-Enrich 264
principled negotiation 223–4
problem solving 9, 46, 219–31, 262; assisted 251; benefits of concrete solutions 221–2; brainstorming 219, 225, 226–7, 231; case examples 54, 55, 231; difficult conversations 197; emotional challenges of 222; encouraging joint 129–30; evaluation 227–9; fairness 223; follow-up 219, 230; hold your 191, 220–1, 225; negative process interfering with 41; practical suggestions for 225–30; PREP problem-solving template 219; problem definition 5, 225–6; projective identification 136; sequencing of interventions 250, 256, 257–8; "solving the moment" 41, 42; stalling 222; structured methods of 20; unsolvable problems 153; *see also* negotiation
Program on Negotiation (Harvard) 183
projective identification 9, 133n4, 134–51; case examples 140–4, 148–9; component steps 135–6; containment 137–8; dating/marrying the problem or cure 144, 145; failure to soften 136; as interpersonal defense 134–5; interventions 149–51; marital polarities as examples of 145–9; recipient's predicament 138; as royal road to success 142; self-acceptance 256; sequencing of interventions 250, 254, 255; as unconsciously enacted scenarios 135
pseudodialogue 65
psychic equivalence 110
psychoanalysis 19, 21n2, 81–2, 97, 199, 213; containment 137; dealing with resistance 15; desire to hurt the partner 93; emotion regulation 207; individual therapy 128, 258; insight 94; nonjudgmental state 210; projective identification 134; sequencing of interventions 253; therapist's mental health 263; transference 116, 123, 130–1, 133n2; *see also* psychodynamics; self psychology
psychodynamic therapy 6, 15, 21n2, 50–1, 96; individual therapy in a dyad 217; mixing with relationship/ educational interventions 259–61;

rules for difficult conversations 203; sequencing of interventions 250, 253–6; transferences 124–5; *see also* psychoanalysis
psychodynamics 9, 81–2, 260, 262; communication problems 253; cyclical 203; emotion regulation 217; hidden issues 85; improv game 50; negative process 42
psychoeducation 71, 102
punctuation of cycles 48
pursuer–distancer couples 61, 62, 63–9, 105, 137, 148, 149, 157, 215

questions to ask clients 97, 100–1, 104

"radioactive" tasks 58, 65
Rauer, A. 205n3
Real, Terrence 25, 45, 121, 187–8, 196–7
reframing 18, 94, 95–7, 99, 128, 254
Reiner, Rob 109
Reis, H. T. 233
relational power 63, 217
relationship education 9–10, 50–1, 181–205, 253, 263; active empathic listening 189–94; counterproductive moves 187; difficult conversations 195–202; guidelines for teaching 184–6; impact of rules 203; mixing with psychodynamic interventions 259–61; modeling 185; performance debate 182–4; rationale for 181–2; sequencing of interventions 256–7; slowing down 187–8
Relationship Enhancement 264
relationship episodes 119–20
religion 83, 242
repair 52
repair conversations 158–60, 202, 214
repetition compulsion 24
repetition of emotional statements 100
resilience 28
resistance 15, 77–8, 94, 99–100, 186, 247–8
respect 86
responsibility: acceptance of 28, 60, 157, 168, 199; admission of 160, 171, 174–5; attribution of 59; defence mechanisms 35n5; emotion regulation 209; excessive guilt 25; fear of accepting 174; homework letters 176; maturity 156; systemic awareness 48

revenge 45, 93, 102; anger as 58; getting even 26; insults 96; mild forms of 166; shame and 165–6; trauma-related 91; unforgiveness 162
Ringstrom, Philip 45, 132, 194
Rohrbaugh, M. J. 62
roles 62, 69; fatal attraction couples 145–6; transference 120; unconsciously enacted scenarios 135
romance 233, 236; romantic wishes 23
Rosen, I. C. 167
routines 222, 237, 241
Rubin, Edgar 115n1
rules 182, 184, 185, 188–9; co-captains problem 31; for continuing difficult conversations 199–202; emotional challenges 193; impact of teaching 203; for listeners 190–2, 205n6; mutual regulation of emotion 212; for opening difficult conversations 195–7; for recovery conversations 160; for speakers 195, 202, 205n6, 260; timeouts 213–14; too many? 202; unenforceable 164–5

sacrifice 30, 155, 156, 157
safety 17, 18, 77, 92, 95, 162, 163, 240
same-sex relationships 6–7, 244n5
Satir, Virginia 13
scapegoating 74–5, 142
Scharff, David 133n4
scheduling, importance and benefits of 236
Scheinkman, Michelle 50, 133n4, 249
schemas 81, 82, 102, 133n2
Schnarch, David 93, 240
secondary emotions 95–6
Seedall R. B. 130
self-acceptance 156, 256
self-awareness 27–8, 34n4, 81, 93, 99–100, 156
self-control *see* emotion regulation
self-criticism 88, 121, 171, 173
self-disclosure 132, 234
self-discovery 82
self-esteem 26, 27, 28, 66, 188; attacks on 167; blaming others 59; case examples 143, 217; dominating–submitting couples 70, 78n2; fear of shame 88–9; injuries to 57; maturity 156; positional bargaining 223; pursuer–distancer couples 68; revenge 45

self-evaluation 134
self-exposure 28
self-fulfilling expectations 118–19
self-images 45
self psychology 31, 88, 92, 107n4, 122, 131, 137
self-soothing *see* emotion regulation
sequencing of interventions 249–61
The Serenity Prayer 154
sex 3, 9, 47, 240; absence of 234; after affairs 177; case examples 11, 53, 54, 55, 104, 106, 142–3, 144, 243–4; co-constructed desires 92; comfort with sexuality 28; constraints to 235; control over 70, 222; explanatory interpretations 99; high expectations 23; incompatibilities 30; lack of interest in 175; positive experiences 233; psychodynamic perspective 81; punctuation of negative cycles 48; pursuer–distancer couples 66; restoring intimacy 258; scheduling time for 236; sequencing of interventions 250; sex drive 26
shame 16, 91, 93; abusers 207; apologies 171; blaming others 59; case examples 54, 142–4, 215; constraints on empathy 104; defenses against 25; emotion regulation 209; fear of 88–9; forgiveness and 167, 178n3; grievance stories 164; helping the offender 173–4; hidden behind anger 57–8; perpetrators of transgressions 163; personal responsibility 28; projective identification 142–4, 147–8; psychodynamic perspective 81; pursuer–distancer couples 67–8; revenge and 165–6; self-images 45; systemic awareness 48
Shapiro, David 15
sibling transferences 132n1
Siegel, Dan 205n4, 208, 210
Singer, J. A. 120, 235, 242
Skerrett, Karen 120, 235, 242
skills training 7, 9–10, 181–205, 260, 262; active empathic listening 189–94; counterproductive moves 187; difficult conversations 195–202; emotion regulation 206–18; guidelines for teaching 184–6; impact of rules 203; modeling 185; performance debate 182–4; rationale for 181–2; sequencing of interventions 250, 256–7; slowing down 187–8; *see also* relationship education
social isolation 242–3
soft start-ups 189, 225
softening 94, 101, 102, 128, 181, 260; blamer 67; constraints on empathy 103; gradual 218n1; projective identification 136
Solomon, Marion 208
"solving the moment" 41, 42
Sparks, J. 264
speaker–listener technique 205n6, 219
specialized treatment 250, 252
sports psychology 207, 211, 212
Sprenkle, Douglas 153, 253
Spring, Janice 169–70, 172, 178n2
stalling 60, 222, 254
standards 228
Stanley, Scott 133n3, 205n2, 205n6, 234
Stone, Douglas 181, 194, 197
stonewalling 40, 96, 193
The Story of Us (film) 109
Stosny, Steven 176, 207, 215, 218n4, 240–1
stress 23, 28, 32–3
subjectivity 28, 43, 44, 109, 155
substance use 5, 7, 17, 143, 154, 172, 252
systemic awareness 48
systemic therapy 5–6
systems view 9, 17, 39–40, 97

taking sides 16–17
Talk To Each Other (TTEO) Model 8, 12, 13, 15–16, 17–21, 82; *see also* Couple Therapy 1.0
talking: attitudes about 64; daily reviews 237; pseudodialogue 65; "talking like friends" 236–7
team-mates 31
Terman, Lewis 27
terminology 8, 40
therapeutic alliance 16, 21, 75, 132, 234, 247–8
therapy 5, 8–9, 262–3, 265; blaming of therapist 76; collaboration 247–8; individual 77, 95, 128, 177, 217, 258; integration 5–6; upgrades 9; *see also* behavioral therapy; psychoanalysis; psychodynamic therapy
"third story" 197, 204, 205n8, 223
three choices, when faced with adversity 154

Three Cs (calm, curious, and caring) 51, 187, 204, 205n4, 215, 248
Three Rs (reveal, revalue, and revise) 112
time alone 93
time constraints 235
time famine 32
time limits 195–6
timeouts 202, 211, 212, 213–14, 216, 257
tone of voice 60–1, 93, 201
transference 9, 116–33, 254; acceptance 157; allergies 121, 122, 126, 157, 188; challenge of disconfirmation 127–8; containment 137; emotion regulation 209; evoked by marriage 117; as expectations 118–19; fears about therapist bias 16; interlocking transferences 122–3, 127, 128, 136; negative 45, 77, 116–17, 118–19, 121, 122–3, 127, 131, 138, 203, 221; positive 116, 123–4, 131; projective identification 135; psychodynamic therapy 124–5; relationship episodes 119–20; roles 120; sequencing of interventions 250; towards therapist 130–1; triggers 126–7; varieties of distortion 117; wishes and fears 116–17
translation 17, 18–19
trauma 24, 84, 91, 163, 164; dating/marrying the problem 144; family of origin work 255; transferences 118; uncomforted 122
triangulating couples 61, 74–6, 78
triggers, reality 126–7
trust 31, 102, 144, 162, 256; extramarital affairs 60; identified-patient couples 77; loss of 168–9; major betrayals 160, 252; positive experiences 222; psychodynamic perspective 81; slow return of 176
truth 108, 149, 191, 199
"turning toward" each other 237

unbalancing 16–17
unenforceable rules 164–5
unforgiveness 162–3, 167, 169, 178n2
unhappiness 4, 9, 11; disclosure of 56; fatal attraction couples 146; Gottman's work 40; uncovering 15
unified detachment 47, 159, 205n8
unrealistic wishes 22, 23–4; reframing 96–7

unsolvable problems 153, 155
upgrades 7, 9, 39, 262
Ury, William 41, 219, 223
usable object 109

Vaillant, George 35n5
valences 62
validation 99, 122, 190, 198
vengeance *see* revenge
veritas, in vino 61
victim blaming 166–7
victim mentality 27–8
vilification 44, 155, 178n1
violence 7, 31, 91, 154, 161; case example 214, 215; dominating–submitting couples 69, 70; emotion regulation 207; fear of shame 89; forgiveness of 167; helping the offender 172–3; revenge 45; siding with the least likeable partner 17; specialized treatment 252; timeouts as prevention 214
vulnerability cycle 40, 42, 133n4; *see also* negative interaction cycles
Vulnerability-Stress-Adaptation model 34n1

Wachtel, Ellen 133n5, 139
Wachtel, Paul 21n2, 133n4, 133n5, 139, 183, 203, 244n2, 260
Wallerstein, Judith 46
"we-ness" 34, 242
Weeks, G. R. 6
Weingarten, K. 92, 237
well-being 4, 31, 136
whining 17, 65
White, Michael 47, 102, 171, 190
White, Robert 93
Wile, Dan 51, 68–9, 97, 102, 133n4; conflict-avoiding couples 73; "contingency contracting" 220; criticism "levels of attack" 44; dominating–submitting couples 71; doubling technique 14, 98; listening 195; mind-reading 199; multifaceted clients 100–1; "nice-guy backlash" 159–60; skills training 183; "solving the moment" 41; taking sides 17; witnessing 171
win-win situations 223
wishes *see* desires
witnessing 102, 105, 170–1
worry, polarities of 146–7
Worthington, E. L. 178n2